Valuable Law Books.

JOHN GRIGG,

No. 9, NORTH FOURTH STREET,

Has published the following valuable Law Books.

BLACKSTONE'S COMMENTARIES, by Christian, Archbold & Chitty, 2 vols. 8vo.

CHITTY ON CONTRACTS, a new and practical Treatise on the Law of Contracts, not under Seal, and upon the usual Defences to actions thereon; with corrections and additional references of recent English and American Decisions, by Francis I. Troubat, Esq., second American edition, in 1 vol. 8vo.

All persons of business will greatly benefit themselves by an attentive perusal of this valuable work.

FONBLANQUE'S CELEBRATED TREATISE ON EQUITY, a new edition, with considerable additions, by A. Lausatt, Esq., in 2 vols. 8vo.

PETERS' CONDENSED REPORTS OF CASES in the Supreme Court of the United States, containing the whole Series of Decisions of the Court from its organization to the commencement of Peters's Reports, at January Term, 1827. With copious Notes of Parallel Cases in the Supreme and Circuit Courts of the United States, in 6 vols. 8vo.

The reported decisions in the Circuit and District Courts of the United States, upon similar points, are also collected and digested in the work, as notes; and abstracts of those Cases, and also of the collateral decisions of the Supreme Court, are given; so that the Professional Gentleman and the Student, will be in possession of all the adjudicated Law of the courts of the United States, in an authoritative, condensed, and arranged form.

PETERS' REPORTS.—Reports of Cases argued and determined in the Supreme Court of the United States, by Richard Peters, Esq., Reporter of the Supreme Court of the United States, in 4 vols. royal 8vo.—These Reports are published annually, in July.

"There is at Washington a power, which has neither guards, nor palaces, nor treasures; it is neither surrounded by clerks, nor overloaded with records. It has for its arms only truth and wisdom. Its magnificence consists in its justice, and the publicity of its acts. This power is called the Supreme Court of the United States."

No Law Library can be considered as complete unless the Decisions of the Supreme Court of the United States occupy a place in it.

SAUNDERS' REPORTS, in 3 vols. royal 8vo. The fourth American, from the fifth London edition.—This edition contains one third more matter than any previous one.

In the case of Bullythorp *vs.* Turner, Willis's Reports, 170, Lord Chief Justice Willis having cited the authority of Saunders, observed, "that he was so very learned a man, and so well skilled in pleading, that no other authorities need be mentioned after him."

TOLLER ON THE LAW OF EXECUTORS AND ADMINISTRATORS, with notes and references to American authorities, by Ed. D. Ingraham, Esq., in 1 vol. 8vo.

The above work is not only absolutely necessary for every gentleman of the Bar, but will be found a very valuable guide to every individual who is left an executor or administrator. The copious notes added to this edition by the American editor, render it very valuable.

RUSSEL'S REPORTS OF CASES in the High Court of Chancery, during the time of Lord Chancellor Eldon. 1 vol. 8vo.

CONDENSED ENGLISH CHANCERY REPORTS.—The Reports which begin the series of Condensed English Chancery Reports, are those of Messrs. Simons and Stuart, commencing in 1821, and containing, in two volumes, the cases decided in the Vice-Chancellor's Court from that period to 1826, when Mr. Simons became the sole Reporter.

In the same volume will be included the second of Mr. Russel's Reports of Cases decided in the High Court of Chancery, in the years 1825 and 1827. The first volume of Mr. Russel's Reports has already been re-published in this country, and may be procured of the principal Booksellers in the United States.

The second volume of the Condensed English Chancery Reports contains the first and second Simons's Reports of Cases in the Vice-Chancellor's Court, and the third and fourth Russell's Cases in the High Court of Chancery; thus bringing down the whole series of Decisions to 1828, inclusive.

The subsequent volumes will contain the whole of the later Chancery Decisions in the High Court of Chancery and in the Vice-Chancellor's Court *condensed;* they will be published here, immediately after their appearance in England.

This Work will be invaluable to the American Bar.

As a limited number of copies will only be printed, those who wish to possess the work, can secure a copy by an early subscription. Booksellers, generally, in the United States, will receive subscriptions for this Work.

The price, to subscribers, will be $5 per volume, handsomely bound in calf; to non-subscribers, $5 50 per volume.

LAW LIBRARIES supplied on the most favourable terms, and all orders thankfully received, and promptly attended to.

All the new Law Books for sale as soon as published.

𝔙𝔞𝔩𝔲𝔞𝔟𝔩𝔢 𝔐𝔢𝔡𝔦𝔠𝔞𝔩 𝔅𝔬𝔬𝔨𝔰, &𝔠.

PUBLISHED BY J GRIGG,

NO. 9, NORTH FOURTH STREET, PHILADELPHIA,

And for sale by the principal Booksellers in the United States

THE PHARMACOPŒIA of the United States revised edition, by authority of the National Medical Convention, which met in Washington, in January, 1830 in 1 vol 8vo

All persons ordering this work will please say "the Philadelphia edition of 1831"

VELPEAU'S ELEMENTARY TREATISE ON THE ART OF MIDWIFERY, or the principles of Tokology, and Embryology, in 1 vol 8vo Translated from the French, by Charles D Meigs, M D &c

This is a new work, and is said to be a very valuable one, by many who are eminently qualified to judge

COOPER'S FIRST LINES OF THE PRACTICE OF SURGERY designed as an introduction for students and a concise book of reference for practitioners By Samuel Cooper, M D With Notes by Alexander H Stevens, M D, and additional Notes and an Appendix, by Dr S M'Clellan Third American, from the last London edition, revised and corrected With several new plates and wood cuts, in 2 vols 8vo

This work is highly esteemed by all the distinguished of the medical profession, and, in many of our Medical Schools is used as a Text Book

EBERLE'S PRACTICE OF MEDICINE A Treatise on the Theory and Practice of Medicine, in 2 vols 8vo By John Eberle M D Professor of Materia Medica and Obstetrics in the Jefferson Medical College, Philadelphia

This is one of the most valuable works on the Practice of Medicine, that has ever issued from the American Press

A TREATISE ON THE MATERIA MEDICA AND THERAPEUTICS, in 2 vols Third edition, improved and greatly enlarged By John Eberle, M D Professor of Materia Medica and Obstetrics in the Jefferson Medical College, Member of the American Philosophical Society, Corresponding Member of the Medico-Chirurgical Society, &c.

A TREATISE ON THE ANATOMY PHYSIOLOGY, AND DISEASES OF THE BONES AND JOINTS, in 1 vol 8vo By S D Gross, M D

MANUAL OF GENERAL ANATOMY containing a concise description of the Elementary Tissues of the Human Body From the French of A L Bayle and H Hollard By S D Gross, M D

MANUAL OF THE ELEMENTS OF OPERATIVE SURGERY arranged so as to afford a concise and accurate description of the present state of the Science in Paris From the French of A Tavernier, Doctor of Medicine of the Faculty of Paris, late Surgeon to the 3d Regiment of Artillery, &c &c By S D Gross, M D

MANUAL OF PRACTICAL OBSTETRICS arranged so as to afford a concise and accurate description of the Management of Preternatural Labours, preceded by an account of the Mechanism of Natural Labour From the French of Julius Hatin, Doctor of Medicine of the Faculty of Paris, Professor of Obstetrics, and of the Diseases of Women and Children, &c &c &c By S D Gross, M D.

ELEMENTS OF CHEMISTRY including the recent discoveries and doctrines of the Science By Edward Turner, M D Professor in the London University, F R S E &c &c — With important corrections and additions, by Franklin Bache, M D Professor of Chemistry in the Franklin Institute

HUFELAND ON SCROFULOUS DISEASES 1 vol 12mo

BICHAT ON PATHOLOGY, in 1 vol 8vo

RUSH ON THE MIND, new fine edition, 1 vol 8vo.

This work is valuable and highly interesting for intelligent readers of every profession, it is replete with curious and acute remarks, both medical and metaphysical, and deserves particular praise for the terseness of its diction

SCHOOL BOOKS.

Torrey's First Book for Children
—— Spelling Book or Second for Children
—— Pleasing Companion
—— Moral Instructor
Smiley's Arithmetical Tables
—— Arithmetic in Dollars and Cents
—— Key to ditto, for Teachers
—— Geography and Atlas, improved
Grimshaw's History of the United States
—— History of England
—— History of Greece
—— History of Rome with Questions and Keys to each
—— Ladies' Lexicon
Conversations on Chemistry
—— on Natural Philosophy.
Grigg's American School Atlas
Walker's Dictionaries
Murray's Exercises and Key, 12mo edition
Horace Delphini
Virgil Delphini
Clark's Cæsar Delphini
Hutchinson's Zenophon with Notes and a Latin translation under the Greek in each page
Life of General Marion
Life of General Washington, &c &c

Valuable Works,

PUBLISHED BY J. GRIGG, PHILADELPHIA,

And for sale by the Booksellers, generally, in the United States.

THE AMERICAN CHESTERFIELD, or Way to Wealth, Honour, and Distinction.

"We most cordially recommend the American Chesterfield to general attention; but to young persons particularly, as one of the best works of the kind that has ever been published in this country. It can not be too highly appreciated, nor its perusal be unproductive of satisfaction and usefulness."

BIGLAND'S NATURAL HISTORY OF ANIMALS, 12 coloured plates.

BIGLAND'S NATURAL HISTORY OF BIRDS, 12 coloured plates.

PERSIA, A DESCRIPTION OF. By Shoberl, with 12 coloured plates.

These works are got up in a very superior style, and well deserve an introduction to the shelves of every family library, as they are very interesting, and particularly adapted to the juvenile class of readers.

BENNET'S (Rev. John,) LETTERS TO A YOUNG LADY, on a variety of subjects calculated to improve the heart, to form the manners, and enlighten the understanding. "That our Daughters may be as polished corners of the Temple."

Much of the happiness of every family depends on the proper cultivation of the female mind.

CARPENTER'S NEW GUIDE. Being a complete Book of Lines for Carpentry, Joinery, &c., in 1 vol. 4to.

The Theory and Practice well explained, and fully exemplified on eighty-four copper plates, including some observations, &c. on the Strength of Timber, by Peter Nicholson. Tenth edition. This invaluable work superseded, on its first appearance, all existing works on the subject, and still retains its original celebrity.

HIND'S VETERINARY SURGEON, or Farriery taught on a new and easy plan, being a Treatise on all the diseases and accidents to which the Horse is liable. With considerable additions and improvements, adapted particularly to this country, by Thomas M. Smith, Veterinary Surgeon, and member of the London Veterinary Medical Society, in 1 vol. 12mo.

The publisher has received numerous flattering notices of the great practical value of this work. The distinguished editor of the American Farmer, speaking of the work, observes—"We can not too highly recommend this book, and therefore advise every owner of a horse to obtain it."

MALTE BRUN'S NEW AND ELEGANT 4to ATLAS, exhibiting the Five Great Divisions of the Globe, Europe, Asia, Africa, America, and Oceanica, with their several Empires, Kingdoms, States, Territories, and other Subdivisions, corrected to the present time; and containing forty Maps, drawn and engraved particularly to illustrate the Universal Geography by M. Malte-Brun.

The Atlas is particularly adapted for Colleges, Academies, Schools, and Private Families. There is no work that ever was published in this country which has received more numerous and flattering recommendations.

NEW SONG BOOK.—Grigg's Southern and Western Songster: being a Choice Collection of the Most Fashionable Songs, many of which are Original, in 1 vol. 18mo.

Great care was taken in the selection to admit no Song that contained, in the slightest degree, any indelicate or improper allusions. The immortal Shakspeare observes—

"The man that has not music in himself,
Nor is not moved with concord of sweet sounds
Is fit for treasons, stratagems, and spoils."

SENECA'S MORALS.—By way of abstract to which, is added a Discourse, under the title of an After-Thought, by Sir Roger L'Estrange, Knt., a new fine edition, in 1 vol. 18mo.

CONVERSATIONS ON NATURAL PHILOSOPHY, in which the Elements of that Science are familiarly explained. Illustrated with plates. By the author of "Conversations on Chemistry," &c. With considerable additions, corrections, and improvements in the body of the work; appropriate Questions, and a Glossary. By Dr. Thomas P. Jones.

The correction of all the errors in the body of the work, renders this edition very valuable; and all who understand the subject, consider it superior to any other in use.

CONVERSATIONS ON CHEMISTRY, in which the Elements of that Science are familiarly explained and illustrated by Experiments and Engravings on wood. From the last London edition. In which all the late Discoveries and Improvements are brought up to the present time, by Dr. Thomas P. Jones.

All preceptors who have a sincere desire to impart a correct knowledge of this important science to their pupils, will please examine the present edition, as the correction of all the errors in the body of the work, renders it very valuable.

A DICTIONARY OF SELECT AND POPULAR QUOTATIONS, which are in daily use; taken from the Latin, French, Greek, Spanish, and Italian languages: together with a copious collection of Law-maxims and Law-terms; translated into English, with Illustrations historical and idiomatic. Sixth American edition, corrected, with additions. 1 vol. 12mo.

In preparing this Sixth edition for the press, care has been taken to give the work a thorough revision, to correct some errors which had before escaped notice, and to insert many additional Quotations, Law-maxims, and Law-terms.—In this state it is offered to the public, in the stereotype form.

A

TREATISE

ON

PATHOLOGICAL ANATOMY.

BY

WILLIAM E. HORNER, M. D.

ADJUNCT PROFESSOR OF ANATOMY IN THE UNIVERSITY OF PENNSYLVANIA,
SURGEON AT THE INFIRMARY OF THE PHILADELPHIA ALMS HOUSE,
MEMBER OF THE AMERICAN PHILOSOPHICAL SOCIETY, &c.

PHILADELPHIA:

CAREY, LEA & CAREY—CHESNUT STREET.

1829,

GRIGGS & DICKINSON, PRINTERS.

ANALYTICAL INDEX.

CHAPTER I.

General Considerations on Disease,   -   -   -   -   9
     Causes.
     Progress.
     Termination.
     Diagnostic.
     Treatment.

CHAPTER II.

On the Form of Disease,   -   -   -   -   -   -   19
     Alterations of Tissue.
     Irritation.

CHAPTER III.

Phenomena of Irritation,   -   -   -   -   -   -   23
     SECT. 1.—Phlegmasia.
          2.—Hæmorrhage.
          3.—Sub-inflammation.
          4.—Nervous Irritation.
          5.—Secretory Irritation.
          6.—Nutritive Irritation.

CHAPTER IV.

Sympathies,   -   -   -   -   -   -   -   37

A

Jn? Brooks
Sept. 16th
1833

CHAPTER V.

Irritations of Cellular Tissue,   -   -   -   -   -   45
    Phlegmasia.
    Chronic or Sub-inflammation.
    Secretory Irritation.
    Nutritive Irritation.

CHAPTER VI.

Irritations of Serous Membranes,   -   -   -   -   60
    Phlegmasia.
    Chronic or sub-inflammation.

CHAPTER VII.

Irritations of Mucous Membranes,   -   -   -   -   78
    Phlegmasia.
    Pseudo-membranous Inflammation.
    Pustular Phlegmasia.

CHAPTER VIII.

Chronic Inflammation of Mucous Tissues,   -   -   94
    Ulceration.
    Gangrene.

CHAPTER IX.

Mollescence of Mucous Membranes, -   -   -   -   105
    Fungiform or granulated condition.

CHAPTER X.

On the healthy and diseased Appearances of the gastro-in-
    testinal Mucous Membrane.

CHAPTER XI.

On Follicular Inflammation of the Gastro-intestinal Mu-
    cous Membrane,   -   -   -   -   -   -   117

CHAPTER XII.

Dissections illustrating the Pathology of the Abdomen,   191

CHAPTER XIII.

Irritations of the Pulmonary Tissue,   -   -   -   225
    Hypertrophy.
    Atrophy.
    Emphysema.
    Œdema.
    Peripneumony.
    Abscess.

CHAPTER XIV.

Phthisis Pulmonalis,   -   -   -   -   -   -   243

CHAPTER XV.

Irritations of Heart,   -   -   -   -   -   -   260
    Pericarditis.
    Hydro-pericarditis.
    Pneumo-pericarditis.
    Carditis.
    Mollescence.
    Induration.

CHAPTER XVI.

Irritations of Heart continued,   -   -   -   -   276
    Dilatation.
    Hypertrophy.
    Ossifications.
    Polypi.

CHAPTER XVII.

Irritations of Heart continued,   -   -   -   -   289
    Ossifications of Valves.
    Vegetations of Heart.
    Ruptures.

CHAPTER XVIII.

Dissections of Thorax,   -   -   -   -   -   -   299

CHAPTER XIX.

General Pathology of Nervous System,   -   -   -   326
    Sect. 1.—Experiments.
        2.—Sympathies.

CHAPTER XX.

Irritations of Encephalon,   -   -   -   -   -   351
    Phlegmasia.

CHAPTER XXI.

Irritations of Encephalon continued,   -   -   -   358
    Sub-inflammation.
    Cancer.
    Hydatids.
    Tubercles.

CHAPTER XXII.

Mollescence of Encephalon,   -   -   -   -   -   371

CHAPTER XXIII.

Irritations of Medulla Spinalis,   -   -   -   -   389
    Phlegmasia.
    Mollescence.
    Dissolution and Removal.

CHAPTER XXIV.

Irritations of the Nerves,   -   -   .   -   -   405
    Phlegmasia.
    Sub-inflammation.

CHAPTER XXV.

Dissections illustrating the Pathology of Nervous System,   408

PREFACE.

University of Pennsylvania.

THE following work is intended more especially for the use and guidance of practitioners of medicine. Its appearance from an institution, which, whatever may have been its former sterility in this respect, has left but little room for animadversion at its want of fecundity in authorship in latter times, calls perhaps, for an exposition of the motives and qualifications of the writer; especially as it treats of a department in our science comparatively strange to the mass of medical men, and for which there is no sufficient provision by the plan of instruction, in any of the numerous colleges of our country.

Pathological anatomy, by the recent organization of the most improved schools of Europe, has taken a high and commanding attitude. The numerous observations which have been made in it, and the increased skill arising from various and accumulating experience, have at length enabled its cultivators to systematize its facts, and to make a close and instructive application of them to nearly every case of disease, which they are called upon to treat. It is

B

now almost universally conceded to be the light and test of every opinion in medicine; and when the latter fails to harmonize with it, whatever may be the ingenuity of the opinion, it is not likely to obtain either permanent attention or consideration, and must perish in that oblivion which has buried so many medical theories. The modern pathologist has ceased to consider *disease* as an independent existence, which may insinuate itself into the human body; and whenever its name is mentioned, he invariably associates with it the existence of a change or lesion in the structure of some part of the body, which in fact, is the disease itself.

The disgusts inseparable from a course of morbid dissections, the peculiar opportunities which it requires, its extent and the great length of time demanded for its full prosecution, and for the collecting and preparing morbid specimens, have been and will still continue to be obstacles sufficient to prevent physicians generally, and teachers in medicine, from attaching themselves to Pathological Anatomy, notwithstanding its extreme importance, and the universal admission of its advantages to the accomplished practitioner. In my own case, without any desire to pervert facts, or to represent them in more imposing colours than they are entitled to, it is, nevertheless, only fair to mention the circumstances which have led to this work. For fifteen years my attention has been turned with some intensity, and for the greater part of the time, almost exclusively to the cultivation of anatomy in all its relations.

A medical position in the army of the Niagara fron-
tier, in 1814, opened to me a field of pathological
observation of unusual extent and instructiveness,
from the frequency of the combats with the enemy,
and from their very sanguinary character, for the
most part.   To this may be added the diseases
insepaiable from militaiy movements in inclement
seasons.   Peace being restored, an almost immediate transition fixed me in the anatomical department of this institution, under the direct guidance
of that celebrated anatomist, the late Dr. WISTAR.
There profiting by the lessons of experience and of
cultivated intellect, in which he abounded, and was
so free in communicating, the opportunities presented to me were cherished and improved.   The death
of this estimable individual in 1818, was followed
by an association with one not less distinguished in
the professional annals of our country, and who has
been justly and emphatically called the father of
American surgery: I need scarcely mention the name
of Dr. PHYSICK. Aided by his advice and encourage-
ment, and I may say stimulated by the example of
that lustre of character which attends the decline
of a life spent in undeviating integrity, in benevolent
exertions, and in successful attempts for the advance-
ment of our profession, I have still pursued my original course.

The situation of prescribing surgeon at the Philadelphia Alms House Infirmary, where a vast number of cases of disease of a most interesting character. are annually treated; has also contributed in

no small degree, to the general stock of pathological observations made by me.

In this, my progress through anatomy, to the present time, in addition to the numerous dissections of the University, it has been my gratification to assist continually in the post mortem examinations of the physicians of the city; and many of the observations and preparations in the Anatomical Museum, which I prize most, have been obtained through that channel. The gratification was to me double; first, that of advancing a step in knowledge; and secondly, in finding myself on such good terms with the body of my profession, that the most secret and confidential operations of its members, were spontaneously exposed to me. I know in fact no higher mark of the confidence which one physician reposes professionally in another, than an examination subsequent to treatment: the errors and misconceptions of the prescriber are there fully exposed when they have occurred, and his reputation stands more or less committed. Happily for our profession, breaches of confidence on this point are very uncommon: in my own personal observation, I have never known of one, and such a betrayer would be justly held in so great abhorrence, that his first treachery would also be his last.

                                    W. E. HORNER.

July 25th, 1829.

INTRODUCTION.

It has been said very properly, that there exist two classes of diseases: in the one they present an evident lesion of one or more organs, and are therefore called *organic diseases;* and in the second, they leave such indistinct traces of altered texture, that the latter is, at most, conjectural; this class is called *nervous diseases.* I have no doubt, myself, that the mechanism of life is sometimes impaired in such an invisible and impalpable way. that the injury is not cognizable to the senses; at the same time, I think the latter class has been very much overrated, judging from the facility with which I detect morbid alterations now, where formerly I did not suspect them. It is evident that pathological anatomy can alone give us certain information in regard to *organic diseases*, and, by a process of induction, afford instruction on such as are *nervous.* For example, we all know that difficulty of respiration attends the organic diseases of the lungs and heart; if a patient should die with that symptom, and a sufficient cause of death could not be found in the altered structure of the lungs and heart. or other viscera, the conclusion is left, that the disease was a purely nervous one, at least, according to our ideas of nervous; it being such as to escape our scrutiny. . .

This example shows the close connexion between physiology and pathology, that symptoms and morbid alterations should always be studied in alliance, so as to become mutual interpreters, and that an eminent pathologist* has reason for saying that Pathological Anatomy would only be a study of pure curiosity, if it were limited to the description of morbid alterations.

Physicians from the time of Galen, have sought in the vivisection of animals, an illustration of the problem of life; and no period has been more distinguished than our own, in those sacrifices of living beings, which, for the time, seal up the sympathies of our nature, and make us insensible to the cries of agony and to the fair claims to life. I have myself assisted rather often, to be fully vindicated in those assumptions of power over the comfort and lives of God's creatures. It appears to me, however, that this cruelty in the cause of science is diminishing considerably; that the artificial state in which animals are placed by severe experiments in mutilating them, and the introduction of poisons, confessedly tends to destroy the rigid accuracy of result which has been looked for, and that opposite theories and observations are generated under precisely the same course of experiment placed in dif-

† Lallemand Recherches sur l'Encephale, p. 280

ferent hands. Happily the truth begins to glare upon us, that humanity and science are not opposed, and that the cruelties of the profession have been the most fruitful source of its deviations from sound doctrine. On the contrary, the subjects of *pathological anatomy* are those whose sensitive existence has been restored to that ocean of life from which it was first drawn, and they are the perishing and insensate remains of a matter, which, in a short time, must be resolved into the elements which compose it. It is pathological anatomy, aided by an observation of symptoms during life, which will reveal to us the mysterious relations of different organs in the human body, will assign the respective grade of importance to each one, and will determine the degree of alteration of texture within which they can execute their functions, and beyond which they must die. It is this study which will finally explain the ever varying combinations of symptoms, which prevent any two cases of sickness in different individuals from being exactly alike.

Without pathological anatomy it is very possible for a physician to be fully instructed in the literature of his profession, to be versed in the theories of all the celebrated teachers from Hippocrates to the present time, to have an intellect perfectly sound in the processes of induction, to be continually exercising his judgment and skill in the treatment of diseases; yet if he has not accurately depicted on his mind, the morbid lesions which are going on in the system, it is impossible to exercise his calling as a science. and as has been pithily observed,* he will have seen many patients, but no diseases. Execute dissections, and a new horizon is unfolded to view: the darkness which hung over his path becomes a brilliant and a shining light; the uncertainty which attended his steps is converted into assurance; the mistakes of prognostic which compromitted his character, are converted into the prophecies of a superior intelligence. Such is the difference between the practical and the speculative physician; between the man whose studies have been chastened by a continued reference to the evidences of dissections, and one who has resisted or neglected them.

The salutary influence of pathological anatomy upon criminal jurisprudence, is continually felt where the scales of justice are nicely balanced. The Germans have so far admitted its importance, that they have applied it especially to legal medicine, under the name of Anatomia Forensis. A judicious opinion on a trial for life or death sometimes rescues the innocent from undeserved punishment, and surrenders the guilty to the violated laws of humanity and religion. It perhaps would be exceptionable to indicate cases where much of the sentence pro or con, has turned upon the evidence of physicians; they occur annually, and unhappily there are too many where the deficiencies of this evidence, defeat the ends of justice, which are to protect the innocent and to punish the guilty.

Important, then, as this branch is in its medical

* Cruveilhier, Anat. Pathol. p. 10.

and forensic relations, it is not a little remarkable that it has only assumed the shape of a science, since the beginning of the present century. There has been an evident anxiety on the part of anatomists, for more than a century and a half, to contribute largely to it by a report of dissections and of observations, and to give some system and consistency to them. The attempt, however, failed for want of some few plain principles to guide the undertakers; the materials for the building, though sound and abundant, could only be amassed in a confused and disordered pile; no sound foundation could be laid, no symmetrical plan executed, and the prostrate materials of one edifice constituted the wavering foundation of equally short-lived superstructures. The masterly and brilliant idea of Bichat, of the elementary tissues of the body, so well developed by him, that he has left nothing to be added, and nothing of consequence to be detracted, furnished exactly those principles for pathology, of which it had stood in need. He foresaw the influence which these principles would exercise in giving harmony, unity, solidity, and endurance to a design, and himself sketched the outlines of it in a work on Pathological Anatomy.*

A glance at the several stages of this important and interesting science will not be inappropriate, as it will enable us to see what has been done in it, and what is its state at this moment.

---

* Anatomie Pathologique dernier cours de Xavier Bichat, Paris, 1825. This work has been translated by Dr Togno, of Philadelphia

Thomas Bartholin published, in 1674,* the first special treatise on Pathological Anatomy.

Theophilus Bonetus, in 1679, presented to the world his celebrated work, " The Sepulchretum," in which all the facts of preceding ages are recorded and associated with the original observations of the author himself. This work is one of the monuments of the anatomy of the seventeenth century; and, though abounding in faults and defects, is rendered venerable by a recollection of the limited lights and opportunities under which it was written: its materials were excellent and copious, and have served more or less for the principal works that have appeared since. The best edition of it was published at Leyden in 1700, with notes and additional observations by Mangetus.

The interval of time before the appearance of any other work of high authority was more than eighty years. The celebrated Morgagni then published, in 1761, in Venice, his famous work on the Causes and Seats of Diseases, as revealed by Anatomy; the reputation of which, for accurate description and variety of observation, has been handed down undiminished to the present day. It is indeed justly styled one of the most precious monuments of our art, and its dissertations, couched in the form of letters, abound in the most profound and judicious criticism united to the most exact observations of nature. Morgagni appeared on the theatre of medicine at a time well suited to elicit something of

---

* Consilium de Anat. Pract. &c. Hafniæ, 8vo.

value from a gifted and aspiring mind. Special anatomy was in a state of high cultivation, having then approached almost to those confines, beyond which we now find it so difficult to extend it. Physiology, under the guidance of Haller, seemed (but fallaciously) settled on an indestructible basis: surgery, under the administration of Dessault, seemed also to have approached its ultimate point. The edifice of medicine, to be complete, required a finished column of Pathological Anatomy, and that one was presented to it by Morgagni. Now that the stream of time and additional experience have swept us beyond the influence of great names, we may leisurely survey their works, point out their defects; and in following the progressive improvement of the human mind, criticise their errors for our own benefit, and for that of our successors.

The leading objections to Morgagni's work are a periphrastic style, whose profuseness, almost suffocates the sense; an insupportable minuteness in the detail of collateral and unimportant circumstances; a tedious repetition of observations; and an artificial division of diseases into those of the head, of the thorax, of the belly, and into the chirurgical and universal disorders. It is evident, that under this topographical arrangement of diseases, all system must be lost, that the analogies of deranged texture arising from a similar elementary tissue in different parts of the body, are neglected and cannot be approximated; and that it is impossible to lay down, under these circumstances, any general rules which shorten the

path of study and lighten the burden of the memory.
These things are said with the utmost deference to
the memory of this celebrated man, and I do not consider him as guilty of offence in being thus obnox-
ious to them. The fault was that of the age in
which he lived, and not of the author, and in spite
of all, it is confessed that this work has exercised
the most extensive and beneficial influence in the
art of curing diseases. It has substituted in pathology a deranged texture of organs as a cause of disease, in the place of the gratuitous theory of a radical heat and radical moisture, so humorously sa-
tirised by Le Sage, in his sketch of Dr. Sangrado.

In a short time after the publication of Morgagni
on the Causes and Seats of Diseases, there appeared
in 1767 the treatise of Lieutaud of Paris, entitled
Historia Anatomico-Medica. This work is a collection of pathological observations derived principally from the various authorities and communications up to the date of its publication; the remainder is from the author's personal observations. The
arrangement is nearly on the same plan with Morgagni's, depending upon the regional or topographic
distribution of the body. The facts are stated in a
concise way, the inferences are few, and there are
no digressions or disquisitions. As a mere collection of cases, it possesses great value, but its merits
do not go beyond this point. It has no pretensions
as a system of pathology, neither would it be possible to elaborate it into one, as none of the facts are
founded upon the great theory of modern medicine,—

the distinctions and the analogies of tissue,—and the elementary changes which they undergo, either in approximating other tissues or in adopting abnormal combinations.

In 1803, M. Portal, professor of medicine in the College of France, published, in five octavo volumes, " The Course of Medical Anatomy; or, Elements of the Anatomy of Man, with Physiological and Pathological Remarks." The plan of this work is a distribution of descriptive anatomy, under the usual heads of osteology, myology, angeiology, splanchnology, and so on. At the end of the description of each organ or apparatus, are added many valuable remarks on their physiology and pathology, derived from the regular treatises on these subjects, from the detached communications of individuals, and from the personal observation of the author. This work abounds in the learning of the day in which it was published, and is a most excellent addition to our stores of Pathological Anatomy; yet, not being founded on the principles of general anatomy, the same objections bear upon it as upon preceding treatises.

Anterior to the publication of M. Portal's work, appeared in England, in 1793, Baillie's Morbid Anatomy, a work universally esteemed for the correctness of its plates, and the succinctness and accuracy of the text. Most of the organic alterations known up to that time are delineated in it. The writer enjoyed in its composition unusual advantages;—a highly gifted and cultivated mind,—an indefatigable

zeal,—and a close connexion by consanguinity with
the two Hunters which opened to him, when a young
man, the treasures of their experience. The just celebrity of this work carried Dr. Baillie rapidly into the
best and most lucrative business of London, and he
continued to enjoy there, till the day of his death in
1824, the reputation of being the first physician of
the British empire. It, also, as a system is defective; its facts and observations not being connected
with any leading principles or rules.

It was while the science was advancing by these
slow degrees, that Bichat gave the course of lectures alluded to; and about the same period M. Dupuytren, the present celebrated surgeon of Paris,
being then the dissector in chief of the School of
Medicine, undertook a similar course. Availing
himself of the vast field in which he was placed, and
collating the labours of his predecessors and contemporaries, he executed a scientific course, in
which, abandoning the routine of special anatomy
and of nosological classifications; he adhered simply to the nature of the altered texture and to its
symptoms, and thereby produced a complete and
detailed classification of organic lesions. It is
stated,* that from this course were obtained the
fundamental ideas of Bayle and Laennec on the
classification of morbid structures and tumours.

While those contributions to pathology in general have been going on, the science has obtained the
most distinguished assistance from particular trea-

Cru lbier. p 20

tises, the objects of which were more circumscribed.

In 1763, Avenbrugger, a physician of Vienna,
published his work on percussion, as a mode of detecting the diseases of the thorax. By a very singular fatality it remained unknown or in obscurity
till 1808, when Corvisart, physician to Napoleon,
brought it to light by a translation of it from Latin
to French, attended with copious commentaries.
About the same period Corvisart published his celebrated work on the diseases of the heart, for the
distinguishing of which he became so famous. These
two writers, Avenbrugger and Corvisart, may be
justly considered to have led the way to the highly
finished and unequalled work of Laennec in 1819,
on the diseases of the thorax, entitled a Treatise on
Mediate Auscultation and the Diseases of the Lungs
and Heart, where the use of the stethoscope is set
forth so advantageously.

Other works also of great merit have appeared
within the last ten or twelve years. Time will not
permit me to do more than designate them: they are
Bayle on the Pulmonary Consumption; Bertin on the
Diseases of the Heart, and Large Vessels; Andral
on the Diseases of the Gastro-Intestinal Mucous
Membrane, Billard on the same subject; Rostan
on the Brain, Lallemand on the same subject; Ollivier on the Spinal Marrow; Gendrin on the Anatomical History of Inflammations, and many others.

In addition to this catalogue of admirable writers
on pathology in the French school of medicine. I

may now state that M. Broussais, in his History of
Chronic Inflammations, has, in my opinion, rendered
a service to pathological medicine, of the utmost importance; and no one ought to consider himself as
having accomplished a proper course of professional
study, who has not perused it with such deep attention as to be thoroughly impregnated with his principles. Commencing his professional career with
an earnest desire to understand thoroughly all the
vital and morbid phenomena of pulmonary consumption; he assembled the facts on the subject reported
by different authors, expecting by their approximation to draw some sound general conclusions. He
was, however, disappointed; he found in his mind
an immense void, which compelled him to ascend
to the first source for himself, and by interrogating
nature there, to learn from her those operations,
which, in the uniformity of her laws, she never ceases
to present.

Under this impulse, he became charged with a
military service of great extent, where crowds of
soldiers were labouring under the disease which he
wished to explore. In these circumstances he had
the resolution to collect and to digest for himself
the history of each individual case, to set down its
symptoms from day to day, with its treatment, and
to observe its progress till its termination, either in
a perfect return to health, or in death. When the
latter occurred, he executed or superintended the
dissection of the patient for himself. Pursuing this
course rigidly for three years, 1805–6–7, in the midst

of the brilliant campaigns of the French in the north
of Europe; he found himself at length in possession
of all the facts that he desired, in regard to both
chronic inflammations of the lungs, and of the abdominal viscera. The first edition of this work appeared
in 1808, since which three others have been published, the two last in rapid succession. The result
of the inquiries of Mr. Broussais is, that the cellular
tissue is the leading seat of inflammation in most organs, and that the activity of the inflammation seems
to depend very much upon the relative quantity of
this tissue. That the analogies of chronic inflammation in all the organs of the body are very strongly
marked, but that it is modified by peculiarities in
the texture and composition of organs. That the
principles of inflammation being uniform both in the
acute and in the chronic stage; with an allowance
for differences of texture, one may apply to all the
organs of the body what he has narrated concerning
the progress and production of inflammations, in the
abdomen and thorax. That the period when one
made especial beings of the disorganization of the
lungs, of the bosom, of the testicle, of the neck, of
the uterus, was one of superstitious darkness in our
profession, and which has given way to the lights of a
physiological doctrine. That an osteo-sarcoma, a
spina ventosa, a chronic peripneumony or gastritis,
recognise the same original principles, and exhibit
results differing from one another, not in the essence of the disease, but from peculiarities in the
tissue assailed. That chronic inflammations of or-

D

gans essential to life, destroy more individuals than
pestilence and the sword added together, and that
these sorts of derangements have been very much
overlooked or not properly appreciated by any of
his predecessors.

I have now made a rapid sketch of the state of
pathological anatomy as a science, and it is evident
that much has been done for it; much, however, remains to be done in verifying and correcting the observations of others, in adding new ones, and in the
sound deduction of consequences.

A glimpse of the route to be followed having been
presented, a few preparatory hints before entering
upon it will not be amiss. Bichat has, with his usual felicity, stated, that the modes of death of all individuals are resolvable into three, each of which
impresses with its characters the organs of the body.
They are sudden death; death from an acute disease; and death from a chronic disease.

In sudden death while the individual is in a state
of health, the proper physiological appearance of the
organs, generally, is retained. The exterior of the
body preserves its plump and rounded contour, frequently the cheeks retain for some days a blush of
redness, and the mouth seems almost in a speaking
attitude. The mucous membrane of the stomach
and bowels is of a light pink colour; the muscles are
red, firm, contracted, and closely packed one upon
another, their relative situations being exactly observed. The violence which occasioned death will
be found most commonly upon one organ, as an

apoplectic effusion upon the brain, a rupture of the heart, or a congestion of blood in the lungs; from these several organs being such as require an incessant and uninterrupted exercise of their functions, for the support of the mechanism of life.

Acute inflammations which come to a rapid termination in death, alter sensibly the body from its physiological state. After the organ which is the seat of the inflammation, the principal alteration is in the sub-cutaneous adipose substance, which disappears very rapidly. If the disease be somewhat protracted, the muscles become emaciated more or less, and lose their redness and firmness. Other alterations in the body are not very perceptible. Putrefaction is disposed to take place quickly.

In the third case, where the mode of death is lingering, besides the disorganization which has occurred in the organ assailed, the whole mechanism of man is in a state of emaciation or marasmus. The plumpness of the exterior of the body has disappeared, the skin is shrivelled, and sticks closely to the parts beneath, the angular projections of the bones are readily seen under the skin, and even defined, the limbs and trunk are deprived of their fat, cellular substance and muscular matter; even the bones themselves diminish in size and lose their marrow, the place of which is supplied by serum in great part. The expression and extreme emaciation of the face, with its sunken, hollow eyes, collapsed cheeks, and open mouth, indicate strongly the misery from which the individual has escaped, and the blessings of death, where all pain and sorrow cease. Even the internal organs are affected by this general marasmus: the gastro-intestinal tube becomes thin and diaphanous; the liver and spleen are both shrunk and diminished much in size; and, from the general diminution of volume in the viscera of the abdomen, its muscles are drawn so far backwards that the projection of the spine in front through them is very conspicuous. The colour of parts, owing to the destitution of red blood, becomes much lighter, the brain is almost entirely white and firm, the muscles become yellow, watery, and like loose rags, infiltrations of serum are seen in various parts of the body. The fibrous membranes and structure, and the nerves, seem to suffer less diminution and change than any other organs, yet even they are affected.

Such are the effects of a chronic irritation on the human body tending to its dissolution. But the change is not confined to the solids, for the fluids themselves experience it also. The blood is abundant in sudden death, or, in that from acute disease, diffluent for the most part and black, diffused in the body, and well proportioned in its three constituents of serum, lymph, and red globules; but in chronic affections the two last disappear almost entirely, especially the red globules. This fluid, such as it is, recedes from the peripheral parts of the body, and is found principally in the heart and the large veins emptying into it; and, what is very common, the fibrine or lymph is collected into clear lumps scarcely tinged at all with red particles, and filling up the heart and its vessels with the concretions called polypi. It would seem, indeed, to be a law of the blood, that in proportion to the diminution of red particles so is the tendency of the lymph to assemble into these clots; hence it is in chronic affections with marasmus, that the blood often exhibits the buffy coat on being drawn,—a fact not sufficiently understood by practitioners, and frequently misinterpreted, to the great injury of patients.

Another remarkable feature in chronic diseases of long continuance is, that the affection is seldom confined to the organ primarily assailed; but most frequently excites chronic inflammation in others, principally such as are of most importance to life. Thus, in pulmonary consumption we almost invariably find chronic ulcerations of the mucous coat of the intestines, and the reverse; in chronic inflammations of the brain, we find both intestines and lungs with chronic inflammations; in chronic inflammations of the bones and joints, pulmonary consumption follows. In fine, the brain, the lungs, and the intestines, seem to be the three sentient points of the system, readily taking up primary diseases, and always responding to the diseases of one another, and to those of other organs.

PATHOLOGICAL ANATOMY.

CHAPTER I.

GENERAL CONSIDERATIONS ON DISEASE.

THE changes in the natural organism of the body, designated by the term disease, have their origin generally from
the influence of the physical agents, by which we are surrounded. Some of these agents act but feebly, and seem
rather to predispose to disease, than actually to excite it;
others are so energetic as not to leave a perceptible interval between their application and its consequences: while
others, again, are of so obscure a nature, and have such uniformity in their effects, as to be considered specific agents or
causes.

The most frequent sources of disease, are the agents the
most indispensable to animal life; as air, water, caloric,
light, electricity, and aliments. Any one, or all of them, by
being applied in an excessive or diminished degree, produce a deranged action; from which it appears that man on
all occasions has to observe the middle course, and to avoid
extremes in his physical as well as in his moral relations.
Under these circumstances, an exact scale for the conduct of
life is much to be desired; yet it is difficult, perhaps impos-

sible, to form it on immutable principles suited to every individual: for the degree of susceptibility to morbid impressions, is variously influenced by habits of life: age, sex, temperaments, and hereditary conformations.   Infancy disposes
to diseases of the brain, puberty to those of the thorax, middle life to disorders in the digestive organs, old age to diseases of the urinary apparatus, and the female sex to nervous affections.   In addition to these predispositions, almost
every individual has some place or point of his organization
weaker or more liable to undue excitement than any other,
or rather all other parts; so that when the general physical
causes just mentioned act somewhat beyond their customary
force, this point or place feels first the irregularity and is frequently thrown into disease.

Under all these infinitely modified circumstances, depending upon the variety of physical agents, of susceptibilities, and
upon the variety of organs that may be affected, the general
traits of diseased action are very analagous.   Thus its first
symptom is an increase of sensibility of the part, which, if
the disease be external, disposes one to feel the place and to
relieve its itching by gentle rubbing.   This symptom increases until it is evolved into the full and distressing sensation of pain (dolor;) frequently incessant, and most generally augmented by those excitants, which during the state of
health produced no appreciable impression.   There is also
an afflux of fluids (fluxus) to the part, by which its volume
is augmented: swelling, therefore, becomes another of the
symptoms of disease.   Other symptoms will be manifested,
according to the office which the organ affected executes in
the apparatus or machinery of life, and the more or less complete suspension of the duties of this organ.

The symptoms of disease are briefly all the departures
from the usual standard that occur in the form, in the size
and texture of organs; and especially in their actions.   The
symptoms, whose boundaries are circumscribed by those of
the affected organ, are termed *local*. those which are mani-

fested in organs not the seat of the disease, are called *sym-pathetic*. And again, there is a class of symptoms of a more diffused kind, which are called *general:* these are an acceleration of pulse, heat of skin, dryness of the tongue, shivering, and loss of muscular power.

On the Progress of Disease.

The order in which symptoms arise and follow each other constitutes the progress or march of disease. The progress is said to be *continued,* when there is no interruption to it from beginning to end; it is *intermittent* when the symptoms appear and disappear at intervals; it is *remittent* when, without disappearing entirely, its intensity is diminished at intervals, it is *acute* when it hastens to a termination, and *chronic* when the symptoms are slow in their developement.*

The continued progress is more common than any other; it is, however, seldom so uniform, but what occasional diminutions or augmentations may be observed: the augmentations, for the most part, occur during the night, the diminutions by day. Continued diseases also frequently are observed to augment for a time, then they remain stationary for a succeeding time, afterwards they decline and disappear.

---

*As the object of the following preliminary remarks on the morbid changes of the human body, is to prepare the reader for understanding more completely the convictions and language of the author in regard to the nature of these changes, he thinks it due to candour to state that in point of professional faith, he is an avowed adherent to the modern school of physiological medicine, at least in its doctrines. He has, therefore, both in the classification of subjects, and in the ideas inculcated, used freely the publications emanating from that school To the reader who is fond of such comparisons a reference to these works will show a common origin. Those which have been most serviceable are the Examen des Doctrines Medicales par F. J V. Broussais. Goupil Exposition des Doctrines, Boisseau Pyretologie Physiologique, Roche et Sanson Nouveaux Elements de Pathologie

These phases are technically called periods: the first is that of augmentation, (incrementum;) the second that of violence, (status;) the third, that of decline, (decrementum.)

In many cases of disease these periods are so abridged as not to be distinguished from one another, and are terminated either by sudden death, or by a very abundant discharge of sweat or urine, or by a copious spontaneous hæmorrhage.

The intermittence or periodicity of disease is one of the common forms of it. Each successive re-appearance of the symptoms is called by the collective term of *attack*, which, for the most part, begins with a shivering, followed by heat, and ends with a copious perspiration. The time intermediate to any two proximate attacks, is called apyrexia or intermission.

If the attacks be renewed every day, the disease is a quotidian; if every two days, a tertian; if every three days, a quartan; if every four days, a quintan; if every five days, a sextan.

Remittent diseases occupy the position intermediate to continued and to intermittent, and incline at one time to one, and at another time to the other.

Diseases may last from an hour or two, or even a shorter period to many years; this difference in duration has produced the distinction into acute and chronic. A disease may, according to some, be called acute so long as it has not exceeded forty days, afterwards it becomes chronic: nothing, however, can be less true, and indeed more unreasonable in medicine than this distinction, for the differences of tissues alone cause immense differences in the active stages of their diseases. An inflammation of the brain passes into a chronic state in less than twenty days, while one in the bones is still in the period of augmentation at the expiration of that time.

Of the Terminations of Disease.

Diseases terminate in several ways, of which that by metastasis and by crisis are the most remarkable. The cure by
metastasis occurs when the tissue primitively affected, ceases
to be the seat of the disease, and the latter is transferred to
another tissue; this displacement of the diseased action occurs spontaneously in many instances: on other occasions,
however, it is obtained by the interference of art, and is then
called revulsion. It sometimes happens under this disposition
of the animal frame, that a purulent collection of a distant
part of the body is suddenly removed from the place of its
formation and transported to the intestines, or bladder, with
the natural contents of which it is discharged. A circumstance worthy of attention in those cases is, that when fluids
or deposites of any kind are thus transported, they are generally thrown upon excrementitial surfaces, by which they
can be readily discharged from the body.

Crisis frequently assumes the appearance of metastasis,
but most commonly it is manifested by the copious return of excretions, which had been suspended previously.
These excretions are chiefly urine and sweat. The explanation given of this phenomenon is, that so long as the organ suffering was in a state of disease, the sympathy of the
skin and kidneys did not permit a free elaboration of their
secretion, but upon the removal of the primary disease, the
restriction was of course taken off from them.

Diagnostic.

The art of distinguishing diseases from one another, is called diagnostic, and to possess it to much extent the physician must have not only profound anatomical and physiological views, but that tact or experience which is derived from frequent observation of diseases at the bed-side of the patient.

In establishing our diagnostics, one of the most simple rules, but of the utmost importance, is, that when certain functions of the body are troubled, the symptoms depend upon a disease situated in the organ itself seeming to be disturbed. Thus, if there be difficulty in respiration, cough, deep seated pain in the thorax, purulent bloody expectoration, and a flat sound upon one side of the breast when it is struck, we infer that the patient has a diseased lung. The inferences in this case consist in a plain and direct reference of the symptoms, to the organ thus locally pointed out.

But it frequently happens that symptoms are not so easily referred to a diseased organ, either because they are not very intense or because the difference is so slight as not to be applicable between those which arise directly from the affected organ, and such as are merely sympathetic. This difficulty occurs in most chronic complaints, and in order to remove it, the proceeding is as follows. A superficial examination is first made of the head, neck, thorax, and abdomen, in order to obtain the general indications, of what organs or tissues are diseased in them and what are sound. A second examination is made, in which the consideration of the sound organs is left out, and such are marked as seem to be diseased; another exclusion is then made by which such organs are left out as seem to be merely sympathetically affected, and those of a doubtful kind are reserved for ulterior examination. Finally, in a third investigation, all the tissues or organs whose lesion does not afford sufficient cause for all the symptoms observed, are omitted successively, and a conclusion is made by fixing the disease upon one organ. Sometimes the symptoms are found to arise from two organs which shows a case of *complication.*

Cases, however, are occasionally so obscure that we cannot apply their symptoms to any one or more organs. The patient complains of only a feeling of general indisposition without local pain or uneasiness, and the most diligent and attentive examination does not serve to elucidate the disease. As the indisposition progresses the patient may become a victim to it, without the proper interposition of art. To disentangle the symptoms and to give more prominence to such as emanate from the diseased part, to destroy indeed the equilibrium which has been established among them, it is recommended to administer a strong stimulant; for, although this stimulation is received upon the stomach, yet it excites more strongly the organ really diseased, as in gout, pulmonary consumption, and other affections.

These several methods of diagnostic are so sure, that they are generally sufficient to indicate the seat and nature of diseases. For under their application the envelope of the body is rendered almost perfectly transparent, to the instructed physician.

Of the Prognostics of Diseases.

So many circumstances influence the progress and termination of diseases, that our judgments on these points are very apt to be incorrect; but the requisitions of patients and of their friends render frequently, the expression of opinion upon critical cases unavoidable. If the prognostic be confirmed by the death of the patient, we obtain the verdict of having passed a most enlightened judgment upon him; if however he recovers contrary to the prediction, though his restoration may have depended solely upon our advice and cares, yet ignorance is imputed to us. The greatest caution is therefore useful, and there should also be always connected with an expression of opinion, the expression of doubt and certain reservations. The leading precepts of prognostics are as follows:—

1. Disease is serious and threatening according to the importance of the organ assailed by it; to its intensity; to the age of the patient; to his constitution; his habits of living; to the state of mind, whether it be depressed by long mental exertions or by afflictions.

2. The more those unfavourable circumstances are numerous and complicated, the greater of course will be the danger; and the less numerous they are, of course the less will be the danger.

3. The favourable symptoms are, the usual state of the countenance being preserved; sprightliness. hope, a feeling of security; free respiration; tranquil sleep, from which the patient can be easily awaked; a soft moist skin; spontaneous bleeding from the nose, anus, or uterus.

4. Unfavourable symptoms are, extreme agitation or an unvarying immobility; rapid emaciation, in chronic affections; night sweats, in diseases of the lungs; great alteration in the physiognomy; infiltration of the limbs; gangrenous spots on the skin; partial or general convulsions; delirium, especially in adult persons; abundant sweats, especially when they are cold.

5. When restlessness succeeds to immobility in an acute affection, it is a mortal sign, especially if the patient make useless efforts to rise from bed. The same is the case in regard to the sardonic laugh, twitchings, a sudden and profound alteration of the countenance, carpology, loss of voice and muttering in acute diseases, the sudden cessation of acute pain with a profound alteration of the countenance, discouragement, despair, fatal presentiments, an exaltation of the intellectual faculties succeeding to delirium, spontaneous swoons and faintings, a voracious appetite appearing sudden-

ly in the course of an acute disease without a diminution of other symptoms: (This sign commonly announces death within twenty-four hours;) the passage of liquids through the esophagus as through an inert tube; hiccough, intermittence or suspension of the pulse, cold in the external parts while the internal are burning with heat; the want of effect in sinapisms and vesicatories; loosening of the skin or its ungluing where leeches have been applied.

Extreme debility is considered by many as a very unfavourable symptom; the observation of modern writers has, however, taught us that it is only so in chronic diseases, for as to acute, it is sometimes present from the beginning, and does not add to the unfavourableness of the prognostic.

After this enumeration, it should yet be borne in mind that none of these symptoms are absolutely unequivocal; for patients have recovered while they were present in greater or less number.

Of the Treatment of Diseases.

The principal general precepts under this head, are to remove the cause which has produced the disease, and then to keep the affected organ in a state of perfect inactivity or repose.

The first of these is such an obvious appeal to common sense, that it would, perhaps without suggestion, occur to the mind of every one. Thus the individual afflicted with intermittent fevers should be withdrawn from marshy or miasmatic places; one affected by an epidemic should be withdrawn from the focus of it. A foreign body should be extracted; displaced and divided parts should be restored to their primitive position. It frequently happens that by such management the patient is restored immediately to health: in a majority of cases, however, the physician is called too late for such rapid restoration, and has to resort to other means.

There is no rule of medical treatment of more general and useful application, than that of the perfect repose of a sick organ; we have, therefore, to forbid all deep meditation to a sick brain, all vision to a sick eye, all conversation to an inflamed larynx and lung, all motion to an irritated and inflamed muscle, and to fractured or dislocated limbs. It is under the judicious and general application of this rule that Dr. Physick has illustrated frequently his own unusual professional sagacity, and wrought many of his most unexpected and famous cures. As in all other things, there is a time for its useful application; and there is a time when it ceases to to do good, and may do harm. For example, a joint which is on the eve of an anchylosis should be moved from time to time in order to prevent it; a brain threatened with imbecility or fatuity, should be put on the moderate exercise of its faculties; an insensible eye or ear should in like manner be exercised.

When the several gradations and epochs of a disease have been passed through, it still remains to the physician, by a course of aliment, exercise, and amusement, to shorten the period of convalescence in a patient.

CHAPTER II.

ON THE FORM OF DISEASES.

As diseases consist in alterations of the tissues of our bodies, the observation and study of these alterations or in other words, pathological anatomy, is of the greatest importance. The alterations in the same tissue differ from one another, but when they are not characterized by a difference of symptoms during life, the simplicity of medicine, for the most part, requires that they should be considered as identical, at least in their general characters. Without some such restriction, different grades and mechanical forms of the same affection would be considered as different diseases; for it is well known, that the tissues, though the primary irritation be the same, present subsequently different physical and chemical changes or conditions, depending upon the duration of the disease, its intensity, its rapidity, the period at which death from it occurred, and some other circumstances.

The natural succession of alterations of each tissue, should be diligently noted from the commencement to the termination by death, and the first changes in an especial manner, as they are the principal and most important ones; such, indeed, as lay the foundation of all the others.

The alterations of the different tissues are as follow:—*

1. "Redness, injection, swelling, and loss of cohesion in the tissues. It is commonly called inflammation, and is by far the most frequent of all the primary changes, and the cause of many consecutive ones."

2. "Red indurations, granulations, vegetations, fungus, polypi."

* Roche et Sanson, loc. cit.

3d, " Vesicles, pustules, suppuration, erosion, ulceration, perforation, gangrene."

4th, " Thickenings, granulations, opacity of tissues naturally transparent, adhesions, effusions of serosity, false membranes."

5th, " Conversion of one tissue into another, such as into the cartilaginous, the osseous, the fibrous, the mucous, the dermoid, the serous, the cellular, the erectile."

6th, " White induration, gelatiniform degeneration, tubercles, encephaloid matter, cancerous matter. These alterations succeed often to inflammation, but they are sometimes primitive: they are called in mass sub-inflammations."

7th, " Contraction, obliteration or dilatation of natural canals."

8th, " Accidental canals, fistulæ, accidental tissues, cysts."

9th, " The developement of gaz in the midst of organs."

10th, " Living bodies developed in the midst of organs."

11th, " Effusions of blood; collections of this liquid. These alterations are called hæmorrhagies, which are most commonly indicated by an effusion of blood externally during life."

12th, " Productions which are cretaceous, stony, hairy, horny, melanose. The mode of formation of these alterations is not fully known."

13th, " Changes in form and position, as wounds, ulcers, distensions, lacerations, ruptures, fractures, and dislocations."

14. " Foreign bodies."

15. " Vicious conformations."

" We as yet are unacquainted with the alterations of which liquids are susceptible; it is asserted that they may be altered primitively: others maintain that their alteration is always consecutive, to a previous alteration of the organs charged with their preparation. It nevertheless appears that in scurvy, the composition of the blood is altered primitively. Perhaps it is also the case in other diseases; but to this day the proof has not been exhibited; and in the existing state

.of the science, it is not permitted to admit the primitive alterations of the blood and of other liquids but as possibilities. On the opening of dead bodies, the blood is found more or less liquid, of a natural or black colour, putrified;—the bile green, yellow, black, pitchy, corrosive;—the mucus is white, yellow, green, purulent, pultaceous, glue-like, membranous;—the serosity is limpid, turbid, thick, inodorous, fœtid. But all of these alterations are without a known value, the greater part of them depend evidently on a primitive alteration of the tissues, and the same is probably the case with all."

The obscurity which prevails over the real nature of the morbid alterations of the solids and fluids, leaves much to be desired in fixing them upon just and unexceptionable grounds of classification, and the difficulty is increased by certain morbid conditions of the organs, being wholly inappreciable to the eye and touch of the observer, and leaving indeed much to mere conjecture. The following classification adopted by the modern school of pathology serves at least to bring under general heads nearly all the features of a deranged organism, and is, therefore, recommended to us for its simplicity and facility of application to our reasonings and observations in medicine.

Class I.—*Irritations.*

Alterations of tissues, consisting in an unusual afflux of the habitual fluids of the part, and in an augmentation of irritability.

Class II.—*Asthenies.*

Alterations of the tissues, consisting in a diminished afflux of the habitual fluids and in a decrease of irritability.

Class III.—*Lesions of Continuity.*

Fractures, wounds, &c.

Class IV.—*Lesions of Relative Situation.*

Dislocation.

Class V.—*Dilatations.*
A partial dilatation of natural canals.

Class VI.—*Contractions.*
Strictures of natural passages.

Class VII.—*Obstructions.*
Obstruction of natural passages.

Class VIII.—*Accidental Passages.*
The formation of openings and of new passages.

Class IX.—*Morbid Productions.*
Tumours, excrescences.

Class X.
Disorganizations.

Class XI.—*Partial Death.*
Death and gangrene.

Class XII.
Vicious conformations.

Class XIII.—*Foreign Bodies.*
The presence of foreign bodies in the midst of the tissues.*

Irritation.

The full execution of all the phenomena of life, requires a perfect state of health, or integrity in its organs, and the action of stimulants upon them. The condition whereby they are permitted to feel the impressions of the latter, is termed irritability. They are all; and, perhaps in virtue of this irritability, pervaded by fluids, and the seat of the process of composition and of decomposition.

---

*A work having for its object the filling up of this outline would comprise every thing in medicine, I must, therefore, disclaim any such intention my principal object is to deal with the first class or that of irritations, by a report of its phenomena in many of the tissues and organs of the body.

These latter processes, common to all organs, but under circumstances modified more or less in each, may be termed the *organic action* of a part, in order to distinguish them from the *functions* of the same part, by which we mean the particular duty which any organ has to perform in the operations of life. For example, the testicle, and the liver probably have their organic actions, their operations of composition and decomposition very much alike, but their secretions and their functions are essentially different; the one being intended for the propagation of the species, is not indispensable to the individual; whereas the liver cannot be dispensed with. Therefore, when either of these organs is put in contact with a stimulant, if the stimulant be more than it is accustomed to, or if the irritability of the organ be above its common standard, the organic action is augmented; the fluids are drawn to the organ in unusual abundance, and the action of composition and decomposition, or its interstitial action is augmented; but, while this is going on, the functions of the organ are executed with a difficulty and embarrassment proportionate to the increase of the interstitial action.

While the interstitial or organic action is kept within certain bounds, it is very compatible with health, and is a mere excitation; so that it is not every degree, even to the smallest, of increased interstitial action, that interferes with the functions of an organ. When, however, it is brought to the latter point, it constitutes disease or morbid irritation, which is the most general fact in morbid or pathological anatomy.

Morbid irritation being then only an augmentation of the natural interstitial actions of a part, is of course governed by the same laws. We thus find that as interstitial action is harmonized over the whole body, by means of the unity of the latter, or its sympathies, so morbid irritation extends its influence in the same way. Organic, or interstitial action is caused to languish and decrease, by withdrawing the usual stimulants from the body; morbid irritation does the same.

Irritation is always local in the first instance: it cannot ex‐ ist at the same moment in all parts of the body. It may, however, occupy two or three organs, or even a larger number; but, in such case, the suffering of one commonly conceals that of the others. "Duobus laboribus simul exis‐ tentibus, vehementior obscurat alterum," says Hippocrates. It is only in mild diseases, that several points of irritation can exist to the same degree at the same time. Sometimes they alternate in their intensity; on other occasions, when the dominant disease has run its course and terminated, the suppressed one is evolved, and then runs its course.

Irritation is presented under various degrees in each of the various tissues, and may be arranged into *mild, mid‐ dle,* and *intense.* It is acute, when many sympathies are developed, and it passes rapidly through its course; it is chronic under other circumstances; continued when its course is uninterrupted, but progresses regularly from be‐ ginning to end; intermittent, when it disappears for a time, and returns periodically, as in one, two, three, or more days; and it is remittent, when the two last forms of it are blend‐ ed, to wit, when though its course is uninterrupted it is yet under exacerbations and declensions of the symptoms.

The intensity of an irritation depends upon the intensity of its cause, and upon the irritability of the tissue affected. Hence, if a light cause operate upon a tissue of but little ir‐ ritability, the irritation will be slight; but, it will be severe if the tissue be naturally irritable: and we of course have the highest possible point of irritation, when the irritant is severe upon an irritable tissue. It will be easy to imagine a great number of cases depending upon these two circum‐ stances, the grade of irritability of the tissue, and the grade of the irritant.

An uninterrupted course is the most frequent form of ir‐ ritation, and it arises from this, that when the afflux of fluids to a part is once established by an irritant, it is kept up by the irritation itself, notwithstanding the primary cause be withdrawn, so that the two actions, increased irritability and an increased afflux of fluids, tend mutually to a continuance, at least for a time, until the disposition in the body, to re-establish an equilibrium of action with other parts, succeeds.

All irritations which exist under a continued form, may also exist under an intermittent one. The latter has been supposed to depend upon the causes themselves of these irritations being intermittent,* or applied with a sort of intermittent force to the bodies of persons exposed to them. I doubt this theory, because many individuals have intermittent fever, who were exposed but once, and that only for a short time, to its causes. It is more probable, that the intermittence is an effort of the system to restore its own equilibrium, in the same way that remittence is; or even the full and complete arrest of irritation, in any disease whatever. I do not however deny that marsh effluvium is more active by night than it is by day, for its activity seems to depend upon, or to be connected with the quantity of sensible moisture in the atmosphere; and it is, perhaps, precipitated from a state of perfect solution in the air, just as water is, by a lowering of temperature during the night. In this way it becomes an intermittent cause of disease. The effluvium of a dissecting room is always more easily and intensely perceived in a spell of cloudy weather; and is then indeed frequently almost intolerable, until a perfect solution of the moisture in the air, is accomplished by lighting fires. A still stronger example of the effect of moisture in increasing the perceptible quantity of effluvium, is found in the intensity of that, which rises in the vapour of a boiling skeleton. The effluvium from meats, immediately after cooking, is always more disagreeable from its being attended by the vapour that exhales from them.

The influence of sun-set or night in giving effect to marshy exhalations is within both popular and professional experi-

* See Roche et Sanson, vol. i. p. 35, 36, 37, &c.

ence. An illustration of the best kind is found in the Pon-
tine marshes near Rome, which may be passed with impunity during broad daylight, but after six o'clock in the afternoon become dangerous beyond measure, by causing a disease like the yellow fever of our country. Doctor Boisseau has mentioned, that an army apothecary whom he
knew, for several days in succession, at mid-day, had stirred
up the mud of the marshes and remained in the midst of
their exhalations, without suffering from them.

There are six different forms in the local condition of Irritations.

The most numerous of the six, is where the seat of the
irritation becomes painful, warm, swollen, and red from the
increased afflux of blood into its capillary system. This form
of irritation constitutes *Inflammation,* or *Phlegmasia.*

Another form somewhat more unusual is, where the part
thus swollen and heated, permits blood to be discharged either
from its surface or in its centre. This constitutes the *Hæ-
rhagic form,* or *Hæmorrhage.*

A third form is when neither the heat, the redness, nor
the pain of the part is much augmented, and the swelling
is produced by an afflux of the white portions of the blood
only, into the capillary system of the part. This constitutes
Sub-Inflammation.

Sometimes there is neither an augmentation of heat, of
swelling, nor of redness, but only of pain. This constitutes
a *Neurosis,* or *Nervous Irritation.*

In a fifth form the irritation, augmented but very slightly above the healthy standard of vital actions, is manifested only by an excessive growth or nutrition of the part.
This is *Nutritive Irritation.*

And lastly, irritation is sometimes manifested only by an
increase of the natural secretion of the part. This constitutes the *Secretory Irritation.*

Though, in many cases of irritation, the forms of it just

mentioned are kept entirely distinct, yet in many others they are blended. The first form is more common in deep-seated parts, as in the muscles, in glands, and in the interstitial cellular substance. The hæmorrhagic, seems to be more common to the mucous membranes, as of the lungs, the nose, the bowels. The excretion of white matter is more common to serous membranes, as in the pleura and peritoneum; in whose irritations coagulating lymph and serum are both thrown out abundantly, and sometimes even the red particles of blood also.

As each of these six forms of irritation may be light, middle, or intense; acute or chronic; continued, intermittent, or remittent; we have thus the foundation laid for a large majority of diseases. And when we reflect that additional modifications are imposed by the diversity of tissues, temperaments, idiocrasies, ages, sex, climate and seasons; we shall readily understand how an immense seeming variety of diseases will spring from varied combinations of these causes, though they all have a unity in one respect, being all dependant upon irritation.

The six forms of irritation are supposed to be identical, and merely to differ in the degree of intensity.* A strong objection, however, to this opinion is urged by M. M. Roche and Sanson, to wit, that hæmorrhagies, inflammations, and neuroses have each degrees of intensity also, from very mild to very severe forms, and that it is far from being demonstrated that a very severe neurosis, is below the lowest degree of sub-inflammation.

* Boisseau Pyretologie Physiologique p. 27, Paris, 9824.

CHAPTER III.

PHENOMENA OF IRRITATIONS.

SECT. I —PHLEGMASIA.

Acute inflammation, or phlegmasia, is by far the most frequent form of irritations; for it probably constitutes the beginning of ninety, out of every hundred cases of disease. When situated on the external surface of the body it is recognized by redness, swelling, heat, and pain. In parts generally, these symptoms will be presented in different degrees, according to the intensity of the irritation. Their relative proportions to one another, are also modified in a very striking manner by the nature of the tissue affected. In the naturally vascular tissues, the redness is very much augmented in a short time; in such as are of a loose texture, so as to permit an easy distention by the afflux of fluids, the swelling is considerable, but in ligamentous structures, as they are of a hard unyielding texture, the swelling is comparatively inconsiderable, while the pain itself is very severe.

Acute inflammation terminates in several ways. Sometimes the blood which had been accumulated in a part, disappears in a short time from it, and leaves no visible traces; in this case the probability is, that the blood was confined to its regular vascular channels, and that they alone were distended by it. This termination constitutes *delitescence.*

On other occasions the red blood is infiltrated into the affected parts; either by a rupture of the vessels, or by an over distention of them, which permits a lateral percolation.

In such cases, a longer period is required for its removal; and when this is finished, the inflammation is said to have terminated by *resolution.*

Again, it frequently happens, that the vital action of the parts not being sufficient to accomplish the removal of the effused blood; the latter is retained in a fluid state, while the parts affected take on a secretory action, and discharge pus. When an abscess is opened under these circumstances, the discharge is at first fluid blood; mixed with pus more or less completely elaborated, according to the period at which the opening is made; afterwards the secretion of the part is seen in a more unmixed state, and finally perfectly pure pus: being then whitish, milky, inodorous, and insipid. The termination of inflammation here, is said to be by *suppuration.*

In many cases where a surface is the part inflamed, a regular suppuration fails to be established, and a superficial erosion follows. such erosion increases in depth and in extent for a time, and then heals. This termination of inflammation is said to be by *ulceration.*

On other occasions the afflux of blood to the part ceases very gradually, the pain disappears in the same way, and also the increased heat; but the tumefaction continues to augment slowly and regularly, by a deposite of the white portions of the blood, and an indurated mass is finally left This termination is said to be by *induration,* or *scirrhus.* And if the induration remains red, as it sometimes does in the highly vascular tissues, the termination is called red induration or hepatization. In either of the last cases the inflammation is said to have ended in a *chronic state.*

Finally, the inflammatory action of a part is sometimes so excessive that none of the preceding terminations occur, but the part affected is absolutely killed or deprived of life. This is called the termination by *gangrene.*

Pus varies in its colour somewhat, according to the texture of the part producing it; it is therefore whitish, grey, like the leys of wine, or blackish; also it is frequently fœtid:

this I think occurs most commonly in empyema. Albumen is always a constituent of pus, so as to form its basis; besides which it contains some neutral salts, whose proportion varies according to the different varieties of this secretion. The presence of pus in any tissue whatever, may be considered as a conclusive proof of inflammation subsisting, or having subsisted there.

The vestiges of acute inflammation are diminished upon death, and in some measure in proportion to the rapidity of its progress during life. Besides which, it has been remarked that these traces are more readily lost in some tissues than in others; for example, more readily in the skin than elsewhere, more readily in serous membranes than in mucous. The permanency of the vestiges of inflammation in the same tissue, is also affected by certain localities; for example, they disappear from the face more readily after death than they do in other portions of the skin; from the internal coat of the stomach, more readily than from that of the intestines. They disappear also more readily after the moveable and intermittent irritations, than after such as are fixed and continued.

In a very great majority of dissections, the traces of acute inflammation are satisfactorily manifested by redness, tumefaction, softening, suppuration, ulceration, induration. And in chronic inflammations there are other marks; such, for example, as a brownish colour in mucous membranes; purulent collections, adhesions, accidental tissues, and the developement of tubercles, and morbid ossifications.

SECT II.—HÆMORRHAGES.

In regard to hæmorrhagic irritation, the same causes are productive of it, as of the others, yet it would seem to require a certain predisposition, or a nervoso sanguineous temperament, which means, a well developed arterial system, readily obeying the impulses of nervous excitation. Like

other irritations it may be acute or chronic, continued or intermittent. When it exists it is most frequently manifested
by a discharge of blood externally, but sometimes the hæmorrhage is not seen, and then its symptoms are more equivocal.

Acute hæmorrhage is almost always preceded by a feeling of tumefaction, heaviness, heat and pain of the part
which becomes the seat of it. The congestion of which
these are the symptoms, is called by writers the *molimen
hæmorrhagicum;* and, when considerable it is attended by
chilliness, shivering, paleness of the skin, and a contracted
pulse. It is principally upon the absence of these phenomena in some hæmorrhagies, that authors have admitted
such to be passive; that is to say, produced by a relaxation,
a feebleness, and a gaping of the capillary vessels. M.
Broussais has rejected the idea of passive hæmorrhagies except in a very few cases: such as effusions under the skin,
and mucous membranes in scurvy; and such as are produced by mechanical injuries to the vessels. I doubt,
whether facts will bear him out entirely in this opinion;
for it is by no means uncommon to see small spots, and indeed sometimes considerable ones, of red blood effused in
the thickness of muscles in the last stages of dropsy, evidently, I think, proving a passive hæmorrhage. Also, in
pregnant women whose habit of body is delicate, we not
unfrequently see spots of ecchymosis in the legs.

It is owing to the very superficial course of blood vessels
on mucous membranes, that hæmorrhage occurs most frequently in them. The process of injecting a subject affords
sufficient illustrations of this fact; and also that hæmorrhagies occur from membranes, very much in proportion to
the density of their structure. For example, in throwing a
fine injection into a young subject from the arch of the aorta,
so as to fill all the arterial system; the injection will at first
come colourless from the nose and mouth, then it will bring
along with it the colouring matter, so that at length it will

Q

exude in very much the same state, in which it is passed into
the aorta.   But in regard to the serous membranes, as the
pleura and the peritoneum, though much of the injecting
matter escapes into their cavities, yet it it always strained
off from the colouring ingredient.   The same takes place in
the cellular substance.   From this it appears that hæmorrhages of red blood, will occur more readily from mucous
membranes, than from serous; probably both on account of
the greater abundance of red blood vessels in them, and on
account of the superficial positions of those vessels.

SECT. III.—SUB-INFLAMMATION.

Sub-inflammation is a very common form of disease, and
carries off an immense number of victims annually; there
are but few dissecting-room subjects which do not manifest
it in some of their organs.   The same causes may produce
it, as produce any other form of irritation or inflammation,
and it may be either in a chronic, or in an acute state.
It sometimes, indeed frequently from the very beginning,
has only its own peculiar symptoms, such as the afflux of
white fluids to the part, yet, perhaps, in the majority of
cases, it commences by symptoms of common inflammation,
which subside into those of sub-inflammation.   It is attended
at first with but little heat or pain; and few or no symptoms arise from it for some time.   But finally, if the tumefaction goes on regularly increasing, the sympathies of
other parts of the body are strongly excited, and produce
great distress; as, for example, in scirrhus of the uterus,
ovaria, &c.   The temperaments most exposed to this form
of irritation are where the lymphatic system predominates,
as in women and in children.

Sub-inflammation may terminate in several, or indeed in
all of the ways belonging to common inflammation, or
phlegmasia, that is, by resolution, suppuration, ulceration,
gangrene.   It does not, however, seem as yet to be a de-

cided point, whether it ever terminates by delitescence.
When this irritation has gone on for some time, it produces
those changes and disorganizations in the tissues, and organs
of the body known as scirrhi, tubercles, encephaloid matter.   These sometimes remain for a long period without exciting severe sympathies; but finally they become like extraneous bodies, and then the disturbance of the system is very
great.   Cancer is one of the consequences of those sub-inflammations.

Resolution from sub-inflammation may of course be viewed
as the most happy mode of termination, but it is a very long
time in being brought about.   Scirrhus may be considered a more common consequence, and would be a sufficiently salutary termination, provided it remained stationary for
ever afterwards; but as scirrhus is disposed finally to become acutely inflamed itself, exceedingly painful, to suppurate and ulcerate; the efforts of nature to remove it, excite disease in contiguous parts, and not unfrequently cause
death.   Gangrene is a very rare termination of sub-inflammation, but may become a very salutary and speedy one; for
a violent inflammation suddenly attacking a scirrhus mass, its
life is destroyed at once, and it being thrown off, the cure
becomes perfect.   It is on this principle that very stimulating articles applied by quacks to scirrhous tumours, sometimes remove them; but if their strength and action are not
sufficient to accomplish such a degree of irritation, they then
act simply as excitants, and rather exasperate than relieve the
disease.

" The leading anatomical characters of sub-inflammation,
whereby it may be known; consist in a white tumefaction
or engorgement of the tissues, with induration; and the deposite of concreted lymph in the middle of the substance of
organs.   The tissues thus affected, are also converted into
homogeneous masses, white or greyish, in which no organization is recognized."*

* Roche et Sanson, vol. i. p. 53

SECT. IV.—NERVOUS IRRITATION, OR NEUROSIS.

Nervous irritation, or neurosis, is most frequently manifested in females, and individuals of a delicate irritable frame
of body and mind, and also in young persons.   The causes
which produce it are not always very obvious, but they are
frequently found in a neglect of exercise, and of exposure to
the open air; luxurious habits of life, over-stimulating or un-
suitable articles of diet: solitary habits, whereby the mind,
like the body, loses that tone which can only be derived from
an active and bustling intercourse with the world.   If a comparison can be instituted on such an occasion, I would say
that the nervous fluid of both mind and body, is so accumulated for the want of the ordinary means of drawing it off,
that like a highly charged Leyden jar, its surplus of electric
matter is quickly manifested on the approach of the most
delicate tests to it.   In this overcharged state, the least important events or occurrences of life are sensibly felt.   A
light breeze of air, a light shower, a slight neglect of a friend
or acquaintance, a slight mortification or disappointment,
obstacle or insult; make an impression upon an individual
thus circumstanced, quite equal to causes of much greater
magnitude, operating upon one whose intellectual habits are
more suited to sound health and good tone of body or mind.
According to this rule, or condition, our sensibilities are generally proportionate to our habits of luxurious indulgence,
and they increase with the latter.   Such being the law of
our natures, it is not surprising that persons not kept in
subjection by the salutary precepts and humiliation of a proper life; are almost invariably disappointed in not realiz-
ing the happiness they had hoped for; when they are transferred from laborious and necessitous industry to a state of
affluence and self-indulgence.

In regard to the physical condition of nervous irritation.
It may be presented in any of the forms of the preceding

irritations; to wit, chronic, acute, intermittent, remittent
or continued: and these states may run into one another,
so as to give a very great irregularity to the phenomena of
the disease. Pain, which is frequently of a very acute
kind, seems to be the only local symptom of this irritation; for, unlike the others, it is deficient in augmentation
of heat, of redness, and in tumefaction. When the irritation is seated in an interior organ, the presence of pain there
with the absence of heat in the skin and of a more frequent
pulse, will serve to denote the nature of the affection; notwithstanding the apparent disorder into which the functions
of the organ may be thrown.

In some parts of the nervous system, for example in
the brain and in the spinal marrow, their functions may be
very much impaired, and yet there is no local pain; and
upon post mortem examination no appreciable change of organization exists. But if the neurosis has subsisted for a
long time in a continued state, (for most frequently it is
intermittent,) then the affected tissue is perceptibly inflamed.*

A neurosis seldom is succeeded by hæmorrhage, by sub-
inflammation, by suppuration, by resolution, or by gangrene.

SECT. V —SECRETORY IRRITATION.

The secretory irritation does not seem to be peculiar to,
or more disposed to show itself in one temperament, or at
one age than another. It is most frequently a symptom
of some other irritation. Its states also may be chronic, or
acute, intermittent, remittent, or continued.

It is manifested neither by increased heat, by pain, by
redness, nor by tumefaction of the organ which is the seat
of it, but simply by increased secretion. The fluid secreted
will therefore, present itself under several varieties depend-

* Roche et Sanson.

ing upon the affected source, and also upon the modified secretion of each viscus at different periods.   Marandel was
one of the first to point out the secretory irritation and its
varieties. When death follows this irritation, it is commonly
preceded by the inflammation, or the sub-inflammation, of the
affected organ.

SECT. VI.—NUTRITIVE IRRITATION.

The nutritive irritation is the least approximated of any
to a morbid condition, and is simply the excess of nutrition in a part, giving it an increased and unusual size.   It
is, consequently, attended neither by heat, pain, nor redness; and it seems to be a disease principally when by its
size and its gravitation, it encroaches upon adjacent parts,
or pulls them out of place.   There are some cases, also,
where an increased nutrition, troubles the functions of the
organ in which it is situated.

CHAPTER IV.

OF SYMPATHIES.

EACH organ of the body exercises a marked influence upon the others, which becomes very obvious in disease, and has obtained the appellation of sympathy. It is very clear that this mutual dependence of organs must prevail both in health and in disease, and is absolutely necessary to the unity and harmony of the body.

This sympathy, which exists continually between the organs, becomes more prominent and well marked in proportion to the irritability of the individual, the intensity of the irritation, and the importance of the organ affected. When the organ is of the first consequence to the preservation of life and the irritation of it severe, many other organs are found to participate strongly in its affection; and thereby to produce a very general disturbance in the system. The order of importance, in the organs of the body, is thus set down: "The nervous system is that which provokes the greatest number of sympathies; the mucous membrane of the alimentary canal is the second; the heart is next; then the skin, the lungs, the serous membranes, the articulations, the uterus, the testicles, the kidneys, the bladder, the liver, the muscles, the cartilages. The pancreas, the spleen, the thyroid gland, and the bones, are the lowest in the scale, and on nearly the same elevation."*

Channels of Sympathies.—Sympathies have generally been supposed to depend upon the nervous communications

* Roche et Sanson, vol. 1. p. 56.

between organs, for the reason that if the nerves of a part
be cut, its sympathies are interrupted. But it is very difficult
to settle this question by accurate and exact observations,
for the same importance may by the same experiment, be
attributed to the blood vessels.   There can be no doubt of
either a direct or an indirect communication, of nerves from
each point of the body to all other points: so that we have
no difficulty from anatomical arrangements merely, in admitting the nervous theory of sympathy, to its fullest extent.   It is not entirely clear what nerves execute this
office; whether the nerves of the brain and spinal marrow, or those of the ganglionic system, or both together.
M. Broussais thinks that the sympathies of the organs of
animal life are kept up through the intervention of the brain
and medulla spinalis; for the reason, that when its parts
are paralyzed by an affection of these organs, their sympathies cease.   But the intervention of the brain is not necessary to the sympathies of the organs of organic life, inasmuch as they receive their nerves from the sympathetic. As
some of them, however, receive a partial supply of nerves
from the brain and spinal marrow, the intervention of those
organs is partially useful.

Baglivi believed that the membranes were the channels of
sympathy between different parts of the body, because he
considered that all the membranes came from the brain.
Bordeu saw in sympathies only a series of oscillatory movements propagated by the cellular membrane.   The vascular
system has also been considered by some as the channel of
sympathies; as many of them, it was supposed, could be
explained by the anastomoses of arteries; for example, the
junction between the internal mammary and the epigastric
arteries, would explain the seeming connexion between the
mammæ and the uterus.

Sympathies of Particular Tissues.—As a general rule,
it may be stated that each elementary tissue of the body has

a general alliance of sympathy between all its parts. The examples of this are very numerous.

1. In regard to the Nerves or the Nervous System. The alliances of its parts are multiplied and various, existing not only between fasciculi coming from the same root, but between very distant fasciculi, even those on different sides. The sympathy of the two optic nerves is notorious, even to common observation. The several branches of the trigeminus are allied very closely by sympathies; of the pneumogastric; of the Trisplanchnic or Great Sympathetic.

Some of the most remarkable sympathies have been enumerated by Mr. Gall; for example, those which connect the cerebellum and the organs of generation. Castration, it is said, arrests the developement of the cerebellum, and reduces it to a state resembling atrophy. Hippocrates has observed, that wounds behind the ears, rendered the semen unfruitful. Larry mentions the example of a man, who at nineteen years old having received a blow on the back of the neck, his testicles gradually dwindled almost away.

2. The sympathies of the muscles are very manifest in tetanus from wounds. In a rupture of the diaphragm, one of the most remarkable symptoms is the sardonic laugh; the mouth being sometimes most hideously deformed.

3. The sympathies of the skin are very numerous and striking, not only between the different parts of this tissue, but between it and other organs. A partial application of cold to it, causes a general shivering.

Sudden suppression of a copious perspiration, produces an inflammation of some internal organ. The skin is sometimes extremely painful to the touch just over an inflamed organ; as, for example, over the abdomen in inflammations of the stomach, of the peritoneum, of the uterus, &c. Petechiæ, miliary eruptions, and tetter, are often indicative of internal inflammations. The yellow colour of the skin, is also a phenomenon of jaundice and of yellow fever.

3. The sympathies of the different parts of the vascular

system, the heart and arteries, with each other, are sufficiently manifest in aneurism of the arteries, and in dilatations
and ossifications of the heart.   They also sympathize very
readily with the affections of all the other organs, and from
their being subject to comparatively few diseases, are rather
the seats, than the points of departure for sympathies.

4. The sympathies of the serous membranes are very remarkable, both with one another and with the other tissues
and distant parts of the body.   An inflammation of the pleura
is apt to supervene upon operations of a considerable kind in
any part, and to be followed by the death of the patient.   In
such circumstances, a considerable quantity of pus mixed
with serum, coagulating lymph in the pleura and adhesions,
have been observed on one side of the thorax.   About fifteen
years ago, Dr. Physick extirpated a large tumour from the
neck, of a middle-aged woman.   During the operation, the
primitive carotid, the internal jugular vein, and the adjoining nerves, were laid bare.   The woman died of pleuritic
inflammation a few days afterwards.

Latterly, a lady of middle age, fell with a tooth brush in
her mouth, it was driven with considerable force backwards
so as to lacerate the pharynx, and narrowly escaped the
large blood vessels and nerves in the upper part of the neck.
It was followed by pleurisy and inflammation of the lungs,
ending in consumption; of which she died in seven or eight
weeks from the period of the accident.   Excessive pain and
an almost insurmountable difficulty in swallowing were
among the early consequences of the injury: these were succeeded by a large abscess under the insertion of the sterno
cleido mastoid muscle, which at one time communicated
with the pharynx: hence an impression prevailed that the
head of the brush had been driven in that direction.

5. The sympathies of the mucous membranes one with
another and also with other tissues, are equally well marked
with those of the serous.

The preceding is only a very general account of what the

Sympathies of the human body are, the picture can only be finished by the study of each accident, and each disease respectively. But from what has been said, it will appear that every part of the body may be the point of departure for a series of sympathics, though some points more readily excite them than others. Many observations have been made on this subject, from which the inference is, that most of the organs are held in a well settled and reciprocal sympathy; which, though not evident in perfect health, has its symptoms evolved and displayed during disease. And that besides these regular and common sympathies there are many others, which, though they may take place, are yet not to be looked for as inevitable.

Those organs which excite the greatest number of sympathies, also receive the most. Their sympathetic influence will also excite a sympathy of other parts, so that we have here a sympathy of a sympathy; and perhaps the chain of sympathies may have still more links in it. For example, headache is very frequently the indication of the brain sympathizing in the affection of some other organ; and this sympathy may be so much excited as to produce delirium and convulsions, as happens in children, in women, and in irritable persons. This occurs more frequently in phlegmasia of the mucous membrane of the stomach and bowels, than in other affections: it is indeed rare in the latter. Hence, a rule has been laid down in practice, that where delirium and convulsions attend an inflammation of the lung, they are rather indicative of an idiopathic affection of the encephalon, than of a sympathetic one; and so of many other diseases.

The readiness with which the mucous membrane of the stomach and bowels, sympathizes with the accidents and diseases of other organs, is a very remarkable fact in its history, and highly influential upon the principles of pathology. This sympathy is manifested in all severe inflammations of the skin, of the cellular membrane, of the articulations, and other parts of the body;—in all wounds and severe accidents. Its evidences are, the appetite being lost, nausea, heat and pain in the epigastric region, strong thirst, and a redness of the tongue at the edges and point; general heat and dryness of the skin, and, in one word, all the symptoms that mark traumatick fever.

Another of the leading sympathies that occur on the occasion of any disturbance in the system; is an unusual state of the circulation, manifested by the action of the pulse, at the wrist. In health the pulse is as follows per minute: one hundred for an infant, eighty for puberty; seventy for adult life, and sixty for the aged. In either of these states, when the pulse strikes oftener than usual, it is said to be *frequent*; but when the contrary, it is *slow*. There are also several modifications of the pulse depending on its volume: thus. it is said to be *full* or *large*, when its size is greater than usual, or *small*, if the contrary. With these conditions it may be *soft* or *hard, strong* or *weak, vibrating, quick*. Also the strokes may succeed at regular or irregular intervals; they may be of the same strength, an equal pulse; or of varying strength, an unequal one; certain pulsations may be omitted constituting an intermittent pulse; or additional pulsations may be introduced between the regular ones, an intercident pulse.

Frequency of pulse is the most common attendant on irritations, and seems to exhibit in a considerable degree, the measure of their intensity. It is generally attended with increased heat, and the two together constitute the leading phenomena of fever. It is said that when irritation occupies a considerable fasciculus of blood vessels, the pulse is full; but when it is confined to a membrane, it is then small; but frequency attends each of these modifications of volume.

It has, for a long time, been disputed by physicians, whether symptoms of fever could occur without local irritation, or, in the language of the profession, whether there could be such a thing as an idiopathic fever. The new light which has been shed on pathological anatomy, has reduced very much the number of persons admitting it; and indeed seems to bid fair to remove this notion entirely, as an error founded on our imperfect means of investigation.

The sympathies of the skin with other organs, are principally manifested in the nervous system; in the kidneys, the articulations, and in the pleura and peritoneum. The skin also seems to be the seat of three of the remarkable phenomena of fever; to wit, increased heat, shivering, and sweat. The two first depend upon the state of the circulation; for when the latter is rapid, the heat of the body is more equally diffused, so that at every point it is the same, or nearly so, as at the centre of circulation. Shivering is attended with a very general sensation of cold, and may last from a few seconds to many hours. It is the precursor of almost all violent irritations of the body which come on abruptly. Its own approach is sudden, and is manifested by paleness, contraction of the skin, and an erection of the hairs and papillæ on its surface. It belongs to the phenomena of health as well as of disease; and is exhibited frequently at the commencement of digestion, of strong mental emotions, and also during external cold. The theory of it is, that it will occur whenever there is a sudden and strong concentration upon an internal organ of the vital powers, whereby they are withdrawn from the skin.

Sweating is a phenomena, the inverse of shivering; and in both health and disease manifests the more general diffusion of the vital powers: and their having been withdrawn from an internal organ, to be more equalized in their distribution. When it occurs, therefore, spontaneously, during an internal inflammation, it may be considered as a propitious sign, provided the inflammation is acute. Under other circumstances, as in chronic diseases of the lungs and of the joints, it is not favourable; but is indeed rather one of the evil accompaniments of such affections.

The muscles of locomotion also sympathize with the affections of many of the internal organs, so that they become frequently too weak to be used. The more severe the internal irritation is, the more is muscular debility apparent and considerable: there are, however, some exceptions to this rule. More consequence has been attributed to this symptom of muscular debility, than it deserves; or rather it has been much mistaken, and has led to very false modes of practice in fevers, called typhus.

Wherever sympathetic irritation may show itself, as it is of the same nature with the primitive irritation, it not unfrequently becomes a disease of the same character as that from which it arose. It is inflammatory, if it has come from an inflammation; hæmorrhagic, if from hæmorrhagy; sub-inflammatory, if from sub-inflammation; nervous, if from a neurosis; secretory, if from an undue secretion; and nutritive, if from undue nutrition. Upon this is founded diathesis, or one general condition of the body, by an extension of its sympathies from a single point or place. There are, therefore, as many diatheses as there are irritations; to wit, six: the inflammatory, the hæmorrhagic, the sub-inflammatory, nervous, secretory, and nutritive.† So long as the sympathies are confined to the same elementary tissue in which the primitive affection occurred, the rule holds good; at least in a large majority of instances. But when other tissues participate in the affection, the latter is modified in them by their peculiar structure and tendencies. Thus an inflammation of the skin or of the mucous membranes, will produce a sub-inflammation of the lymphatic glands. A pustulous phlegmasia of the skin seldom retains its character, when it affects the mucous membrane of the stomach and bowels. This, however, may arise from the deficiency of epidermis on the latter, not affording a confinement to the matter.

* Broussais Examen, 2, prop. 74.　　　† Roche et Sanson, p. 66.

CHAPTER V.

IRRITATIONS OF CELLULAR TISSUE.

THE universal diffusion of cellular tissue or substance, and its great proportionate abundance in most regions of the body, lead us to infer, that it is very frequently the seat of disease; and such is the case. Its healthy characters have been laid down in my Special and General Anatomy, to which I refer for the details on these points.

This tissue, especially that part which is sub-cutaneous, is very frequently the seat of the various forms of irritation; and as its phlegmasia is a subject of easy observation, and marked by pain, swelling, and redness: these several circumstances conjoined, have led pathologists, till later times, into the error of adopting the type of inflammation in it, as the type of inflammation in all other parts. They have, therefore, stumbled and fallen at the very threshold of their inquiries, by expecting identical phenomena in all other tissues, even in those the least resembling it, in composition and mechanical arrangement. This mistake is probably as old as the science of medicine itself, and forms no inconsiderable part of that stupendous fabric of error which has been sapped to its foundation; and is now ready to fall under the influence of general anatomy as developed by Bichat; and of physiological medicine, as explained by the French pathologists of the present day.

The irritations of the cellular tissue may either arise primarily in it, or from the extension of irritations into it, from adjoining organs. In either case the exaltation of action may be so slight as to exist without the consciousness of the indi-

vidual. From this point, there is an almost innumerable
series of gradations to the most exalted; where the symptoms of heat, of pain, of redness, of pulsation, and of tumefaction, along with general constitutional disturbance, are carried to the utmost extreme consistent with life.

The principal pathological states to which cellular tissue
is subject are, acute inflammation; hardening, as it occurs in
new-born children, and which, according to Mr. Breschet,*
depends upon the foramen ovale, continuing open; anasarca,
degenerations of a fibrous, osseous, cartilaginous kind, and
cysts. There are also some of a rarer kind, as the formation of worms, the cysticercus cellulosus, and the filaria me-
dinensis; and in animals, the æstrus.† When organs are
atrophied, the cellular substance which entered into their
composition is still left in great part.

The primary affections of the cellular substance, when severe, exercise upon other parts strongly marked sympathies.
In its phlegmasia, the brain, the heart, the stomach, and the
liver, suffer; a suppuration from it by a seton or issue, frequently retards, and even draws off an irritation from another
organ. It very readily sympathizes in the primary affections
of the heart, the lungs, the stomach, liver, spleen, womb,
&c., which are most generally attended in their closing scenes
with cellular infiltration.

The irritations of cellular tissue, like those of other organs,
are acute and chronic; and though the line is not strongly
traced where one begins and the other ends, and consequently the distinction is more or less arbitrary and exposed to
different interpretations, yet it is serviceable for descriptive
and didactick purposes.

Phlegmasia—Of the Cellular Substance.

Acute cellular inflammation seldom goes beyond the
eighth day, before it terminates in some one of the modes

---

* Beclard Anat. Gen. p 183.   † Id. 155.

which have been stated by writers.   The most usual are either, resolution as suppuration.

In the centre of an inflammation, during its early stages,
there exist small collections of blood.   The adjoining cellular substance is infiltrated with it also; without having its
texture hardened and impaired like the parts, which are actually the seat of the inflammation.   This effusion of blood,
has been called *sugillation*.   The collection of blood in the
centre of the inflammation, may be traced to ruptured, arterial, and venous vessels, of a very distinct size.   In the
abundance of this effusion, attended with a proportionate disorganization of the surrounding cellular substance, exists
the danger of mortification.

In such patients as anatomists have had an opportunity of
dissecting after death, about the sixth day of a large inflammation, the cellular tissue is still red, from the red globules
of blood being extravasated and identified with it; it is hard
to the touch, and at the same time easy to tear; its interstices are occupied with coagulating lymph, blended with
the red globules; it contains a small quantity of serosity
which may be squeezed from it, and it has lost its extensibility and its power of contraction.   These appearances diminish, as they recede from the focus of the inflammation.

From the experiments of Mr. J. Hunter on the ear of
a rabbit,* and from my own experiment on a child who
had died during the eruptive state of measles; there is no
doubt that the vessels of an inflamed part are considerably
augmented in volume, and remain so after death.   This observation, it should be understood, applies, however, to the
capillary trunks and to some secondary ones, but not to the
principal one leading to the part inflamed.   If large nerves
and large blood vessels lead through the part inflamed, the
inflammation affects the superficial cellular coat, but not the
more deeply seated.†

* Treatise on Inflammation.
† Gendrin Hist. Anat. des Inflammations, vol 1 p.15

While the cellular substance remains in a state of inflammation, its cells lose their usual permeability to fluids, or
air forced into them.   It also loses its customary transparency.   These conditions successively decrease as the distance
from the inflamed spot increases.   While an inflammation
is progressing, the cellular substance in the vicinity, if sub-
cutaneous, becomes filled and distended with serosity, which
gives to the skin a shining appearance, and in which the
redness of the inflammation is gradually lost.   This serous
effusion is attended with a dilatation of the corresponding
vessels, showing that its character is an active one; and it
penetrates into the thickness of organs, and between the interstices of muscles.   If an injection according to Mr.
Gendrin, be made of the vessels which are seated immediately within the bounds of this inflammation, their capillaries, though extremely numerous and well filled with red
blood, will not receive the injecting material, except a few
of the larger ones.   This may arise from their being obstructed by the detention of blood in them, which cannot be pushed out by the force of the injection.

The adipose matter adjoining a cellular inflammation,
when the latter is severe, is converted into a substance of a
semi-fluid consistence, and strongly resembling the ·suetty
matter of an enlarged sebaceous follicle in the skin: after a
while it is mixed with the pus of the part, and discharged
along with it.   In moderate inflammation, or, at more distant points, from a severe one, the adeps, instead of undergoing this change, is absorbed and removed; and when the
inflammation has subsided, it is deposited again, though
slowly, by advancing from the circumference to the centre,
This process is occasionally very long in being fully accomplished.

After an acute cellular inflammation has lasted six or eight
days, a secretion of pus begins in the cells occupied by the
previous secretions and deposites.   These cells, on being
squeezed, first yield a few small drops of pus like a perspi-

ration, the pus afterwards assembles into small foci, which finally coalesce into one. In the mean time the redness of the part is disappearing, and it becomes soft and fluctuating. In the midst of the pus of an abscess, are found whitish, elastic, semi-transparent and ropy flakes, (bourbillons,) commonly supposed to be mortified cellular substance; but from the want of analogy with the latter, they are more probably one of the products of the inflammation; to wit, masses of coagulating lymph. In common language they are called the core of the bile, and their discharge is supposed, by the vulgar, to lead immediately to the cure of the inflammation.

When pus is formed, or rather collected into a focus, it is kept from diffusing itself into the adjacent structure, by the matting and impermeability of the adjoining cells; and the cavity which contains it, becomes lined with a coating of coagulated lymph, resembling the false membranes on the pleura, peritoneum, and other serous membranes. If the abscess continue for a long time, and thereby becomes chronic, the lining of it assumes a slate colour, like mucous membranes under the effect of an old irritation.

From the report of the French anatomists, Ribes, Velpeau, and Gendrin, it appears, that in the dissection of persons who have died with purulent collections in them, it is by no means unusual to find pus, in the venous trunks which originate in the suppurated part. This occurs without an inflammation of their internal tunic; which, under other circumstances, might be alleged as the source of it: it is, consequently, absorbed by the radicles of the veins. M. Velpeau has reported the case,* of a female dead from abscesses, in whom he found pus in the deep-seated veins of the leg, in the femoral vein, the iliac, the vena cava, and in the right auricle of the heart. Pus was also found in the lymphatics and in the thoracic duct. Mr. Dupuytren is said to have once found the lymphatic glands and vessels of the

---

* Archives Gen. de Med 1824, tome vi p. 227

abdomen occupied by pus, supposed to have been absorbed from an inflammatory tumour seated in the superior internal part of the thigh.*

The abscesses of cellular substance become much more dangerous by contiguity to organs important to life, whose functions are thereby impeded.   Of this a striking case was presented to me in 1817, in an abscess of the neck; the effect of which, was a spasmodic action of the muscles of the larynx, and finally death.

G. W., aged 28, of a delicate habit and disposed to pectoral affections; after a protracted journey in a cold climate in the middle of winter, was seized with sore throat and occasional fits of coughing.   The symptoms, under the usual treatment, were unabated at the end of three months.   At this period they were exacerbated, and on the occasion of of his attempting to swallow some tea, a spasmodic affection of the glottis supervened, which arrested his respiration for a few moments, and was near killing him.   Relief for the time was obtained by the administration of a dose of ipecacuanha, which vomited him.   The day after, a similar paroxysm occurred, which was relieved in the same way.   Deglutition at this time became extremely painful and difficult; which was manifested by the violent action of the muscles of the throat, and agitation of countenance.

A slight swelling near the left parotid became visible, for which fifty leeches were applied, and repeated twice afterwards in the interval of a day, and of five days.   The tumefaction of the neck, however, progressed, and showed itself on the right side.   The patient became affected by profuse night sweats, with a copious sediment in his urine; but his cough diminished considerably.   His neck continued still to swell until its augmentation, in a few days, had become very considerable.   The swelling extended from the angle of the jaw to within an inch and a half or two inches of the sternum, in a direction anterior to but parallel with the

* Gendrin, parag. 49, 50

sterno cleido mastoideus. The swelling was indurated, and seemed to arise from the lymphatic glands of the neck.

An obscure fluctuation was next felt over the thyroid cartilage, but not sufficiently distinctly to indicate the puncture of the part. The difficulty of swallowing was still great, and the voice much impaired. It may be remarked also, that though a large morsel or mouthful could be swallowed, a small one produced with such difficulty as to threaten instant suffocation. A distress of respiration had also supervened latterly, which the patient said seemed to arise from an impurity in the air of the chamber, preventing the full benefit of respiration. A small tumour became perceptible on the right side of the pharynx, just behind the posterior half arch of the palate. For these several symptoms, a blister on the neck was resorted to on two occasions, and a course of mercury instituted, in consequence of the patient having latterly had syphilis.

In three days afterwards a convulsive suspension of respiration for about half a minute occurred, from which the patient recovered, but only to sink in a few hours into the arms of death.

Dissection.—On opening the neck, an abscess containing half a pint of pus was found occupying the space from the os hyoides to the lower end of the thyroid cartilage; on the left side, it extended to near the mastoid process; and on the right, to the angle of the lower jaw. The mucous membrane of the pharynx was much inflamed; that covering the epiglottis and arytenoid cartilages was tumefied to four lines in thickness. The sacs in front of the epiglottis were filled up by the tumefaction. The internal membrane of the larynx and trachea was in a state of considerable inflammation.

Thorax.—There was an universal peripheral adhesion of the lungs to the thorax. The lungs were firmer than usual, and did not collapse much, when their adhesions were torn asunder. Two ulcers were found in the right upper lobe, derived from tubercles just passed into a state of mollescence.

The pericardium contained two ounces of serum. The heart was unusually large, and the coronary veins minutely distended with blood.

Abdomen natural.—Upon a review of the case, it would seem that the frequent fits of suffocation and the difficulties of swallowing, arose from the abscess surrounding the larynx and pharynx, which disqualified their muscles from the execution of their natural actions.

It is rather difficult, in the present state of our knowledge, to affix a precise pathology to erysipelas; yet I am disposed to view it as seated primarily in the cellular substance, and differing from other forms of inflammation principally by being diffused, instead of collected into a focus. It may, therefore, exist in any part of the cellular tissue, but we oftener see it as sub-cutaneous. The skin itself would seem to be the seat of this affection, only so far as it may be influenced by its contiguity to the disease, and by the proportion of the cellular tissue entering into its composition. This proportion, we know, varies at different points; and it is in spots where the cellular ingredient of the skin is most abundant, that erysipelas is most common; as, for example, on the face, neck, and perineum. When the skin becomes affected, the disease passes from the sub-cutaneous into the cutaneous cellular tissue, by continuity of structure. By this rule, we find erysipelas propagating itself along the cellular tissue of even fibrous organs, as the following dissection shows:

A robust black subject, (male,) with erysipelas of the left leg, from its middle to the end of the foot, was introduced into our dissecting-rooms, (1828.) The cuticle was found loose in the whole extent of the disease, and the leg somewhat tumefied. The sub-cutaneous cellular adipose substance was in a state of suppuration equally extensive; there being a mixture of purulent matter and coagulating lymph blended with the masses of fat. The disease went down to the fascia of the leg, and penetrated along with the cellular substance of the vessels and nerves that pass through it. It also penetrated the interstices between the *fasciculi of the ligament of the ankle;* having laid the fasciculi bare and separate like a maceration followed by dissolution of the cellular substance.

From the experiments of M. M. Majendie, Prevost, and Dumas upon the injection of pus into the veins, it appears that it is followed by abundant suppurations in different organs. M Gendrin,* attaching these facts to individuals who die with copious suppurations upon them, from an abscess or from a wound, and in whom there are also found after death inflammations of the lungs, of the intestines, and of the liver, infers that these inflammations come from the absorption of pus by the veins.

It is not yet fully known how long it takes an inflamed spot of cellular substance which has gone into suppuration, to be restored to its normal or physiological condition; for it remains hard, resisting, impermeable, and inelastic, for a long time, if the inflammation has been severe. Chemical tests, when applied to it, show a considerable alteration in its properties; for it becomes by maceration very speedily decomposed into a reddish, fœtid, and ropy mass. When boiled for a long time, it yields a froth in great abundance resembling albumen, and affords much less gelatine than the cellular substance does in its healthy state.†

Chronic or Sub-inflammation of the Cellular Tissue.

When an acute inflammation of the cellular substance has subsided by a diminution in the intensity of its symptoms, without their being wholly removed; it gets into the state of scirrhus, or of a hard tumour, which remains, with but little variation, for an indefinite time. Not unfrequently, such tumours form gradually, without any very well marked

* Gendrin, loc. cit. p. 51.   † Id. par. 53, 54.

symptom of inflammation; being produced by the incessant action of some irritating cause,—as pressure, the lodging of foreign bodies, as gun-shot, splinters, &c., and occasionally without any very evident reason. Sometimes an ulceration of the urethra, by permitting a leakage of urine into the perineum and scrotum, will produce an extensive chronic induration of the corresponding cellular substance of these parts. I have seen it repeatedly, of various extent. The last summer, (July, 1827,) I treated a patient at the Alms-house, who had borne about him for ten or twelve years, a chronic induration of the scrotum, which made the latter as large as a double-fist. It had also extended itself to the penis, and caused an elongation of the prepuce two inches or more beyond the extremity of the glans penis. Sub-inflammation of the cellular substance is also found under chronic ulcers, and forms, most commonly, their basis.

Sub-inflammation is attended with but little discoloration of the skin, unless it be seated partly in the texture of the latter, and then the increased vascularity and circulation, are manifest on the external surface of the body, by a blush in the part. It sometimes forms a round, elevated tumour; and, on other occasions, a flat and extensive thickening. I lately, (November, 1827,) saw in our dissecting-rooms a case of the latter in the loins, under the skin, from the lodgment of several bird-shot there, in a black male subject. Wherever this species of morbid structure may prevail in the cellular substance, it will be found to have the following anatomical characters, when cut into: The cells of the cellular substance have lost their permeability to inflation, and are filled and identified with a fibrinous gelatinous matter, very difficult to cut, and resisting laceration. The part, though vascular, does not present the recent extravasations of blood of acute inflammation: the fluids which supply it seem to be principally the transparent portions of the blood.

In the progress of a chronic inflammation, the moderate degree of redness which it may have had originally, diminishes still more, and indeed does not exceed the vascularity of parts in a state of health; and its resistance, want of elasticity, and impermeability, become still more marked.   The Barbadoes leg is said to present this pathological change in its cellular membrane; and it is likewise the case in old rheumatisms.

The secretions of a chronic inflammation of the cellular substance, are never like those of an acute one: instead of being pure pus, a thin, serous or sero-purulent matter is discharged, sometimes mixed with blood.   If the surface be ulcerated and exposed to the air, it then reddens and becomes injected like an old ulcer.   If there be not an open ulceration, there is frequently in the thickness of it small ulcerated cavities containing a yellowish, muddy serum, with some pus and cheesy matter intermixed.

The parts which are contiguous to, or pass through a chronic cellular inflammation, are for a long time kept distinct and unaffected by it, except from its bulk; but when it ulcerates, then they become irritated, and suffer considerable pain.   If the chronicity be but a few grades below active inflammation, or phlegmasia, the contiguous cellular substance is not unfrequently infiltrated with serum.

When a mass of cellular substance under chronic inflammation is macerated, it is converted in a short time into a soft fluid pulp, but not so speedily as in acute inflammation; and its original cellular structure is by no means made evident, as in the case of acute inflammation.

The time is indefinite for the removal of such affections: they may last for months and years, with but little alteration. It sometimes happens, that after a long duration of indolence they assume an active inflammation, become penetrated with red blood, softened, and very humid, and present at places throughout them collections of an imperfectly formed pus. Under such circumstances, they are not so ready to be discussed or removed as to get into a large foul ulcer, which does

not heal until the indurated mass is wholly removed. It is
in this way that lymphatic indurations in scrofula and venereal most frequently heal.

The cellular tissue presents some varieties in its disposition and habits of disease, depending upon its varied position and usages. That under the skin is most subject to
acute and chronic inflammations, from its greater exposure to
injuries. The sub-mucous cellular tissue is much more compact and dense than the first; and though it is sometimes
found in a distinct state of disease in the alimentary canal,
yet it is not very common: that under the serous membranes
is not unfrequently the seat of purulent depots, as in lumbar abscess.

In the ulcers of the several tissues of the body, their cellular membrane performs the most important part, as it is
the source of the secretion of pus.*

Secretory Irritation of Cellular Tissue.

Anasarca or serous effusion into the cellular membrane,
as in dropsies, is seldom a primary affection, and is most
commonly consecutive or sympathetic. The tissue is not
altered, as the fluid effused is a superabundance of the common secretion into its cells. This fluid is transparent, and
generally more or less coagulable by heat.

Small patches of blood are sometimes extravasated in the
deep interstitial cellular membrane, without there being sufficient cause to suppose that they arise from mechanical injury.
I think that I have seen them most frequently in anasarca.

Among the secretory irritations of cellular membrane may
be mentioned preternatural tumours, consisting in wens and
in cysts. Some wens contain a matter like curds, intermixed
with hard masses of various consistence and figure: they are
classified under the term atheroma ($\alpha\theta\eta\rho\alpha$, pap.) Others contain a mixture like that of honey and wax, and are called

* Bichat. Anat Pathol. p 146.

Meliceris, (μελι, honey; κηρος, wax.)   Others have their contents resembling suet, hence the term steatoma (σ7εαρ, suet.)
Others, again, are composed of balls of fat; hence their
name of Lipoma (λιπος, fat.)   These tumours, very generally, are formed in the sub-cutaneous cellular membrane,
in various regions of the body; and are surrounded by a
lamina of it, under various degrees of condensation and of
thickness.   In such as are merely fat, the sac is very thin,
and does not seem to have suffered any kind of pathological
change: they, indeed, belong rather to the cases of excessive
nutrition in a part, than to secretory irritation.   Many encysted tumours contain merely a straw-coloured serous fluid,
resembling the serum of the blood.

The sacs of these several tumours are perfect, or without
an opening, and, with the exception of perhaps the lipoma,
have a very strong analogy with the hardened cellular substance of cicatrices.   Bichat* considers them as formed
originally by granulations, and not by the compression and
condensation of cellular substance.   Sometimes bands traverse their interior, and the fluids vary considerably in their
colour and consistence; though for the most part they have
albumen for a basis.

The interior of the cranium, from the very small quantity
of cellular substance there, is very seldom the seat of encysted tumours, if we except the little vesicles so frequently found along the plexus choroides, and occasionally some
small ones adhering to the pia mater on the surface of the
brain, and resembling hydatids.   But in the cavities of the
thorax and abdomen they every now and then occur, and
by their continued augmentation, encroach upon the space
allotted for important viscera.   Under such circumstances,
they are distinguished with great difficulty from the primitive diseases of the viscera, whose actions are interrupted
by them, and they finally produce marasmus and death.

* Anat. Pathol. p. 150

Nutritive Irritation of Cellular Substance.

I was requested on October 22d, 1828, to examine for Dr. S. Jackson, about thirty-six hours after death, a gentleman, aged thirty-two, who died from colick. He was extremely corpulent universally, but especially in the abdomen. A layer of fat half an inch thick was beneath the peritoneum: the several processes of the latter seemed to be so thoroughly converted into fat, that the serous structure was almost extinct, and small drops of oil stood out like a halitus upon all the surfaces of the abdominal viscera. The fat was so fluid and abundant that it had collected in the peritoneum, and ran from it in a stream when the abdomen was opened. The body was emphysematous, from the commencement of putrefaction.

The remains of active inflammation of the gastro intestinal mucous surface, of a high grade, could be distinguished, though impaired by the putrefaction, and the whole mucous coat of the stomach and duodenum was coated with bile, which he had thrown up in great quantities before death.

The liver was enlarged, and yellow universally, which might have been suddenly produced. There was no bile in the gall bladder. He was said to have lived freely. The lungs were surcharged with blood all over, and emphysematous under the pleura.

The heart was enlarged and covered with fat. Vessels taken for lymphatics, and of a very light yellow colour, were seen radiating all along the small intestines. As he had not eaten any thing since Sunday the 18th, it is not likely that the lacteals contained chyle, but as the mucous coat of the intestines was tinged with a quantity of bile which had passed down them, it is more probable that the lacteals contained it, and were thereby discoloured.

The exhibition which we have just had of what was called the Canadian Giant, a man aged 62, is a strong example of the nutritive irritation in cellular substance. This individual, who stood six feet four inches high, weighed upwards of six hundred pounds.   The circumference of each leg is about three feet at the calf, and but little less at the ankle; and what is remarkable, this enormous deposite of fat, making him so much larger than ordinary men of the same stature, has been chiefly on the body below the thorax, and in the lower extremities.   Such an oppressive load of fat is equal to an extraneous body attached to him, and makes him walk with the utmost difficulty.

A few years ago, (1820) a mass of fat, which filled a large wash tub was exhibited at a public Museum in Market Street.   It had been taken from a bullock and surrounded its kidney; it was not stated that the animal suffered obvious inconvenience from it.   Being held out as a subject of popular curiosity it was erroneously advertised as an enormous kidney; it was, properly speaking, an enormous mass of fat surrounding the kidney.

In regard to the morbid sympathies of the cellular membrane: it is very apt to be affected by contiguity and propinquity, to other parts labouring under disease.   This is manifested in phlegmons, in fractures, contusions, strains, peritonitis, pleuritis; when it tumefies, and receives an additional quantity of fluids into its interstices.   In intermittents, and organic affections generally, we find it to take on this leucophlegmatic habit.   In affections of the lungs and some others it emaciates.   In acute affections it becomes flaccid and does not resume its natural elasticity till restoration to health.   It also becomes flaccid in old age.

CHAPTER VI.

IRRITATIONS OF SEROUS MEMBRANES.

THE serous membranes form a very considerable part of the area of the internal surface of the human body, by lining its large cavities, reflecting itself over their viscera; making the bursæ mucosæ; and constituting the interior periphery of the moving articulations. From this great extent of surface it may be readily inferred, that they are frequently diseased from different causes; and that from their varied application, the symptoms must not only be general or common, from the common nature and composition of these membranes; but special and varied, by the nature of the parts over which they are reflected. The normal condition of serous membranes has been pointed out in my Treatise on Anatomy,* and I therefore pass over the consideration of it at this place, referring the reader to what has been said there. It is sufficient here to state, that, consisting in condensed cellular substance, they present a very strong analogy with it in their pathological changes.

The serous membranes are subject to acute and to sub-inflammations, to hæmorrhagic, and to secretory irritations; and they also present transformations of their appropriate tissue into one which is fibrous, cartilaginous, bony, &c.; all of which may be attributed to a slow irritation.

The purely nutritive irritation is very uncommon, and would seem to be almost inconsistent with the common character of serous membranes.

* Vol. ii. p. 7. et seq.

The sympathies of the serous membranes are readily excited. These sympathies are first of all, with the affections of the organs or parts which they cover, then with one another, and finally with distant organs. The most usual form in which this sympathy manifests itself, is by an undue accumulation of the serum in their cavities, but sometimes by more unequivocal marks of inflammation, as redness and the effusion of coagulating lymph. Bichat* has made a remark which, I think, frequently applies to our cadaverous autopsies; that if in acute diseases we could see the serous membranes as we do the skin, we should find them, like it, undergoing signal changes in their secretions, by being more ' or less moist and replete with them, and more or less dry, according to the stages of the disorder. If death occur while the exhalation is more abundant, we find it collected in a large quantity; but if the absorption be paramount, those membranes are dry.† In the same way, if the exhalation from the skin were collected into a sac, instead of being absorbed by the atmosphere, or by the clothing; we should find after death, the quantity of humidity singularly varied. The probability is, that these exhalations from serous membranes sometimes go on very rapidly. In the case of W. J. Esq., a gentleman who died in a few minutes illness, from ossification of the coronary arteries of the heart;‡ serum had accumulated, in twenty minutes, to the amount of five ounces in the left pleura: at least, from the perfect health that he enjoyed previously, there is good reason to suppose that it was not in the pleura, before the sudden illness which so speedily terminated his life.

The organs which the serous membranes most readily

---

* Anat Gen v ii 569

† It is not uncommon to find the tunica arachnoidea in a half desiccated state, and I have, in two instances of cohck, found the beginning of the colon so dry as to be almost crisp   These cases will be detailed in the progress of this work.

‡ See chapter on the Gastro Intestinal Mucous Membrane

sympathize with are the heart, the lungs, the liver, the spleen, the stomach, and the womb. The serous, or the parts of serous membranes nearest to the viscus affected, take the lead, and the others are brought in consecutively, according to distance, or to some previous affection, rendering their sensibility more quick. In the pathological condition of the heart, the pericardium first feels; in those of the lungs, the pleura; in those of the liver, the peritoneum, in those of the womb, the latter also, and especially that portion of it nearest to the womb, at least, according to my experience from dissections.

It is asserted by Bichat,* but I think in too general a manner not to be exposed to many, I may say, indeed, an undue proportion of exceptions; that, whenever the accumulated serosity of those membranes arises primarily from the diseases of other organs; this fluid or serosity is limpid, transparent, and probably of the same nature with that which circulates in the lymphatics: and for this reason, that the exhalents which secrete the fluid have their action increased only by sympathy; or the absorbents which convey it away have theirs decreased by the same cause, and of course the fluid remains in a healthy state, being only changed in quantity. On the contrary, when dropsies of serous cavities depend upon diseases of serous surfaces, as tuberculous inflammation, or a degenerated acute inflammation, &c., almost always the effused serum is altered from a healthy aspect: it is milky, or contains shreds of albumen, coagulating lymph, &c. From this passage, Bichat would lead us to infer, that the sympathetic irritations of the serous membranes, were not the same in their phenomena as the primary ones; and that neither can they be. My own opinion is, that these sympathetic irritations are only inferior in intensity in most cases, to the irritations of the organs that produce them; and that it is very possible, nay, by no means uncommon, for this sympathetic irritation to have the same

* Anat Gen, 2—568

phenomena as if it had been primary. Witness, for example, the peritoneal inflammations of the highest kind, consecutive to those of the mucous coat of the stomach and bowels; the highest inflammations of the pleura consecutive to the developement of tubercular consumption, and not unfrequently putting a sudden termination to the life of the patient.

Phlegmasia of Serous Membranes.

The frequency of acute inflammation in serous membranes, is only surpassed by that in the cellular and mucous tissue; yet these membranes have among themselves some distinction in the facility and frequency with which they take on inflammation, and very nearly in the following order: thus the pleura comes first, then the peritoneum, then the pericardium, then the tunica vaginalis testis, and finally, the arachnoidea of the brain.* The synovial membranes of the joints are left out of this enumeration for the reason, that their inflammations more frequently arise from injuries.

The most common cause of serous inflammation is a sudden suppression of cutaneous transpiration, by cold, either dry or humid. The excitement of the vessels of the skin being transferred to some one or more of the serous membranes; their increased action is attended with the phenomena appropriate to such a condition.

The acute inflammation of serous membranes is characterized by a very sudden invasion; and by an excessive pain of the part, not surpassed by the pain of any other tissue. Its progress is proportionably rapid, for sometimes it finishes its stages in three days, either by a termination in death, in suppuration, or in some other of its modes. I examined once a gentleman, who died in fifty-nine hours after the cause productive of peritoneal inflammation, to wit, an operation for the stone in the bladder had been applied: nothing could

* Bichat, Anat. Pathol 39

have exceeded his sufferings during his illness, or exhibited more clearly the pathological features of the disease.

This inflammation begins by a redness much superior to what one would suppose, from the few blood vessels met with in the normal state of these membranes. As it advances the redness becomes more and more intense, and is disposed into patches of various sizes, from one line to six, eight or even more, having narrow interstices between them. The redness during its first stage has its seat in the sub-serous cellular tissue, which soon becomes penetrated with serosity, and somewhat tumid. As the disease advances, the redness begins to show itself in the substance and on the interior surface of the serous cavity by innumerable red points, looking like the ends of blood vessels, and from which blood itself is occasionally effused. Many of these points are microscopical, others can be seen very distinctly with the unassisted eye. The patches of blood at this time in the sub-serous tissue become darker, and by blending, assume very much the condition of a common ecchymosis, which I believe them to be. While the serous membrane is in this state of vascular injection, it is clear that new avenues to the red blood have been formed, perhaps not so much by a creation as by a dilatation of old passages, which, in the natural state receive only the serous or white part of the blood.

Some serous membranes, however, are not always disposed to become red during their acute inflammations: this is especially the case with the arachnoidea, which, from a state of transparency, becomes turbid, milk-coloured, and somewhat thickened.

The common vascular trunks which run beneath an inflamed serous membrane, augment considerably in volume, and, therefore, seem also to have their numbers increased. This probably arises from such as are habitually invisible, receiving now so many files of red blood abreast at once, that they thereby become distinct. The blood vessels would seem also to be left after death in a dilated state, as an artificial injection readily fills them and demonstrates their abundance. M. Gendrin informs* us that it is impossible to make such injections, arrive in the sub-serous cellular tissue, when the serous membrane first begins to redden. Before this period, mercurial injections reach as far as the serous membrane, but by no means penetrate its texture, unless it is somewhat slightly inflamed. He assures us that repeated experiments on animals have established these facts.

M. Gendrin further informs us, that the distinction between the inflammatory redness of serous membranes and that of mere sanguineous conjestion, is as follows. In the former there is always in the progress of the disease a punctuation with red blood, already alluded to; and subsequently the membrane becomes opaque and of a greater density than is healthy. Also, this redness can neither be removed by pressure, nor repeated washings, whereas that of congestion yields to both of these measures. In some persons who die from suffocation, the pleura presents rose-coloured patches, from the arrest of blood in the sub-serous tissue; but in other respects the texture of the part is unaltered, which alone would indicate the distinction of congestion from inflammation.

The tumefaction of serous membranes under a state of acute inflammation is nearly always inconsiderable; indeed, I may say, not to be appreciated by the eye in many instances, though inexpert observers are very apt to believe and to assert that they meet with it frequently, thickened to several lines. The delusion sometimes arises from their not stripping the diseased membrane from the subjacent parts; hence its thickness is confounded with the contiguous layers of adipose and cellular substance. In other instances a false membrane forming on the interior surface of the serous one, but which may be readily pulled or scraped away, leads to the mistake.

* Loc. cit vol. 1. p 73

In the progress of acute inflammation, a serous infiltration sometimes occurs in the subjacent tissue, and extends itself into the serous membrane itself: this happens more frequently in the arachnoidea, but it may also occur elsewhere. With this reference to the actual condition of the parts, the term thickening is sometimes used and defended as correct.

In some cases of serous inflammation, the red points existing on the surface of the membrane, resemble very closely extremely small petechiæ, which leave scarcely any interval between one another, and have these intervals of a dull cloudy colour. In instances of very violent inflammation followed by sudden death, the redness of the part is very strong: and there exist small ecchymoses in the subjacent tissue, and a small quantity of reddish yellow serosity is effused into the serous cavity.

Fluid secretions from the surface next to the cavity are a common consequence of serous inflammation. These secretions vary: sometimes they are a serosity like that of blood not altered in its sensible or chemical qualities, but abundant: this is very common. Sometimes this serosity is blood, the red blood being in various proportions to the serum. In one case which occurred to me, they appeared to be in equal proportions. Another form of secretion is that of coagulating lymph, and a fourth, pus. One or all of these may happen in the same patient and from the same membrane; so that they seem to be merely gradations of the same inflammation, which, according to my views, stand as follows in the ascent of action:—first, serum, then coagulating lymph, then pus, and then blood; in all of which we see the parallelism with inflammation of the cellular tissue.

From the beginning of acute inflammation the secretion of serum becomes more abundant, but at the same time its absorption is accomplished with proportionate rapidity for some time; hence an accumulation is prevented.   M. Gendrin* asserts that he has established these points by experiments on animals, where he had excited inflammation in the pleura and in the peritoneum. This absorption is not overcome even by the deposite of a false membrane; for we every now and then find the latter existing where there is no accumulation of serum, yet there could be no doubt that the latter had been secreted: an inference arising from our general observations, and not difficult to establish by following the progress of certain cases, with the stethoscope. But if the inflammation be excessive, the secretion of serum is arrested for the time, and consequently absorption ceases to go on. These facts seem to be proved by experiments on animals, and by observations on the progress of inflammations in the pleura, peritoneum, and arachnoidea. The function of absorption, however, seems to be more injured in those cases generally, than that of secretion; for when the inflammation abates, and the exhalents pour out serum, the latter accumulates and forms the dropsies of the respective cavities, in which it is placed.

False membranes, (pseudo-membranes,) as they are called, are a membranous concretion of coagulating lymph, thrown out on the interior face of inflamed serous membranes. In the commencement the lymph appears in very fine drops, resembling a halitus, and distinct from one another: these drops augment, run together and form a net-work, which is converted by the addition of new matter into a continuous sheet or a perfect membrane. If a similar process be going on at the same time on the opposite surface, it ends by the two false membranes agglutinating and becoming identified. In most cases this matter of agglutination is a thin layer not exceeding the thickness of a piece of parchment; but in others it is three or four times as thick, and flocculent. The latter condition prevails more frequently in the pericardium, the former in the pleura and in the peritoneum. M. Bec-

* Loc. cit. I.—70

lard* says, that sometimes the matter of agglutination poured
out from serous cavities is so abundant as to fill them to distention.   I have myself not seen a case of this extreme kind,
though I have met lately with one narrated in a subsequent
part of this work, where there was a clot of fibrinous secretion four or five lines thick in a child of fourteen
months.

It is by no means unusual in our dissecting-rooms to see
the interior surface of serous membranes covered as it were
with a thin pellicle resembling that which forms on the eye in
a moribund state.   But the difference between the two is, that
in the eye, if it be wiped off, it leaves the organ with its natural polish, whereas on the serous membrane, a surface somewhat rough is left, resembling very fine villosities.   This
appearance is very apt to take place where opposed surfaces
are about forming an unnatural adhesion, or have just formed
it, and is an early stage of the secretion of coagulating lymph.
While this process is going on, the probability is, that the
serous effusion of the part is either arrested or blended with
the lymph; for if it proceeded in full force, it would wash
away the lymph, or bedew its surface so much as to obviate
the adhesions which are so common in the inflammations of
serous membranes.   I have had frequent occasion to remark,
that where the peritoneum presented this roughened villous
state with adhesions of its proximate surfaces, that the serosity in its cavity was very trifling, or entirely deficient.

When lymph is first poured out in the form of a false
membrane, its adhesion to the serous membrane is so slight,
that it may be raised up and scraped off very readily with
a knife handle conducted between it and the membrane; but
after it has remained for a time, it is changed into cellular
tissue, in which canals are formed suited to the transmission of blood, and finally becoming perfect blood vessels,
communicating with and conducting the blood vessels of the

* Anat. Gen. p. 195

contiguous inflamed membrane. This vascular metamorphosis of what was an inorganic effusion of lymph, I have seen much more frequently where there was an adhesion of the opposite sides of the inflamed membrane; as, for example, of the pleura pulmonalis with the pleura costalis. Mr. J. Hunter and Sir Everard Home, established the fact that the blood vessels were originally formed in the false membrane, and joined by a process of inosculation to those of the true membrane. It had been previously believed that the latter prolonged its vessels into the first by a species of growth. M. Beclard, who joins in opinion with them,* asserts, that by thrusting at hazard a mercurial pipe into a new adhesion, a set of arborescent canals will be injected, whose trunk is in the centre of the adhesion, and whose branches, like those of the vena portarum, arise at each end, and are directed towards the adjoining serous membranes. The vessels thus primitively formed, do not at that period communicate with those of the serous membranes; but they do subsequently, and then the arrangement is modified by the adhesion, or false membrane, becoming more vascular at the extremities, by which it inosculates, and less so in the centre.

False membranes, or adhesions, vary much in their extent and shape: sometimes they consist of broad, flat, riband-like bands, from one to several inches wide; on other occasions, they are thread-like filaments assembled in greater or less numbers. The two preceding cases present them of the length of an inch or more. Then there is a third form, in which the adhesion is universal, and so close that it does not allow of a separation of its two ends without tearing. This condition is frequently met with in the last stages of pulmonary consumption; and sometimes from pleurisies, where the structure of the lung is sound. The band-like, the filamentous, and the close adhesions are frequently all met with

* Anat. Gen. p. 195.

in the same cavity, and, when ancient, look like normal cellular structure connecting adjacent parts.

It has never occurred to me to ascertain by direct personal observation, whether these false membranes, when once
formed, remained for life.   The question is well worth examining into, with much more attention than has been heretofore bestowed upon it.   I am inclined to the opinion, from
general analogy, that they are sometimes, at least, removed;
because we see the adhesions and indurations of wounds
giving way to the effects of time and of interstitial changes;
and, if this process occur in cellular structure, why may it not
in a serous membrane, whose general parallelism with the
texture and properties of the latter is so complete.   In addition—M. Beclard* is of the same opinion; and maintains it
upon the following observations upon a maniac whom he dissected.   This patient had at different periods inflicted a dozen or more wounds upon himself, some of which penetrated
the abdomen.   In the most recent, the intestine adhered to
the wounded spot; in another, less recent, the adhesion was
by a bridle; and in another, still more remote in time, the
bridle was absorbed in the middle, and thereby broken.

If after the pseudo-membranes have had time to organize
themselves, but while they are yet recent, another attack of
inflammation comes on, they take a part in it, and become
red and infiltrated with blood, which cannot be removed by
a common ablution.   A bloody serum is poured abundantly
into the cavity, and has so many red globules in it, that it
resembles almost pure blood; from which it can be distinguished principally by its not coagulating, and by the colouring matter not separating from the serum.

Pus being also one of the secretions of inflamed serous
membranes, is sometimes found in their cavities without false
membranes, and with little or no serum.   In such instances,
it coats, or is smeared over the surface producing it, and is

* Anat. Gen. p. 197.

sometimes amassed in large quantities.' In the latter case, however, it generally has some filaments of coagulating lymph floating in it. The sub-serous cellular tissue is also disposed to the secretion of pus, and is occasionally much infiltrated with it. When an inflammation of serous tissue continues for a long time, with but little or no diminution, or, when there is an exacerbation during the declining state of inflammation, the purulent secretion is a very ordinary consequence in most of the serous cavities.

The blood which is poured out in serous imflammations, is sometimes pure, or almost so. I have frequently seen it mixed with a large proportion of serum; but never, that I remember, entirely pure as it circulates in the vessels; though I have no doubt of the fact, both from analogy, and from the report of writers.

It is asserted by M. Gendrin, that serous membranes are never inflamed, without the proximate cellular substance being in the same state; and manifesting, indeed, the first pathological changes, by its redness, its infiltration with serum, and the facility with which it tears. Occasionally, air is secreted into its interstices, and it becomes emphysematous. Putrefaction cannot be properly alleged as the cause of the latter, because the emphysema is not attended with the other indications of putrefaction, and is confined to the space suffering from the inflammation; and, moreover, putrefaction is not always attended with emphysema. It is the effusion and increase of bulk in the sub-serous tissue which constitutes the first act of thickening from inflammations in serous membranes. The readiness with which this change occurs depends upon the laxity and abundance of the sub-serous tissue, and upon the facility with which the serous membranes may be resolved by maceration into cellular substance. The arachnoidea standing foremost in these respects, quickly thickens under the influence of even a slight inflammation, by the deposite of serum in it and the adjoining cellular tissue, and not unfrequently is converted into a sort of

gelatinous-looking membrane, containing yellowish serosity
with a slight tinge of red, which may be pressed out with
the fingers:

With the exception of the arachnoidea, this thickening
process seldom, I think, reaches the free or secreting surface
of serous membranes, unless under a long continued chronic inflammation.   This notion has already been advanced,
and, I trust, will not be forgotten, as it seems to form one of
the peculiarities of serous inflammation.

Chronic or Sub-inflammation of Serous Membranes.

The chronic or sub-inflammation of serous membranes
may be either the termination of an acute inflammation, or,
it may result from a mild irritation kept up for a long time
upon them.

Pain is very far from being the invariable concomitant of
it, especially when it comes on without the acute stage; and
though pain frequently attends, yet it is so often absent,
that it cannot be reasonably considered as an indispensable
symptom.

The colour of serous membranes in this condition is frequently altered very inconsiderably from the normal state.
They have a light tinge of red sometimes, which may remain
for a time; but it is disposed finally to subside, and to take on
a brownish hue. Occasionally they become absolutely black,*
in spots of varied magnitude, which are probably the resi-
duum of particles of red blood originally extravasated there;
but their thickness under such circumstances is not sensibly
increased.   These spots have none of the peculiar character of mortification, and therefore are not liable to be mistaken for it, and they are very often attended with a secretion of bloody serum into the serous cavity.   M. Gendrin

* See Gastro Intestinal Mucous Membrane, case of J. Neaman

views them as a union of the hæmorrhagic congestion, with chronic inflammation.*

Chronic serous inflammations very frequently finish life by a repetition or an accession of the acute stage. When the latter has existed a few days, the vessels are found turgid, and the whole membrane of a bright red; which has induced some pathologists to think that it was the appropriate colour of chronic inflammation, from their not reflecting that the patient had perished in a paroxysm of acuteness. Under such circumstances, the redness may be either striated, punctuated, or uniform; and the indications generally are such as manifest the blending of acute with chronic inflammation.

Tumefaction, and an augmentation in density of texture, are among the leading characters of chronic serous inflammation, and especially the second. The former, most frequently, does not seem to be so much an increase in the thickness of the proper serous membrane, (though it does sometimes occur) as an increase in the thickness of the subjacent cellular tissue, which becomes infiltrated with serum and coagulating lymph, and identifies itself with the inflamed serous membrane so completely, that one can no longer define their boundaries. Under these circumstances, the surface of the serous membrane is reduced sometimes to a very thin pellicle, and retains its gloss and colour; but frequently the reverse, also, is the case, and it is roughened and turbid; or may be entirely covered by a false membrane, which has identified itself also with the serous, and undergone such pathological changes, as to make the distinction between the two no longer perceptible.

The augmentation in density of texture, frequently occurs in chronic inflammation, without much increase in thickness. The membrane, though more difficult to tear, and more resisting than either the healthy or the acutely in-

* Vol 1 p. 170.

flamed one, has its extensibility, and its contractility much
diminished: it is also more difficult to tear up strips from it.

One of the pathological changes of structure in chronic
inflammation of serous membranes is the evolution of mul-
titudes of small, closely set pimples, which are whitish, flat,
in various shaped patches, and frequently interspersed with
brownish points.   They project slightly, and are covered
by a pellicle, which shows that they originated in the thickness of the membrane, from which they cannot be picked
out, but are blended with its structure.   When cut, it is
seen that they are an infiltration of whitish matter, of a very
light rose-colour; and that they are surrounded by a moderate degree of vascularity.   According to M. Gendrin, *
they differ from tubercles, which are also one of the modes
of derangement in serous structure.

Tubercles are preceded by a deposite of false membrane,
which becomes organized, but in a very morbid way, and in
the thickness of which they are developed.   They are first
of all seen as small white grains, which are diaphanous,
slightly vascular, and easily separable from the membrane
which surrounds them.   In their progress, the false membrane adheres more and more strongly to the serous, and
finally becomes inseparably identified with it.   The two, by
their union, form a thick lamina, in which the tubercles are
set; and which becomes extremely vascular, with no disposition to puriform secretions.

The false membranes which are found in chronic inflammations, are well organized and tough.   Sometimes they are
almost ligamentous, and are disposed to become cartilaginous, especially on the spleen, according to my own observations.   They are, however, not the inseparable result of
chronic inflammation; for we frequently meet with cases
without them, and sometimes the inflammatory action has
occurred only in the sub-serous tissue, so as to produce only

* Anat. Gen. Vol. i. 166.

an apparent thickening of the whole serous membrane. I am disposed to believe that these cartilaginous changes are more common in the sub-serous tissue than in the serous tissue itself; for in the majority of the cases which have come under my notice, the serous membrane formed only a thin pellicle on their surface.

Chronic inflammation sometimes obliterates entirely the serous cavity in which it occurs, by the agglutination of the contiguous surfaces. It is by no means uncommon in the thorax, and is also met with, but not so frequently, in the abdomen. Partial adhesions are, however, very common in the peritoneum. These adhesions, both partial and general, sometimes keep the contiguous surfaces closely approximated; and, on other occasions, are so long that they permit a separation of from one to fifteen or twenty lines, even more. If the adhesions be in a chronic state, without a recent paroxysm of acute inflammation, they are about as dry and look for the most part like tough cellular substance; but, under other circumstances, they are infiltrated with a serous or gelatinous fluid, giving them a yellowish semi-transparency.

When chronic inflammation has proceeded slowly and from the beginning, as a sub-inflammation, the serous membrane has but little red blood in it, and is frequently found thickened and condensed, by the infiltration of an albuminous fluid. ·

The secretions from serous membranes, in a state of chronic inflammation, frequently accumulate in such quantities as to produce great inconvenience, by pressing upon and interrupting the action of contiguous organs; as, for example, in the dropsy of the pericardium, of the pleura, of the peritoneum, &c. The principal constituent of such secretions is serum, either transparent and yellow, or turbid and milky. This serum contains shreds of coagulating lymph, and frequently purulent matter. In some instances, I have seen it so gelatinous and ropy as to resemble in its consistence a thin size of glue. As a general rule, it may be stated that we meet with the sero-purulent effusion most frequently in the pleura, and the gelatinous in the peritoneum; at least, such has been my experience: in the brain, the effusion is for the most part transparent.

When a serous cavity is occupied by its secretions, it is generally considered as a proof that it is or has been in a state of inflammation either chronic or acute.   I doubt whether this opinion is always correct, though it unquestionably is in the majority of instances.   We every now and then meet with instances where there is no vascular injection, no false membrane either adhering or floating, and no appearance of disorganization in the serous membrane containing the undue quantity of serum.   This is very frequently the case in effusions into the tunica vaginalis testis, and into the ventricles of the brain, and would seem to be instances of the purest secretory irritation.   The reply, however, has been, that an inflammation once existed, but had departed before death.

M. Gendrin remarks, that an invariable evidence of peritoneal dropsies being from inflammation, exists in the following circumstances: to wit, induration, and thickening of the sub-serous tissue about the crural arches, the ischiatic notches and pelvis generally, and about the heads of the diaphragm.   My own observations do not permit me either to confirm or deny this statement, though I am willing to acknowledge its correctness.

In addition to the effects of chronic serous inflammation upon the sub-serous tissue in tumefying and hardening it, other contiguous parts also suffer.   The lymphatic glands tumefy, harden, and sometimes suppurate.   Circumscribed tumours are sometimes produced in the sub-serous tissue, which suppurate and discharge into the serous cavity, thus adding to the general disorder of it.   On other occasions these tumours remain entire, and continue to increase by an internal secretion of serum; and as they enlarge they of course project into the serous cavity, and form distinct cysts upon its borders.   This, I think, more common in diseases of the ovaria.

Instances have occurred of a spontaneous ulceration from the cavity of the serous membrane to the skin, perforating completely the parietes of the part, and discharging externally the product of the inflammation, whatever it may have been.   I have met with one case of the kind in empyema, and also saw a second where I believed it would have occurred if the urgency of the symptoms of oppressed respiration, had not induced an immediate artificial opening with a lancet.   I have never seen a tendency to this perforation except in the thorax.

Chronic inflammations of serous membranes, like acute ones, are susceptible of being cured, but require a much longer time, and are proportionably difficult.   As the disease recedes, the effused fluids are absorbed; and the false membranes, if there be any, become more and more fibrous and hard.   I have seen this winter, (1827–28,) a dissecting-room subject, which presented a strong polished well organized adhesion, extending from near the apex of the heart to the pericardium, almost identical in appearance with the usual arrangement of the alligator's heart; so much so, as to leave me in doubt whether it was a natural or a diseased production.

Both the serous and the sub-serous tissue remain for a long time hard and tumefied in chronic inflammations; and in this state are disposed to run into the fibro-cartilaginous and osseous condition.   They are also subject to steatomatous degenerations.

CHAPTER VII.

IRRITATIONS OF MUCOUS MEMBRANES.

To the venerable and philosophic Pinel, is due the honour of having first given to affections of the mucous membranes, a classification and arrangement depending upon their common structure. Nevertheless, these membranes were not viewed by anatomists in a general and·systematic manner, till Bichat* seized upon their traits of resemblance, and, by the powerful efforts of his genius and industry, demonstrated their identity, and, consequently, the analogies of their physiological and pathological conditions. Anatomists have now very generally adopted his views; a sketch of which will be found in the second volume of my Special and General Anatomy, and to which I refer for an account of the normal state of the mucous membranes.

When we reflect that one mucous membrane lines the whole interior of the alimentary canal, from the mouth to the anus; another the whole interior of the respiratory apparatus; and a third, the genito-urinary: we shall be impressed with the immense extent of their surface, and be ready to acknowledge that they vastly exceed in area the skin, and, indeed, any class of membranes belonging to the human fabric. In like manner we shall be prepared to appreciate the frequency, the variety, and the extreme importance of their morbid derangements.

These derangements are Phlegmasia, Sub-inflammation, Hæmorrhagies, Gangrene, Ulceration, Cysts, Hairs, Horny

* Traité des Memb. an. XIII. 1799

productions, and various degenerations; also, changes in the quantity and quality of their appropriate secretions.

Mucous membranes have a prominent and ready connexion with most other parts of the body, both by the affections which originate in them, and by such as originate in others: or, in other words, the reciprocal sympathies are prompt and numerous. An irritating substance, as a pinch of snuff, put upon the schneiderian membrane, throws into convulsive action, by sneezing, all the muscles of respiration. A sapid substance in the mouth, induces a discharge of saliva from the salivary glands; alimentary matters, in passing over the mucous membrane of the duodenum, excite the discharge into it of the fluid secreted by the liver, and by the pancreas.

These latter are instances of the strong sympathies between mucous membranes and the glands, whose excretory ducts open into them. They are only a few out of a great number of similar examples, which it belongs to the physiologist to quote more at large. We see in them the foundation of what modern pathology has asserted, that the irritations of glands opening along a mucous surface, are generally preceded by the irritation of that surface itself; consequently, glands are seldom primarily affected,* unless from local violence.

Mucous membranes, like other tissues, are much disposed to convey irritations or to suffer them, sympathetically, between their distant points; thus, a stone in the bladder causes pain and itching at the end of the urethra. When the gastro-intestinal mucous membrane is out of order, the secretions of the tongue suffer, and it becomes charged with a mucus, varying in colour and in moisture very much, according to the intensity of the affection within.

Mucous membranes are also in that kind of sympathy with other organs and tissues, that the elevation of their action either depresses or excites the action of the others. Thus, during digestion, when the mucous secretions are at

* Broussais, Prop. 150, &c.

their highest point of normal excitement or action, transpiration from the skin, according to the experiments of
Sanctorius, is diminished to a most notable extent.   On
the contrary, in small pox and other eruptive diseases, the
first lesion or irritation being in the stomach, the skin,
though at first chilly, and its action diminished, yet in a
few days assumes the irritation from the stomach, is covered
by eruptions, has its action elevated and relieves the stomach. But what proves that neither one organ or the other,
can be irritated to a certain point without the other partici-
pating; the stomach, after being quiet and healthy for a few
days, from the vicarious office of the skin, then resumes its
own responsibility, and a secondary fever is lighted up from
its irritation.

It is evident, that a principal part of the practice of medicine, indeed almost the whole of it, depends upon a judicious management of these sympathies of tissues with one
another.   The fact seems sufficiently ascertained that they
always carry on a reciprocal vital intercourse; that sometimes the excitement of one depresses the other, and at other
times stimulates it; and that, on other occasions, the excitement, like the rays of light between two opposed mirrors, is
so rapidly communicated and reconducted, that each organ
may be said to hold the other in a state of excitation.   The
expert physician so manages his stimuli to a sound organ
as to draw off the excitement from a diseased one, and at
the same time avoids increasing instead of decreasing the
excitation.   This, perhaps, is the leading reason why the
same remedies have such different effects in the hands of
different practitioners.

There can be but little doubt that the sympathies of organs and tissues are always active: (life is, in fact, a collection of sympathies, for the removal of any important organ
immediately produces death,) yet we are too much in the
habit of considering them as extinct, unless they are caused
to emerge by disease or accident.   This arises from their ex-

isting for the most part without our consciousness, and from the circumstance being a sign of disease when we do become conscious of them. Generally, we have no consciousness of the presence of clothing upon us, if it fits easily, so as not to incommode: yet the inference would not be fair, that the sense of touch is dormant or suspended, for consciousness is very quickly re-established by a little roughness, or undue pressure or exposure. This proves that our minds or perceptions, and not the interior intercommunications, are at fault. Why this intercommunication should sometimes be at par, and on other occasions to the loss of one organ with the gain of another, and alternately fluctuating, is one of the most inexplicable phenomena of life.

Phlegmasia of Mucous Membranes.

It is said by high authorities in medicine, that if mucous membranes are of all the tissues of the body those in which inflammations are most apt to occur: so are they those in which the characters of such affections being most strongly traced, are rivalled only by those of the skin and of the cellular substance.

The acute inflammations of mucous membranes are presented under three leading traits: these are the Erythemoid; the Pseudo-membranous, or that which is disposed to take on the secretion of coagulating lymph from the inflamed surface, and the Follicular or Pustulous. These different forms of inflammation, seem to depend upon the portion or constituent of the mucous membrane, which is the seat of inflammation; the follicular being situated in the cryptæ and muciparous glands, and the others in the common membrane or derm.

The degree of sensibility of such membranes in a state of phlegmasia is not uniform: some suffer a vast deal of pain, while others go on to disorganization, occasionally without a single sentiment or consciousness of uneasiness. A rule on this head seems to prevail, to wit, that the pain is severe at

11

or near the extremities of mucous membranes, as the conjunctiva, the mouth, the pharynx, the rectum, the urethra
and bladder, the vagina; while it is obtuse in the intermediate places. Bichat* has suggested that the difference depends upon the commencement and end of the mucous
membranes receiving many cerebral and very few ganglionary nerves: whereas the reverse is the case with the
pulmonary and gastro intestinal mucous membranes; for
they receive many ganglionary and but few cerebral nerves:
indeed the intestines are entirely destitute of the latter.
Under equal circumstances, the pain of mucous membranes
arising from inflammation, (if we except that from mechanical irritation, as a calculus in the kidney or bladder) seldom
equals in intensity that of the cellular, the serous, the fibrous,
and the osseous tissues; but in general, when it exists at all,
is dull, heavy, and frequently completely lulled when the
affected part is kept in perfect repose.

Of the Erythemoid Inflammation.

The colour of inflamed mucous membranes, depending
as it does upon the state of circulation of the blood, and the
intensity of the irritation, is heightened beyond the natural standard, so as to present every variety of hue, from a
lively rose-colour to a deep brown. In some cases, it occupies a very extensive surface and is uniform; in others, it is
in parti-coloured patches; in others, again, it is arborescent,
after the mode and place of the vascular ramifications. In
others, again, and especially in the stomach of old drunkards, there are spots of red, which, when examined with a
microscope, are seen to consist of a congeries of very fine
points, as if the red blood had been extravasated by a few
globules at a time, at the very end of the capillaries in the
surface of the mucous coat. These spots, consisting in col-

* Anat. Gen.

lections or aggregations of microscopical points, are insular, and leave meandering interstices between them like the winding of a river among clusters of islands and rocks. The French pathologists mention another form of the redness of erythematous inflammations which I do not remember to have observed upon mucous membranes, to wit, in zones.

The inflammatory redness has seldom an abrupt termination at its margins, but is lost by degrees in the adjacent parts. It is so identified with the structure of the mucous coat that it cannot be removed or pushed from place to place by pressure, like the colour which is natural to parts, or which has come from congestion depending upon an obstruction of the respiratory organs. Maceration in water removes it much more slowly, than it does a redness from mere accumulation of blood. Another evidence of inflammation having existed in mucous membranes, is that the surfaces not occupied by vascular effusions or injections, have their natural pearl colour changed into a dirty yellow, resembling somewhat that of a jaundiced skin; and the membrane, upon being raised up and held before the light, will be found to have lost much of its natural transparency.

Though redness be generally the effect of mucous inflammation, yet if the latter be from some very active cause which produces death in a short time, before the red globules have time to identify themselves with the mucous membrane, or to be extravasated in considerable numbers in its thickness; the redness, in such case, leaves frequently very indistinct and even no traces after death. Some cases of this kind to be hereafter referred to more particularly, have occurred to me. The rule which has been established by M. Gendrin,[*] from an observation upon the conjunctiva of a consumptive patient, and from experiments upon the conjunctiva and trachea of dogs irritated by chemical articles, is that

[*] Loc. cit. I—516.

when the inflammatory redness has reached only to vascular
arborisations not very fine, it may disappear upon death; but
if it has gone beyond this point, it remains.   He also infers
that the vessels of mucous membranes will not admit an injection when they are in a state of inflammatory congestion.

The tumefaction of inflamed mucous membranes is variable according to their situation, and some peculiarities of
structure; and also according to the duration of the malady
with which they are affected.   It is less considerable than
that of cellular tissue under equal circumstances, but exceeds
that of other tissues excepting the skin.   This thickening
appears simultaneously with the redness, or a little before it,
and keeps pace with it, augmenting continually until the redness is at its highest degree.   Such as are most vascular and
have the most loose cellular substance below them, and such as
have the greatest number of muciparous glands and follicles
in or beneath them, tumefy the most.   The obstruction to respiration and swallowing, in the phlegmasiæ of the pharynx
and larynx exemplify this.

Their surface, and especially when covered with papillæ,
becomes rough to a slight degree: the papillæ or villi tumefy also, and erect themselves so as to give a chapped or
fissured appearance to the interstices between them, but they
collapse upon death.

The texture of an inflamed mucous membrane, besides the
tumefaction, is augmented in its density so that it tears or
resists force more strongly than natural, while the inflammation is evolving and progressing: but, when the latter recedes
and the membrane becomes infiltrated with muco-purulent
matter, it becomes much softer than what it is in the normal state; and is sometimes so pulpy and disorganized that the
slightest handling, or even sweeping the finger over it will tear,
it up, from its attachment to the subjacent cellular coat.   This
softened state, (ramollissement,) though common to all mucous membranes, occurs more frequently in the stomach and
bladder; at least, in my proper experience, I have met with

it there oftenest. In such cases the inflammatory redness most frequently has disappeared, and the membrane looks as if the blood had ceased for some time previous to death, to penetrate it.

These circumstances will assist us in distinguishing a mere vascular congestion of mucous membranes and the attendant tumefaction, from the corresponding phenomena of inflammation.

There is, however, one pathological condition of mucous membranes not so easily ascertained: it is where they and the subjacent cellular tissue become largely infiltrated with serum, at the same time that the redness and vascularity are but indifferently marked. This case seems to hold the middle rank between œdema and inflammation, and will lean to the one or to the other, according to the peculiar symptoms being more or less emergent. It occurs among patients exhausted by protracted maladies.

The muciparous glands and follicles of the mucous membranes, are much disposed to participate in their acute irritations: they swell, become softer, and are infiltrated with a fibro-albuminous matter, which is of a red grey colour, and is rendered very apparent by maceration for a few hours.

In the first stages of acute mucous inflammation, the discharge from the surface and from the muciparous apparatus is unusually abundant and limpid, and has changed considerably its composition; but if the inflammation augment to a high degree, this discharge diminishes in quantity very considerably, and becomes much more viscid than natural. At the highest point of the inflammation, the secretion is almost wholly suspended. This state lasts but a short time, when it is followed by an excessive quantity of a viscid discharge mixed with blood, and of a greenish colour, and frequently lasting for a long time, even after the inflammatory redness has disappeared. M. Gendrin, states, that in this period it is that the mucous membrane, is found infiltrated with a puriform or purulent matter.

There are some varieties in the effects of the inflammations of the mucous membranes, depending upon their natural thickness. In such as are very thin, a serous infiltration, and sometimes a bloody one, is found in the cellular tissue beneath them. In some instances there are merely circumscribed spots of blood. In the augmentation and progress of the irritation, the same cellular tissue is infiltrated with pus or puriform matter. When the mucous membrane is thick, the same morbid secretions prevail, in its substance, instead of in the subjacent tissue, and they may be squeezed out as from a sponge.

It is stated by Gendrin, that absorption ceases upon mucous surfaces during their inflammation, at least upon the greater number of them. This fact he tested by the impunity with which he could apply the extract of nux vomica and pure prussic acid, to the conjunctiva; the schneiderian and the vagina of animals, when these parts had been previously inflamed by tincture of cantharides or boiling oil. But the same substances applied to healthy membranes produced death. He ascertained also, that the caustic poisons produced their appropriate phenomena, only after they had burned off the inflamed mucous membrane to which they were applied, and had got beyond its limits. I have no doubt that these facts are correctly stated by M. Gendrin in regard to the articles used as tests, yet it is sufficiently ascertained that watery fluids of a mild kind, are absorbed with great rapidity by inflamed mucous membranes; as, for example, the stomach. The extent, therefore, to which the rule can go, is that the sensibility of mucous membranes, when exalted, causes them to reject articles, which, under common circumstances, would be received; and this, in point of fact, we see illustrated every day in the treatment of intermittent and remittent fevers.

Of the Pseudo-membranous Inflammation of Mucous Tissues.

The phlegmasiæ of mucous membranes are frequently attended with a secretion of coagulating lymph on their free surface, which secretion being one of the varieties of their pathological condition, has been termed the pseudo-membranous inflammation. I wish it to be understood, that I do not present this as a disease entirely distinct from the erythemoid, because they are identical, being merely different states or stages of the same action: the erythemoid may exist and most commonly does exist without the pseudo-membranous, but the latter does not exist without the former. It is treated of under a distinct head, merely that a more lucid description may be given of the pathological phenomena.

Mucous tissues are less disposed to form, during their phlegmasiæ, false membranes and adhesions on their surface than the serous tissues. This is a very sanative and wise restriction in their diseases, because as they are so subject to the latter, and also line those passages (for food, air, and the secretions,) whose permeability is so indispensable to life, we should have under other circumstances, the latter frequently destroyed by a mere obstruction of canals. Notwithstanding this salutary limitation, they are, however, all disposed to pass occasionally such bounds, and to become encrusted with a coat of coagulating lymph. Examples of it occur in the conjunctiva, the lachrymal sac, the trachea and its ramifications; in the stomach and intestines, as well as the upper part of the alimentary tube; in the bladder and urinary passages at any point from one end to the other, and also in the genital canals male and female. The broad inference is hence left, that no mucous surface is exempt. The evil consequences may be felt immediately from the extent and severity of the irritation; and when this inconvenience is passed through, more remote ones may show themselves by

the partial or complete obstruction of canals of varied importance, to the maintenance and perfection of life.

It has been supposed, that only such mucous membranes
are disposed to the pseudo-membranous inflammation, as are
furnished with cryptæ.   Such, perhaps, is most frequently
the case, yet the following observation of the learned and
excellent Chaussier,* proves that it is not exclusively so.   A
chemist, from exposure to the fumes of oxymuriatic acid,
in large quantity, was seized with an abundant defluxion of
serosity from the eyes, nose, and mouth.   The secretion
stopped in a few hours, and was followed by loss of voice, of
smell, and obscurity of vision.   To this succeeded upon the
surface of the eyes an opaque, whitish, membranous layer,
which intercepted the light, and a similar concretion formed
in the nose, pharynx, and, as was supposed, in the larynx
and trachea.   In a few days the false membrane peeled off,
from the eyes and also from the other parts, and their natural functions were re-established.   The preceding is a singular case, and I presume it has happened to very few persons to see a parallel to it.

As membraniform concretions are so apt to be followed by
the adhesion of contiguous surfaces, which, in the case of
the eye, would be still more favoured by the constant contact of the lid and ball, we are struck with the admirable
provision of nature in regard to this organ.   If the con-
junction had been velvety, like other mucous membranes,
friction would have presented an impediment to rapid and
minutely graduated motion; a secretion of pure mucus
would have obscured vision and attracted moats in the air;
and if the membrane had been serous, as it is so frequently
irritated, adhesions of it would have been almost unavoidable.

Since the first observation concerning the concretions of
the trachea and larynx, they have been so repeatedly seen
that the aggregate of cases is now very considerable.   The

* Gend. vol. i. p. 613.

common cause of them is change of transpiration, or catching cold, as it is called.   This concretion is the croup of medical writers, the peculiar pathology of which will be dwelt on, more at large hereafter.   It is the disease of any age, but is much more common in infancy, than in subsequent periods of life.

Membraniform concretions in small patches, are not very uncommon in the alimentary tube; but the cases are rare, I should think, where the whole circumference of a portion of intestine is lined in this way; though there is every reason to believe, that authors have been exact in their reports of such instances.   In the case of an intussusception of an infant, in the Anatomical Museum, there is a thin crust of lymph upon the mucous surface of the gut; and in an erythematous colon from the Alms House, presented to me, Nov. 1827, by Dr Hodge, where there had been an enormous distention with fæces, he and Mr. Chew, resident pupil, were of opinion that there was a lining of coagulating lymph.   It was sent to me at the University, and being in great haste at the time, I overlooked this feature in the specimen; though I have no doubt, from the general precision and intelligence of these gentlemen, that the observation was exact.   The late Dr. Whillden, of this city, discharged a perfect cylinder, either of coagulating lymph, or of intestine, from the anus.   The case has been reported by his friend, Dr. La Roche.

M. Gendrin affirms, that he has often seen such concretions in the stools of persons affected with diarrhea.   In a dissection, he found the whole colon, and a part of the rectum thus lined with a pseudo-membrane.   The most extraordinary case, however, occurred to him in the Hotel Dieu, in 1817, during the prevalence of abdominal phlegmasia among the patients.   In the body of a man, aged thirty, who died on the eighth day of gastro enteritis, he found the *stomach* lined with a false membrane, in the whole extent of the pyloric half: the mucous coat was uniformly

1°

erythematous, sensibly thickened, and easily detached in shreds.

As regards the urinary passages, a preparation of our Museum illustrates the pseudo-membranous formation on the mucous coat of the urinary bladder. Sponius has met with it in the pelvis of the kidney, and Destrees has seen it expelled by fragments from the urethra of a man affected at the same time with intestinal phlegmasia, attended with membraniform discharges to such an extent, that he thought he was disposing of the whole of his bowels.*

In pseudo-membranous inflammation, the tissue affected is red from its injection with blood; and somewhat thickened, but not so much so as occurs in other phlegmasiæ. The papillæ, and the villi increase also in their dimensions and colour, as well as the mucous cryptæ or follicles; the sub-mucous cellular tissue becomes more friable, and permits the mucous coat to be torn off in shreds. In the case of croup, little white spots occur under the epithelium of the mouth, which are apt from their abundance to become confluent; and at the same time, a large quantity of ropy diaphanous mucus is secreted, which becomes still more viscid in adhering to the parietes of the surface producing it.

When a mucous membrane is destitute of epithelium, the false membrane has first of all the condition and appearance of a lamina of viscid mucus adhering to it; and its consistence augments rapidly by its assuming more and more the character of coagulating lymph: until it has fully done so, its boundaries are lost insensibly in the adjacent mucus. Sometimes a perfectly continuous membrane is formed; on other occasions it exists only in patches interruptedly. The latter is much more apt to be the case where there is an epithelium, than where there is not one. According to the report of M. Guersent,† when the concretion is raised up, the mucous membrane is most generally found entire in

* Vol. i. p. 632.   † Gend. vol. i p. 616

croup; being neither excoriated, nor ulcerated on the inflamed surface.

The following is the process whereby these pseudo-membranous formations are detached; when they terminate by
the recovery of the patient.   The inflammation diminishing
in its intensity, a liquid mucus is secreted by the mucous
membrane beneath the false one, which loosens its connexion, until finally its adhesions are all dissolved, and it falls
off, very much softened and diminished in its consistence,
by the incorporation of mucus with it; it therefore is
sometimes ejected entire, and on other occasions in strips
and fragments, depending upon its state of cohesion.   Occasionally, this process of ungluing and softening does not
occur, and the false membrane is worn away or attenuated,
until it resembles a very fine epidermis spread over the subjacent mucous coat.   This condition is more frequently observed in the mouth and pharynx.

As in the pseudo-membranous inflammations of serous tissues, so in those of the mucous, the false membranes become sometimes vitalized by the formation of blood vessels
in them, communicating with the blood vessels of the adjacent parts.   Anatomical preparations illustrating this fact,
are said to be in the possession of the celebrated Sœmme-
ring, and it has been noticed by others; but the cases, I
should think, are extremely rare.   For my own part, I have
never seen it, though I have no difficulty in admitting it, as
the phenomenon is identical, with what occurs in the inflammations of other tissues.

Of the Pustular Phlegmasia of Mucous Membranes.

The term pustular phlegmasia is adopted by pathologists,
in order to express a leading trait in one of the forms of inflammation, to which all mucous membranes, but especially
the stomach and intestines, are liable.   Instead of being diffused like a common erythema over the whole mucous sur-

face, the irritation is primitively seated in the mucous follicles or cryptæ, and resembles little boils of half a line or
more in diameter, studding at various intervals the affected
membrane.

According to Ræderer and Wagler,* the pustules are coincident with an excessive secretion of mucus; and in their
early stages, it is easy to see the affected cryptæ distended
and swollen by this secretion, and placed beneath a thick
layer of inspissated tenacious mucus, adhering strongly to
the mucous membrane.

The pustules, or what is the same thing, the distended
cryptæ, are moderately projecting, and are either separate,
or in clusters; and upon some of them is a black point indicating the natural orifice of the follicle.   Their colour is
white: the mucous membrane in some places and instances
is universally in the affected region injected, very red, and
is tumefied; but it also happens, that a red areola only is
formed around the pustules, and is infiltrated and swollen.

This pustular phlegmasia attends catarrhal fevers, the
small pox, and some epidemics besides, and has been noticed
by a considerable number of writers, both modern and of a
more remote period.

The pustules which exist on mucous membranes arise both
from the follicles and from the glands; which are in a state
of inflammation, attended with a collection of the fluid secreted from them.   In the case of the glands, when it occurs
where they are aggregated, there is a flattened depressed tumour, with inflammation of the villi.   In the case of the
cryptæ, the tumour is small, round, elevated, and somewhat
acuminated or sharpened at the point.   In the state previous
to inflammation, when the cryptæ are only excited, they are
diaphanous, and form a round projection, with a little depression or point in their centre, indicating the orifice of
the gland.   The affection may recede from this state, and

Gend. vol. i. p. 589.

get well; but when inflammation has declared itself, it is manifested by the cryptæ becoming red, injected, opaque, and being elevated upon a phlogosed surface. The disease may, and does from this limitation extend itself to the villi and whole mucous tissue, and to the sub-mucous cellular coat; but in this advanced stage, the original distinction of it is lost, and it is apt to be followed by ulceration.

The aphthæ which are seen so frequently in the mouth and pharynx of children, are inflammations of the muciparous apparatus, cryptæ and glands there, and are instances of the pustular inflammation. They should, however, be distinguished from small ulcers, which sometimes form in the same membrane, and take on the same appearance, from their suppurating and raising up the epithelium. Pustular inflammation, besides existing along the digestive passages, has occasionally been seen in the mucous membrane of the organs of respiration.

CHAPTER VIII.

IRRITATIONS OF MUCOUS TISSUES

(*Continued.*)

CHRONIC INFLAMMATION OF MUCOUS TISSUES.

CHRONIC inflammations of mucous membranes are frequently the consequence of acute ones imperfectly cured; and they also frequently exist without any previously well marked acute stage; having begun and progressed almost insensibly, and being known rather by the disturbance of the functions of the organ affected, than by local pain and constitutional sympathies. A chronic inflammation of a mucous membrane may continue in this insensibly progressive and almost dormant state for years, when all at once some exposure or irregularity·will awaken and evolve all the symptoms of acute inflammation; and after a short duration, end in the disorganization of the part, and in the death of the individual.

A distinction has been drawn between the chronic and the sub-inflammations of mucous tissues, which I have some difficulty in recognizing the value of, as regards their pathological changes. Moreover, there are no symptoms during life enabling us to perceive the difference, and, as for the treatment, it is identical. Sub-inflammation may come on primarily from an afflux of the white parts of the blood to a part: it also frequently happens, that sub-inflammation is one of the consequences of acute inflammation.

The pain attending chronic or sub-inflammation is seldom severe, and consists rather in a gnawing and sentiment of uneasiness: sometimes it is entirely absent. As to the effect which chronic inflammation produces on the system at large, it is varied continually by the character of the organs affected. Such as are of the first importance to life, as the respiratory mucous membrane, manifest this derangement by emaciation and hectic fever; whereas, in such as are secondary, as that of the vagina, it frequently produces but little inconvenience, and seems indeed consistent with perfect health in other regions.

The colour of muciparous membranes under chronic inflammation varies. When the disorder exists in a state somewhat active, they are of a dark uniform red; but in a milder degree and in a more advanced stage, the colour diminishes proportionately, and indeed, becomes perfectly pale; the only evidence of previous vascular injection consisting in veins filled with a bluish or purple blood, serpentine and varicose, and either in clusters or in an arborescent distribution. These appearances I have frequently seen on the stomach; and latterly, I have seen them on the root of the tongue and on the pharynx, in an old man in our dissecting rooms, (January 10th, 1828.) Generally, there is no injection of the capillaries; and the redness, such as it is, seems identified with the tissue, and difficult to remove from it by maceration. These conditions, however, depend upon the age of the phlegmasia and its state of excitement; for if an acute phlegmasia supervene upon the old one, the red colour is vivified and the capillaries are found distended with red blood. This often happens in the stomachs of old drunkards, when they die with febrile symptoms. The blood is sometimes exhaled from the inflamed surface, and may be occasionally pressed from it as from a sponge.

A very common appearance on the free surface of mucous membranes affected with chronic phlegmasia, are bluish or slate-coloured spots from the size of six lines, or less, to

twelve or more; but generally within these dimensions.
Sometimes this blueness or slate-colour is almost universal:
the colon, in its chronic diseases, presents it in this state
every now and then, and also the urinary bladder.   On the
stomach and small intestines it does not generally extend so
universally.   It is commonly attended with a softening of
the part affected.

When such patches on the stomach are examined with
a lens, the colour seems to be most frequently at the ends
of the villi; but sometimes it pervades the whole thickness of the coat   It is seen of a great variety of shades, from
a light slate-colour to a jet black; and I have generally considered it to have been first of all a deposite of red blood.
Sometimes it is deposited in an arborescent way, corresponding in situation with the larger vascular trunks, and forming
a sort of black ground or fringe for a line or two on each side
of them; being extravasated in the adjoining mucous coat,
and in a slight degree in the cellular.   In a morbid stomach
lately presented to me by Dr. Isaac Hays (January 2d, 1828,)
I became more fully satisfied of the nature of this colouring
matter, and that it is the red globules of blood become black.
In this stomach, the trunks of the veins, as well as their extremities, were filled with it; and it was extravasated in ragged
patches in the mucous coat along their margins, following the
anastomoses of the vessels, and thus forming a strongly marked
reticulation.   From its position in the vessels, the softness
of the adjoining texture, and the general appearances, it
seemed to have been just done. I examined it also by raising
up the mucous membrane.   The colour here was almost jet
black.   A question then arises whether the recent is not the
darkest period of this pathological state; and whether, if the
individual lives, it does not become lighter and lighter, until
it is entirely removed, or nearly so.   The most diseased stomachs that I have ever seen, with almost universal degeneration into scirrhus of the mucous membrane, have been
entirely destitute of these slate-coloured patches, and it may

have arisen from their having passed the period of them, at the time when they were seen by me.

It is stated by M. Gendrin,* that after the cure of a chronic phlegmasia, however light it may have been, the vascular branches remain more voluminous, and are injected. This injection, when closely examined, is found to consist in red vessels disseminated in the thickness, or upon the adherent surface of the membrane, and which dividing into fine branches, become at length imperceptible from their tenuity. These red vessels themselves cannot be traced to any trunk, or rather do not seem to belong to it. He considers this last character important in enabling us to distinguish the ramiform injection, the result of a chronic phlegmasia, from passive vascular congestion.

When mucous membranes have remained for a long time in a state of chronic phlegmasia, they frequently become very much thickened, and their free surface cellular, or rather favoid, like a honey comb. When, however, the affection has been light, though long, the thickening is frequently inconsiderable, and is attended with a slight ramiform injection; the cryptæ are more voluminous than natural, and more apparent, and discharge a secretion of mucus somewhat puriform.

The favoid appearance is not the invariable attendant of the thickened state. I have seen instances where precisely the reverse was the case; there being a smooth polished surface, notwithstanding the very increased thickness.

It appears probable to me, that increased thickness sometimes overcomes, by its rigidity and bulk, the power of the muscular contraction of the stomach and other hollow viscera: and when an ejection of their contents occurs, it is accomplished exclusively, or almost so, by the abdominal muscles only.

The augmentation of thickness is attended with an in-

* Vol i. p 639

I

creased density of texture, and a more homogeneous appearance of the part. It is hard, rough, difficult to tear, resists maceration for a long time, and is finally reduced by it into a sort
of powdered pulp. The cryptæ, which, from their enlargement, are so conspicuous during the early periods of a chronic affection, become at length obscured, and indeed, entirely lost in the surrounding pathological changes, and cannot
by any subsequent artifice be made manifest again.

Chronic mucous inflammations being like others subject to
a renewal of, or an accession of an acute stage, the deranged organization, under such circumstances, increases and becomes
changed in its characters. It loses its hardness and consistence, and is converted into a soft pulpy mass, infiltrated with
pus, with small collections of it diffused about, and in the
adjoining cellular tissue. If this stage persist in its duration
and intensity, the membrane ulcerates: if, on the contrary,
it retrogrades, the membrane loses its redness, but remains
swollen. M. Gendrin, who draws a distinction between
mucous membranes and villous membranes, says that in the
case of the former, it becomes friable, and of the latter, softened and almost diffluent.

In some instances of chronic mucous phlegmasia, where
the symptoms are somewhat active, or where they have become so, after being dormant for some time, vegetations or
granulations are formed on the free surface. These vegetations are red, round, or flat, unequal, and rough, and are
formed by fine vessels highly injected with red blood, and
blended with a gelatiniform tissue. After a while they become less red and more dense in their structure, and remain
often even after the cure of the disease from which they
sprang.

Chronic inflammations of moderate intensity, are attended
with a secretion of mucus more abundant than common.
It is viscid, greyish, and by being floated in water, sometimes separates into two parts; one of which, being thick and
thread-like, floats, and the other being pulverulent, sinks. If

there be an exacerbation, a considerable serous exhalation is joined to the mucous secretion, and appears and disappears with the intensity of the attack.

When these membranes have suffered for a long time, the reddish and the brown colour, which seem identified with them, cannot be removed by washing or a moderate maceration. And artificial injections do not penetrate into their capillary vessels, nor into the engorged vessels around and traversing the affected part. *

Of the Ulcerations of Mucous Membranes.

There is no part of the human system which is found more frequently in a state of ulceration than the mucous membranes, and especially that which is extended between the pyloric orifice of the stomach and the anus. This disposition is no doubt dependant upon their great vascularity, their extreme sensibility and vitality, and upon their very complex organization presenting many constituents, glandular, nervous, vascular, absorbent, and so on, exposed to derangement.

Sometimes ulcerations are the immediate and quick result of an inflammation, acute from the beginning; on other occasions they are the consequence of acute inflammation coming upon a chronic one, and then their progress is much more rapid and disorganizing. We meet with them most frequently, as one of the conditions of the usual progress of chronic inflammation, in the intestinal canal. When they come from primary acute inflammation, the edges are red from the injection of red blood, and not much elevated, and are covered as well as the bottom with purulent mucus. When, on the contrary, they proceed from chronic inflammation, the edges are swollen, everted, ragged, and hard, and the bottom of the ulceration is rough and of a dark livid

* Gend. vol. 1. p 639

red.   In acute inflammation entailed upon chronic, the ulcerated surface is swollen, soft, and bleeding.   These several states may be distinguished from cicatrization by the ulcer in the latter having its margins flat, flexible, and converging towards the centre.

The following portions of the mucous tissue are subject
to ulceration: the conjunctiva, the lining membrane of the
mouth and pharynx, that of the larynx and trachea; in some
rare instances that of the gall bladder, and also of the urinary bladder, and then as mentioned, their occurrence in the
alimentary canal is very frequent.   The order of frequency
with which they occur in the alimentary canal is as follows:
the beginning of the colon first, then the ileum, especially
at its lower end, the termination of the colon and the beginning of the rectum, the stomach, the transverse colon, the
jejunum, and, lastly, the duodenum.   In the mucous membranes devoid of epithelium, the ulcer is preceded by a small
reddish tubercle with a dark point in the centre.   It is thought
that these are the cryptæ in a state of inflammation, which
extends itself to the contiguous parts, and is followed successively by the ulceration.   But where the mucous membrane
is covered with an epidermis, a small white pustule is first
seen, which raising up the epidermis ruptures it, and exhibits
a rounded ulcer at the bottom, which is spongy and of a light
red colour.   The ulcer goes on to extend in diameter as well
as in depth, and removes the whole thickness frequently of
the mucous coat.   Now and then, and especially on the genitals, the ulceration exhibits the same sort of precursor in a
reddish tubercle, as it does when there is no epithelium.

The ulcerations of mucous membranes are often attended
with the formation, in the subjacent tissue, of little fistulous
abscesses communicating with the cavity of the ulcer, and
by their situation loosening or ungluing the mucous coat
from its attachments.   These fistulous sinuses sometimes
form a sub-mucous communication between several ulcers,
which, when they are chronic, have their edges everted.

In the alimentary canal the tunics are generally, indeed M. Gendrin says always, thickened previously to their ulceration. So that when the latter occurs successively by communication from one tunic to another, it is preceded by a thickening of the corresponding tunics. The villi disappear in the circle immediately around the ulceration.

Ulcers vary in their depth, from the various degrees of thickening which occur in different places, whence it happens that an ulcer comparatively shallow, may have removed almost the entire thickness of the intestinal parietes, while one much deeper, does not penetrate beyond the mucous coat. Neither is their depth governed by their extent, for commonly such as have a moderate size are the most profound. Ulcers of the intestines are readily recognized, even before the gut is slit open, if they have destroyed more than the mucous coat, for, in such case, the peritoneal surface is of a crimson colour over the ulcer, and on feeling it, one will be very sensible of an increased thickness and inequality along the edges of the ulcer. In addition to which, if the ulcer has almost reached the peritoneal coat, this coat will be rough on its free surface, and either covered entirely with a layer of coagulating lymph, or have little masses of it interspersed over the threatened place. The latter also, if the tendency of the ulcer to complete perforation of the intestinal canal, leave but little thickness of peritoneal covering, will contract adhesions to the contiguous surface of intestines, so that the cavity of the peritoneum will be protected from the contents of the intestines being poured into it. In some rare cases, however, the perforation communicates with the cavity of the abdomen, and gives rise to general acute peritonitis. Of this I have met with an example in the stomach.

Cases are also related, where an adhesion having formed, the ulceration has progressed beyond the limits of the adhesion, so as to open into the contiguous fold of intestine. Pinel met with an instance of communication between the

stomach and the colon; Frank between the stomach and the
liver, and Gendrin between the stomach and the diaphragm.
I have met with the reverse, also, in one instance, where an
abscess in the right iliac region, besides discharging itself on
the thigh, communicated with the head of the colon, and
made for the remainder of the life of the individual, a constant oozing of fæces from the femoral orifice.*

In the case of Mrs. A. G. a lumbar abscess connected with
caries of the transverse processes of the lumbar vertebræ,
besides discharging below Poupart's ligament, formed a fistulous orifice with the rectum.   And I have latterly seen in
our dissecting-rooms a case where a communication was
made with the bladder from a similar cause.*

Another of the effects of ulcerations of mucous membranes
is the enlargement, and frequently the suppuration of the
lymphatic glands through which pass the absorbents of the
part.   Chronic ulcerations and irritations produce this to
a remarkable degree.   I have not long since seen a case
where from disease of the mucous membrane of the stomach and intestines, the lymphatic glands of the stomach
mesentery and mesocolon, were tumefied and consolidated,
I may say, into a single mass almost as large as the head.
Unless from the evidence of the parts themselves, it was
almost incredible that life should have been protracted to
such an extreme of disorganization and derangement.*   M.
Gendrin considers that such enlargement and the suppuration of lymphatics are rare in any phlegmasia of the intestinal canal, except that attended with ulceration.   And his
idea is, that it comes from the pus secreted by the ulcer being absorbed by the branches of the vena portarum, and carried to the glands by anastomosis with the lymphatic vessels; an opinion proved, as he asserts, by his commonly finding pus filling the branches of the vena portarum, or else an
inflammation of them, in intestinal ulcerations.

* See Anatomical Museum for Preparation.

In the intestinal canal, ulceration presents itself under three forms. The first of them is preceded by the erythemoid state, and is so superficial at first, that it consists only in the destruction and removal of the villi. These ulcers are little disposed to become deep; but, when they do so, their edges are elevated, and highly infiltrated with blood, while, at the same time, they remain smooth. The mucous cryptæ give the second form to ulcerations: becoming affected, in the pustular inflammation, they secrete a pus which distends them, and finally ruptures their parietes. The latter become tumefied by infiltration, and a small, narrow, but profound, ulceration is kept up, which commonly penetrates beyond the muscular coat of the intestine. As such an affection is seldom confined to a single crypta or muciparous gland, but is common to several of them, where they are aggregated, so we most frequently see these ulcers in patches.

The pathological history of the third form of ulcers is as follows. In the first stage, flat plates with perpendicular edges, and of one and a-half or two lines in thickness, are raised upon the internal face of the mucous membrane, by the persistance of chronic inflammation in the muciparous follicles, and in the villi. When recent, these plates are red throughout; but they lose their colour in advancing to a greater age, until they are finally of a light gray. The surrounding villous membrane is disposed to observe their colour whatever it may be: but this is not invariable, and is frequently reversed. The surface of these plates is rough, unequal, and presents no villi. The villous membrane, thus tumefied, is soft, spongy, red, and infiltrated with lymph and blood, in the recent state; and with a puriform gelatine in the more advanced. Sometimes only the sub-mucous tissue participates in the affection, and, on other occasions, it is extended to the muscular.

These plates after a while become softened still more; small shallow ulcerations declare themselves on their surface, and, by augmenting and running together, remove the

whole plate. The edges of the ulcers thus formed, are unequal, thick, ragged, sometimes bevelled, and, at others, perpendicular.

Gangrene of Mucous Membranes.

Another form of disease to which mucous membranes are
subject, is gangrene. It occurs frequently in the gums of
children, and is attended with a loosening of all the teeth,
and a dark greenish colour; with the discharge of a black
ichorous matter, resembling blood dissolved in serum. The
first indication of it is the formation of little phlyctenæ, terminating in black eschars. It is more apt to prevail in places
where children are aggregated, and under six years of age.

That form of gangrene which is seated in the mouth and
pharynx constitutes the angina maligna of medical writers. It
has been observed also in the trachea, æsophagus, bladder, and
is thought not to be very uncommon in the gastro intestinal
canal. I have seen one case where it seemed to be almost
universal in the small intestines and large, and had extended its changes to the peritoneal coat. The patient was a
black man, who died with extreme symptoms of a dysentery.

When the gangrene of the gastro intestinal mucous membrane is in patches, the eschar is of a deep slate colour of inconsiderable consistence, and may be easily removed. Sometimes this state extends itself through the whole thickness of the
intestine; and when a slight distention of it, during life, occurs, it gives way, effuses its contents into the cavity of the
peritoneum; and the individual dies with symptoms of inflammation in the latter.   The adjoining portion of intestine
in gangrene is tumefied, much softer than common, and of a
livid red, from the infiltration of a dark red serum. The
fœtor in these cases is considerable.

CHAPTER IX.

IRRITATIONS OF MUCOUS MEMBRANES

(*Continued.*)

SOFTENING OR MOLLESCENCE

To M. Louis of Paris, a pathologist of high distinction, is due the credit of having pointed out to physicians, in a systematic and well digested manner, the softening of mucous tissues, as one of the morbid changes to which they are very much disposed.   In the stomach alone, M. Louis' computation is, that one twelfth of the patients who have died under his care, have had it either as a primitive affection, or as a complication with some chronic complaint.   To this testimony, I may be permitted to add my own, that even before the appearance of M. Louis' memoir, which was in 1824, I had, in 1822, while engaged in injecting the stomach of a subject, found its mucous coat so universally soft and pulpy, that its blood vessels would not retain a wax injection, but that the latter ran out into the cavity of the stomach almost as fast as it could be thrown into the large trunks, through which I was injecting.   I, moreover, observed at the time, that the villous coat, besides being softened, was abraded upon very slight handling.   It is well known to the profession, that Mr. John Hunter many years ago communicated his observations, on the dissolved state of the stomach, in persons who had died suddenly from accident or the law; and that he attributed it to the solvent

14

power of the gastric juice.   As the person whose stomach I
had, was a patient in the Alms House, who had died from
fever called typhus, I could not suppose in him an activity
of the gastric juice sufficient to produce such consequences,
and I was led to believe that they had been caused by
the undue use of volatile alkali.   I communicated my conjectures to the late distinguished anatomist, Dr. Lawrence,
who was much engaged at the time in dissections at the Alms
House, and they were followed by his detecting the same derangement, afterwards, in many other patients.

My next observations on the same subject, were in two
children.   In neither of these instances had volatile alkali,
or any substance of the kind, been administered. it was
therefore plain, that this might be looked upon, as one of the
natural morbid changes of the mucous coat of the stomach.
The substance of M. Louis' memoir became known to me
about this period; and since then, in my own observations
and through the kindness of my friends, I have had frequent occasion to see such pathological derangements.   I
am not, however, like M. Louis, prepared to establish any
thing like an average of its frequency; but think that he has
approximated the truth as it is even in our climate, and with
our habits of life.   Proportionately, I think, I have seen it
more frequently in children; but of this I am not certain.

I may here mention that such changes in the texture and
general condition of the mucous membrane of the stomach,
have been declared only instances of what Mr. Hunter
pointed out, as a dissolution by the gastric juice.   Without
discussing this opinion, there is one unanswerable argument,
which must overwhelm the objection; to wit, that the same
sort of softening has been noticed in the œsophagus, in the
large intestines, and in the bladder, in all of which there is
no gastric juice.   Consequently, it is a bad philosophy, which
would make a parallel phenomenon in the stomach depend upon
so exclusive a cause as the gastric juice: and that too where
the protracted form of disease must have diminished so ma-

terially the activity of the gastric juice, even if the secretion of it had not been entirely arrested.

From the cases observed, it appears, in regard to the stomach, that though the affection is sometimes latent; yet most
frequently it is accompanied with symptoms, suited to the de-
tection, or at least to the suspecting of it during life. The
appetite is for the most part suspended, but occasionally, only
weakened. Nausea is an invariable symptom, and in a majority of cases, is attended with vomiting, and these symptoms, with some occasional remissions, go on increasing till
death; they being excited by the mildest drinks, even su-
gared water. Pains in the epigastrium are an almost universal attendant, manifesting themselves from a slight degree of uneasiness, pricking, and the sensation of a bar
across it, to a severity of suffering causing patients to refer
all their trouble to it. These pains are augmented upon
pressure, but subject to remissions. The tongue retaining
its moisture, is not much affected; with the exception, in
some cases, of redness at the point, and whitish villosities
in the middle.

Diarrhea generally prevails. Frequently, in adults, we find
the lungs in a tubercular state, to a greater or less degree.
The intellectual faculties are not much impaired, neither is
the bodily strength very much prostrated, except the disease passes onwards in a very acute manner. The countenance has the expression of uneasiness, during the epigastric pains, but not when they are absent. Sometimes there
are alternate chills and heats, but they cannot be considered
as an invariable symptom.

The symptoms connected with this disease may last from
a few days, to one year and upwards. In one individual,
examined by M. Louis, and who had consumption for four
months, there was, however, no indication, except a want of
appetite.

M. Louis, with the view of obtaining some standard for
the natural and healthy consistence of the stomach, insti-

tuted experiments upon thirty-two other patients, in whom the stomach seemed to have undergone no morbid change. In twenty-nine of them he found the consistence of the mucous membrane diminishing successively from the small to the large curvature, and still less in the great extremity, (cul de-sac;) which was proved by his being able to tear off strips an inch or two long from the small curvature; half an inch or three quarters from the large; and only three or four lines from the cul de-sac. He therefore draws the inference, that this law of consistency is uniform, and that when we cannot tear up the mucous membrane in strips, there is a lesion in its organization; and eminently so when it is only of the consistence of a viscid mucus.

A very important indication also may be obtained from the relative thickness of the mucous coat of the stomach; for being thicker at the large curvature, it decreases successively from this to the small one, and at the cul de-sac it is somewhat thinner still. Though M. Louis has attempted to establish some positive data upon the absolute thickness of this coat, they are rather objectionable, for the reason that individuals vary in this respect; besides which, an emaciated subject has the stomach in a state of atrophy; and in anasarca, it is thickened by the dropsical affection. His estimate, however, is as follows: from three fourths of to one millimetre at the great curvature; from one third to three fourths of a millimetre at the small; and from one fourth to three fifths of a millimetre in the cul de-sac. He remarks, very justly, that if an alteration either from the natural thickness, or from the natural consistence, indicate a lesion, how much more then will both of those changes united indicate it? Hence it follows, that one of the most important objects in autopsies, is, to remark the absolute and the relative thickness and consistence of the mucous coat of the stomach.*

* From the frequent reference in medicine to the modern French measures, the following will be found useful:—

The general result of the observations made by M. Louis is, that the capaciousness of the stomach varied: but it was more frequently below, than above the natural standard. Its peritoneal surface offered no indication of the changes within; but the mucous surface was of a pale white with a tinge of blue; this colour was either in approximated irregular patches or in long narrow bands, and the part affected was sensibly to the eye, and to the touch, below the level of the adjoining surface. In these places the mucous membrane was of an extreme softness and tenuity, and transformed into a kind of semi-transparent glairy mucus, of

Measures of Distance.

			Inches	
One Metre is equal to - - - - -			39 37100 of an inch.	
—— Decimetre, or one-tenth of a metre, is equal to,			3 93710	
—— Centimetre, or one-hundredth,	do		.39371	
—— Millimetre, or one-thousandth,	do. -		03937	

		Yards	Feet	
—— Decametre, or 10 metres, is equal to		10.	2.	9.00007
—— Hecatometre, or 100 do.	do	109	1	1.00000

		Furlongs			
—— Chiliometre, or 100 do.	do.	4.	213.	1.	10 00002

		Miles			
—— Myriometre, or 10,000 do do. 6	1	156	0.	.00006	
—— Grade, or deg. 100,000 do. do. 62.	1	23	2	00008	

Measures of Capacity.

One Litre   is 2⅛ pints, or 61 02800 of an inch
—— Decilitre — one-tenth of a litre.
—— Centilitre — one-hundredth of a litre.
—— Millilitre — one-thousandth of a litre.
—— Decalitre — 10 litres, 2 gallons, 64 $\frac{44}{230}$ cubic inches
—— Hecatolitre is 100 do. 26 do   4. $\frac{44}{230}$ do.
—— Chiliolitre is 1000 do. 264 do $\frac{44}{230}$ do.

Measures of Weight.

One Gramme is 15444 grains Troy, or 20592 grains Avoirdupois weight: equal to about 3 lbs. 8 ounces   do
—— Decigramme is one-tenth of a gramme
—— Centigramme is one-hundredth do.
—— Milligramme is one-thousandth do
—— Decagramme is ten grammes
—— Hecatogramme is one-hundred do

the thickness of the lining membrane of the colon, and
sometimes less. It presented the delusive appearance of an
entire removal, so that the cellular coat could be seen at
the bottom: in truth, in some cases it was indeed removed.

When this softening has the form of the long and narrow
bands, it is generally spread throughout the stomach; but
in other states, it occupies commonly the cul de sac, and is
sometimes extended to the cardia and the pylorus. Some
stomachs present this disease in all its various stages of
progression; as, first of all, a slight tenuity and softening in
one spot; then more considerable in another; entire destruction of the mucous coat in a third spot; and the destruction of all the tunics in a fourth, with the exception of the
peritoneal; offering, in these several degrees, a very complete picture of the progress of perforations of the stomach.

Sometimes the affected membrane, instead of the bluish
white colour, is a pale opaque white, or grey, or rose, and
blended with red or black spots. In the child of Mrs. ——,
I found it of the colour of glue.

Another remarkable feature in these cases of softened mucous membrane is the entire deficiency of mucus on the disorganized parts; both the surface where the softening has
occurred, and where the mucous membrane has disappeared,
and this, when there is mucus on other parts of the stomach.
In some of M. Louis' cases, he found the adjoining mucous
membrane of a rose colour, or even of a bright red, softened and attenuated; in others it was unequal, with small
knobs or granulations on its surface, attended by ulcerations.

When the œsophagus is affected in a similar way, the
softening has been found most commonly at the lower extremity, and the disorganization reaching to a considerable
depth   Hence, a very moderate traction is sufficient to produce a laceration through the whole thickness of this tube.

One may readily infer, from what has been said, the danger
of catherism, when the bladder has undergone such change;
for the instrument may be unwittingly thrust into the cavity

of the peritoneum, and thus give rise to acute inflammation from the effusion of urine into it. Happily, the softening of the bladder occurs, it is thought, much less frequently than any other.

When the softening of an intestinal mucous membrane is beginning, or in the early and middle stage, M. Gendrin asserts that there is an entire deficiency of vascular injection, both of the point affected and of its vicinity, as well as of the corresponding portion of mesentery. This pallidness is seen by the aid of a lens to extend itself to the villi, which are withered and collapsed.

A mucous membrane, when affected with mollescence, is frequently found in so pulpy a state that the finger passed over it, will abrade it from the sub-mucous tissue; and we then see in the latter the trunks of blood vessels not so abundant or so distended with blood as usual, and also in a flattened collapsed state. I have, in several cases, observed, that the colour of the blood in them was singularly altered to an olive black, and was percolated in the substance of the mucous coat and in the cellular, so as to constitute broad black streaks ramifying and anastomosing according to the direction and arrangement of the vessels. I have never been able to satisfy myself in regard to the cause of this change of colour in the red particles of blood, and have often been struck with the resemblance between it and that of the black vomit in yellow fever. I have also confirmed, by my own observations, the remark of Louis and of Gendrin, that we never find mucus on the softened membrane; its secretion there seeming to be completely arrested. It is not unfrequently coloured yellow by bile, and by articles of medicine or nourishment, as rheubarb, cinchona, and so on; and sometimes by the rupture of a small blood vessel, it assumes from the infiltration of blood, a dark brown colour.

When the soft membrane has, by a natural process, been removed or cast off, the boundaries are marked by clean perpendicular edges destitute of vascularity. If the slough, if such it may be called, is very extensive, the margins are not, however, quite so clearly marked off, but run rather insensibly into the adjoining parts: one perceives, also, insulated remains of the old membrane scattered in patches over the sloughed surface, and of a consistence very much reduced, and indicating also their disorganization.

When such disorganization in the alimentary canal continues its progress, it terminates by perforating the whole parietes of the latter.   In such cases of spontaneous perforation, the edges of it are clean, pale, and not tumefied, indicating thereby the absence of inflammation, if death has followed almost immediately upon the accident.

Pathologists have differed somewhat in opinion on the cause of this softening of mucous membranes; some considering every case of it to arise from an inflammatory action, and others, that it is frequently idiopathic.   My personal means of observation, have not been sufficiently varied and numerous to enable me to adopt with strong confidence, one side exclusively.   It appears to me, however, that in some cases I have not met with the marks of inflammation, at least as usual; and the disease looked as if it were idiopathic. The symptoms related by M. Louis in his cases, are, for the most part, the attributes of inflammation; such as pain in the epigastrium, want of appetite, frequent vomiting. M. Gendrin, who advocates the doctrine of an idiopathic softening, has argued the point with much force and effect on the subsequent grounds; to wit:

No mucous inflammation in the stomach and bowels commences without marked increase of vascularity, and the vessels of the part, so far from being diminished, as in softening, are not only enlarged and engorged there, but also in the proximate portion of mesentery.   The villi, themselves, far from being withered and collapsed, are expanded and erect, the mucus is abundant, and very tenacious; and strips of the mucous membrane may be torn off: whereas, in the mollities, there is a want of sufficient consistence to execute this process; and its capillaries have completely disappeared. In phlegmasia, moreover, in its early stages, there is an evident increase in thickness, density, and also in roughness: on the contrary, in softening there is diminished thickness, a loss of tenacity, and a soft pulpy feel, besides an arrest of the mucous secretions.

M. Gendrin positively denies* that in the first stage of this softening process, it has been generally attended with incontestable marks of inflammation, such as redness of the softened part, tumefaction, and injection of the bottom and edges of the affection. Cases of this kind, worthy of credit, he reduces to four only, including two narrated in M. Lewis' memoir. In others, supposed to be of a similar nature, he is inclined to believe that the inflammation has merely been coincident, but not necessarily connected. If, however, the patient survive the first stage of softening, an inflammation is then developed over the solutions of continuity; and it becomes sometimes impossible to distinguish whether the softening has been primary or secondary. If primary, the edges are only very slightly injected and swollen, the softened matter is merely tinged with red, and there is a complete deficiency of pus, and of any thing like a pseudo-membranous formation.

M. Gendrin has further informed us, that in such instances of softening as are the effects of inflammation, the affected portion loses all traces of its primitive organization; its villi disappear, and the softened part is slightly elevated by its tumefaction. And being red, from the congestion of its capillaries, this colour decreases gradually to its boundaries, where the inflammation being less intense, there is an augmentation in density, instead of a decrease of it. In idiopathic or primary softening, on the contrary, the mucous membrane arrives gradually to such a pathological condition: it becomes successively thinner and thinner, paler and paler.

* Gend. vol. ii. p 575

Its blood vessels, not distended or injected from the beginning, are one after another effaced and collapsed, and it is only when the last stage is come, that one sees neither villi nor cryptæ.   There is, even when both are accomplished, a difference in their consistence· the idiopathic softening is mucous, diaphanous, and viscid, and approximates the condition of cellular substance in the fœtus, the inflammatory mollescence is friable and opaque.

M. Gendrin,* by way of commentary on this well drawn distinction, says, that it is found also to prevail in other tissues.   That, if the softening be idiopathic, they become mucous, ropy, gelatinous, and without trace of redness, injection of blood, or suppuration: but, if inflammatory, they are harder and more compact to the touch, notwithstanding the extreme facility with which they lacerate; and exhibit always an infiltration and injection of blood, blended more or less with pus.

Fungiform or Granulated Condition of the Mucous Tissues.

The mucous coat of the stomach and also that of the small and large intestine, is, from chronic inflammation, subject to a derangement, in some measure the reverse of mollescence.   To M. Louis, whose account of the latter disease is so satisfactory and good, are we indebted also for the first exact and systematic description, of the one that now occupies our attention.†

In this affection the mucous coat of the stomach loses its velvety arrangement on a surface of variable extent in different individuals; and, in place thereof, there appears one formed from rounded projections, each two or three lines in diameter.   These projections, are separated by superficial furrows, are somewhat varied in shape, and bear a resem-

---

* Gend vol. ii p 579
† Memoires Anat. Pathol 1826, p. 110

blance to granulations on the surface of a sore.   In addition
to these furrows, one sometimes meets with such as are longitudinal, a line or so wide, and an inch and a half long:
having the mucous membrane over them, not more than one
fourth the thickness of that which is contiguous.   Ulcerations not extending through the whole thickness of membranes so affected, are also another feature of this disease
very frequently, and they are from one to several lines in
diameter.

This disease most frequently occurs along the great curvature and the contiguous portions of the stomach, in the cul
de sac, the lesser curvature, and the pyloric extremity.   It
does not seem to be connected with any invariable size of
the organ; for it has been observed both where the latter was
of double volume, and where, by force of dieting, it was reduced to the diameter of the colon.

In this lesion the colour of the mucous membrane is altered from its natural tints, to a rose or red, and frequently
to a gray.   Its consistence is frequently somewhat impaired,
but the most striking feature is in its increased thickening,
which is at once obvious, when the disease is circumscribed.
For then an immediate contrast exists, between the depressed
sound, and the elevated morbid parts.   In a great number of
cases there is a want of mucus upon the sound parts, while
it is spread over the diseased, and when it exists upon the
former, it is less viscid and less abundant than it is upon the
latter.

I have as yet seen this malady in but one stomach: it had
the evidence of chronic or sub-inflammation from its universal induration and thickening.*   M. Louis also seems decidedly of opinion that it is one of the results of inflammation; being marked by redness and by ulceration.   Further-
more, when it affects the colon, the mucous membrane of the
latter is red and tumefied; and its surface granulated, and

* See Anatomical Museum

sometimes covered with a soft, pultaceous membrane of coagulating lymph.

M. Louis has never met with this disease except complicated with others, from which the patients died. Its peculiar
symptoms, therefore, have not been ascertained very satisfactorily.   Such as are known, are common to it with other
stomach complaints: they are anorexia, nausea, vomiting, and
occasional epigastric pain.   Commonly, however, its progress is so slow, that it remains latent till examination after
death.   No indications during life have been remarked in
connexion with it, which have not also existed where the mucous coat of the stomach was found unimpaired after death;
and in every respect healthy, in colour, consistence, thickness, and general appearance.

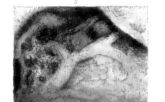

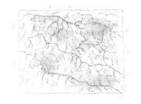

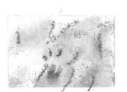

CHAPTER X.

ON THE HEALTHY AND DISEASED APPEARANCES OF THE GASTRO-INTESTINAL MUCOUS MEMBRANE.

The want of some standard, whereby the healthy and diseased appearances of the stomach and bowels may be distinguished, has been felt, perhaps, by all who have engaged in researches into the pathology of these organs. Though much has been written on the subject, yet the vagueness of the language used by authors, and more especially the great inaccuracy with which they employ the terms representing colours, have opened one of the most extensive fields for disputation, in pathology.

We owe much, however, to the labours of M. Billard,* in presenting this subject more in extenso, and in a more satisfactory manner than any of his predecessors. It has given me much pleasure to find, that the inferences to which I was led by my own observations, are generally confirmed by his, both in regard to the healthy, and to the pathological appearances of the gastro-intestinal mucous membrane.

In the numerous post mortem examinations which I have made, both for myself, and my professional friends, I have frequently found that the most opposite conclusions were drawn from identical appearances in the organs under consideration; and there existed no available experience or authority, by which the correctness of these conclusions could be tested, and the truth determined. These circumstances

* De La Membrane Muqueuse Gastro-Intestinale, Paris, 1825.

induced me to institute a series of observations on the gastro-intestinal mucous membrane, illustrated by drawings; and
by coincidences entirely accidental, I was so fortunate as to
obtain in a few months a description of information, that in
the ordinary current of events is not acquired in years.

Three unsettled questions present themselves in this inquiry:—1st. What is the healthy condition and appearance of
the gastro-intestinal mucous membrane? 2d. What is its appearance in congestion from the agonies of dying? 3d. What
is its appearance in genuine red inflammation?

It is necessary in the commencement of this discussion,
to settle the signification of the terms used. This I shall do,
not in an arbitrary manner, but according to the meaning
attached to them in conversation generally. The inferences
of conversation are unavoidably resorted to, because the de-
finitions of our dictionaries are very unsatisfactory; indeed
the terms are there used promiscuously. Thus, for example,
Parr says, that congestion is a swelling that gradually arises
and slowly ripens, in opposition to that defluxion which is
quickly formed, and terminated. In the Dictionnaire des
Sciences Medicales, congestion is defined to be a humoral
collection which is formed slowly in some part of the body,
increases gradually, and finishes by an intumescence of a
variable size. The fluids which form it may be blood, serosity, pus, fat, bile, urine, in one word, any of the fluids belonging to the body. It is thus evident that Parr alludes to
the sub-inflammation of modern pathology, and that the
other has no specific meaning. I now therefore state that
by Congestion, I mean an accumulation of red blood in any
part or organ of the body, without irritation or mechanical
violence; and by Red inflammation, the accumulation of
red blood which attends a local irritation.

1. *Of the Natural Colour of Mucous Membranes.*

When an animal is bled to death, the stomach being empty, the mucous membrane of the latter, and of the intestines, is of a yellowish pearl colour, presenting at a short distance the lightest possible tint of pink, and few or no marks of blood exist, even in the large vessels under the peritoneal coat.

Experiment 1*st, April,* 1827.—At a butchery in Spring Garden, a sheep, which had fasted for twenty-four hours, was slaughtered in the usual way, by cutting the throat, and immediately afterwards dividing the spinal-marrow in front between the occiput and first vertebra. As soon as life was extinguished, we examined the abdomen. The internal membrane of the stomach was of a pearl colour, slightly yellow, approaching to what artists call a light tint of bright brown, and the intestines were almost exactly like the stomach. Neither stomach nor intestines exhibited their blood vessels, even of the largest size, except very faintly, and there were no red patches in either.

Experiment 2*d.*—Was a repetition of the first experiment, and was followed by precisely similar results. These two experiments, or rather observations, were executed by Dr. La Roche and myself.

If an animal be killed with a full stomach by puncture of the medulla spinalis, at its commencement, the mucous coat of the stomach will retain on the surface, where the food was in contact with it, a light lake colour, approaching vermilion, from the detention of blood in its capillary system. The following experiments proved this:—

Experiment 3*d, June,* 1827, at the University.—A full grown female rabbit, of the white kind, was fed upon green cabbage leaves. In about three hours afterwards, she was killed with a saddler's awl, by a puncture of the medulla spinalis, between the occiput and the first vertebra. Immediately upon the introduction of the instrument, the body was seized with a spasm, the extremities were drawn together and convulsed; the animal gaped two or three times, but there was no inspiration. In five minutes after the puncture, the abdomen was opened, and the circulation found by pressure upon the veins, to be going on but languidly in the parietes of the abdomen, and in the abdominal viscera I waited five minutes more, when it seemed to be completely stopped.

I then cut out the stomach, laid it open along its great curvature, and washed away with a stream of water its contents, which presented the appearance of having been well boiled and bruised. The food would have measured probably about an ounce, and was principally in the left half of the stomach: though there was no hour glass contraction of the latter. The mucous coat of the left half of the stomach was of a uniform light lake, approaching vermilion, without blotches or shades of difference, and firm; but the mucous coat of the right half was almost destitute of vessels or injection, and had the dull pearl colour of the stomachs of the sheep bled to death. The mucous coat of the small intestines was the same colour as the stomach, but much lighter.

The vermicular motion continued for ten or fifteen minutes in the intestines, after the abdomen was opened. I observed that the same occurred in the horns and body of the uterus, quite as clearly as in the intestines; and that it could be produced at pleasure by puncture, by clipping, and by stirring. On the uterus being slit open from one end to the other, it flattened itself out, and the internal surface corrugated precisely as in the small intestine. The capillary system of the liver bled freely half an hour after death, upon being punctured with the scissors.

Experiment 4th.—A full grown female rabbit—Opened the abdomen, by a cut from sternum to pubes—intestines became very highly injected with blood, in a few minutes after being exposed.—Laid open the colon and irritated the

internal coat by rubbing—it took on a bright scarlet lake colour, approaching to vermilion;—on the external face of the
same intestine, an anastomosis was manifested resembling
a very fine honey-comb.   The stomach was laid open by a
section along its greater curvature, and the bouillie like contents, consisting of green vegetable matter, turned out.   The
internal coat of the stomach was highly suffused with blood,
and of a deep crimson lake colour.   The stomach bled very
profusely from the cut surface; in consequence of which, it
began to clear up, by its colour becoming less intense.   Applied some alcoholic solution of corrosive sublimate upon
one spot of the internal coat of the stomach, about ten minutes after the commencement of the experiment—it did
not seem to produce any impression, perhaps owing to the
hæmorrhage.   Killed the animal in twenty-five minutes after
commencement, by puncture of the medulla spinalis behind
occiput; then cut out the stomach.   The cardiac half was
of a light tint of lake colour, the pyloric half was of a yellow pearl colour.   The stomach after death, in this experiment, corresponded with experiment No. 3, in the colour
being uniform, not motley.   Peristaltic movements were observed again in the uterus and its cornua.   After puncturing,
gasping occurred, with the usual cessation of respiration.

Experiment 5th.—A full grown rabbit.   Punctured medulla spinalis, at commencement, respiration stopped immediately.   In five minutes opened abdomen, capillary circulation, as well as that in the larger vessels, brisk.   In twenty
minutes, capillaries of liver, spleen, and kidneys bled on being punctured with a saddler's awl—stomach and bowels
did not.   Cut open the stomach along its greater curvature,
and turned out its contents; then removed and washed it well
immediately.   The left half of a lake colour, approaching
vermilion, uniformly diffused as in experiments 3d and 4th,
(see Pl. 1. fig. 1,) the right half of a dull pearl, as in the
same experiments.   (See fig. 2.)

From the great number of blood vessels distributed through

16

mucous membranes, they are, during life, of a very bright red colour, on many of the viscera, as the stomach, the small intestines, the lower end of the large, on the vagina and nose; in many other parts they are much less vascular, as in the lining membrane of the sinuses of the nose, the mastoid cells, and in the excretory ducts generally. The nostril and the vagina, in a robust, healthy person, will probably be found to represent correctly the shade of colour which, in life, belongs naturally to the gastro-intestinal mucous coat. There is a very considerable vascularity of the mucous membrane of the bladder, as I have had an opportunity of ascertaining by injections, and in an infant where there was a congenital deficiency of the pubes and of the fore part of the bladder.

Observation 1*st. Living colour of the healthy Mucous Coat of Colon,* 1827.

There is now a female in the Surgical Ward of the Philadelphia Alms House, who suffered some time ago from prolapsus ani, which is said to have protruded about six inches: the protruded intestine sloughed off, as well as the sphincter ani and the adjoining integuments. This new state of the parts affords a distinct view of the internal coat of the colon, near the sigmoid flexure. The perineum has cicatrized and united to the end of the colon, but the surface is kept excoriated, by the continued excrementitious discharges; from the want of a sphincter. In this patient, the mucous coat is of the colour of the vagina, or of a recently blistered surface of the true skin.

Observation 2*d. Sudden death from ossification of coronary arteries, exhibiting natural colour of Gastro-Intestinal Mucous Membrane.*

July, 17, 1827. Mr. W. J. aged fifty-five, of remarkably temperate, regular habits: for some years previous to his death, was troubled with a shortness of breathing, upon ascending a flight of stairs.   His principal treatment was regularity and abstemiousness.   Last night about 10 o'clock, just before he went to bed, he took, as was not unusual, a glass of cream, which he always considered to agree remarkably well with him.   About 4 o'clock, A. M. he was seized with extreme difficulty of breathing, complained of most violent pain in his loins, said that he was dying, and in a short time expired.   From the commencement to its termination, this attack occupied twenty minutes, during which his senses remained unimpaired.   Dr. Edward Jenner Coxe was present; he found his pulse regular, but small.

At 4 o'clock this afternoon I examined him, assisted by Drs. Dewees and Coxe.

Exterior appearance.—Stature five feet seven inches, square, robust and well set, middle corpulence inclining to obesity.   Skin clear and fresh; features placid; some blueness about the neck from settling of blood; lips pale; pupils middling size; no putrefaction; sub-cutaneous veins bled on being cut.

Thorax.—Lungs perfectly healthy in their structure; soft, elastic; on being cut into, discharged a great deal of frothy mucus and serum.   Right lung adhering in its whole periphery by old adhesions of coagulable lymph.   The left pleura contained five ounces of straw-coloured serum, no remains of coagulable lymph to be seen about it; perhaps there might have been more serum which was removed by absorption after death, an idea advanced by Mascagni.   Vascularity of pleura not considerable; but I could not judge very satisfactorily on this point, from the difficulty of throwing the light in a proper manner upon it.

Heart larger than usual by one-third, covered with fat; only a few drops of synovia in pericardium.   Right cavities healthy and filled with fluid blood, had no coagula in them. Left side contained only a small quantity of fluid blood; left auricle healthy; moderate hypertrophy of the left ventricle:

semi-lunar valves undergoing the earthy degeneration so common in advanced life, with very small ossified points, here
and there, the aorta had also undergone, as far as the arteria
innominata, the degeneration preceding ossification. Sinuses
of Valsalva, twice or thrice as large as natural. Mitral valves
somewhat degenerated also.

Coronary arteries of the heart for two inches after their
origin, and also the branches leading from them, ossified into
rigid inelastic tubes, like the arteries of the extremities in
certain cases.

Cartilages of ribs perfectly ossified.

Abdomen.—Liver healthy.   Spleen, coats of, interspersed with white patches giving it a parti-coloured look;
healthy in other respects.

Stomach of middle size; contained two ounces of mucus,
some of which was loose; while the other formed a white
transparent coat adhering to the sides, but which could be
scraped off easily.   Rugæ of mucous coat elevated, but not
unusually so; whole internal surface of mucous coat on the
summits and sides of rugæ of a very light warm sienna, or
bright brown colour, which was produced by innumerable
microscopical points of red blood remaining in the capillaries.   In the depressions between the rugæ, the stomach of
a dull pearl colour.

The jejunum was of a deeper sienna, and of a more uniform tinge than the stomach; contained feculent matter, consisting of mucus, yellow bile, and cream, all reduced to a
homogeneous and digested mass.   Its lacteals were distended
with chyle, and were seen converging in their ramifications
to the mesenteric trunks, which were also filled.   The lacteals were not perceptible in the ileum.

The colon presented its mucous coat of a dull pearl colour, and contained soft healthy fæces adhering to its sides.

Peritoneum entirely and unexceptionably healthy.   Brain
not examined, as there had been no symptoms of apoplexy
or cerebral disease.

I never, on any occasion of my life, found the abdominal viscera in a state which seemed indicative of more perfect health, or more suitable as a standard of observation; the case I consider in this respect as invaluable.   See Pl. I fig. 3 and 4.

Observation 3d.—Gastro-intestinal Mucous Membrane perfectly healthy.

A man aged seventy, a resident of the Alms House, died suddenly, Sept. 19th, 1828, without previous illness or complaint; and, was examined about twenty-four hours after death.   No particular cause of death was found: the heart was enlarged, and there was some ossification about the valves.   Articles of food undigested were in his stomach, and the mucous coat of the latter, was about the colour of that of W. J. (Plate 1st fig. 3.)   His brain was universally softer, and more pulpy than common, with some congestion.

Observation 4th.—Death from Rupture of the Aorta. Gastro-intestinal Mucous Membrane perfectly healthy.

The subject of this was a criminal in the state Penitentiary on Walnut street, who had been committed for sixteen years, in consequence of robbing a milk cart, and violence done to its driver.   He was of middling stature and well made   For several months he had been complaining of uneasiness in the præcordial region, palpitation, an irregular bounding pulse, and some distress in his respiration.   July 26th, 1828, shortly after taking his dinner, which according to prison discipline, is 12 o'c. M.; he was found in the last agony in one of the corridors of the prison.   At 6 o'c. P.M. the same day, I examined him along with Dr. Bache, the physician of the institution.   It was sultry; the thermometer stood at about 85°.

Exterior Aspect.—General pallidness, no congestions of blood about face or neck: thorax, on percussion, yields a heavy fleshy sound along sternum and in the region of the heart.

Thorax.—On raising the sternum the pericardium was found enormously distended; occupying the whole length of the sternum, and protruding considerably into the left cavity of the thorax. Having slit it up in front, three gills or more of a straw-coloured serum escaped, and some ounces of a bloody serum were afterwards removed with a sponge. The examination progressing, we found a pint of recently coagulated blood, forming a thick layer all around the heart. The aggregate quantity of serum and blood amounted to about one quart, and compressed the heart.

There was no indication of inflammation of the pericardium. The heart was somewhat larger than common; and the left ventricle was dilated with hypertrophy of its parietes, and harder than usual. The right auricle contained an ounce of coagulated blood, and the right ventricle had also a little in it. The left auricle and ventricle were almost empty.

The aorta, from its root to the top of the curve, was in a state of aneurismal change, and dilated about half a diameter beyond the natural size. In its left side, just beyond the semi-lunar valves and in the aneurismal region, there was a small thin pouch the size of a pea, the summit of which pouch was ruptured into an orifice as large as a crow quill. This orifice emptied into the pericardium, and was the channel of the hæmorrhage. On the fore part of the root of the aorta, immediately at its valves, and showing itself to the right of the pulmonary artery, there was another aneurismal pouch, of a hemispherical shape and about an inch in diameter.

The lungs were of a deep blue and much congested. There were some slight old pleuritic adhesions on both sides. In the summit of the right lung there were two or three old tubercles, which were in a callous calcareous state, and surrounded by healthy pulmonary structure. The texture of the lungs generally, was in a state of perfect soundness.

Abdomen.—All its viscera perfectly healthy. The stomach presented a most satisfactory instance of that erythema, or vascular injection of the capillaries of its mucous
coat, which attends digestion.   It is to be observed that the
patient died in half an hour after a hearty meal, there
having been no previous disease of the stomach.   This
viscus was found with a quart of food in it, composed of soup,
bread, and potatoes, very much in the state in which they
had been swallowed.   The whole mucous coat of the stomach was of a crimson lake colour, more intense on the left
half, and subsiding gradually into a dull pearl, as it approached
the pyloric orifice.   The blood in the capillaries of the mucous coat which communicated this colour, was seen very
distinctly not to be in the slightest degree extravasated or
ecchymosed; but was confined to the vessels of the villi,
the number of which communicated the tinge: therefore,
where they were less abundant, the colour was less intense.
When examined in detail, the colour or tinge looked like
what might be communicated to a surface, by touching it in
innumerable places with the point of the finest cambric needle dipped in blood.   An almost exact representation of the
colour of this stomach may be seen in fig. 1st, and 2nd;
plate 1st.   The small intestines resemble fig. 4 of the same
plate, being of a sienna colour.

   There was no hour-glass contraction of the stomach, but
the right extremity was not dilated so much as it is upon
inflation after death; hence the food was contained principally in the left half.

   The head and spine were not examined, owing to the heat
of the day being so oppressive, and to darkness coming on.

   We have now ascertained the colour of a healthy gastro-
intestinal mucous coat, in death from hæmorrhage after fast-
ing; in death from puncture of the medulla spinalis with a full
stomach in life; in sudden death without the probability of
a diseased digestive apparatus, the stomach being empty;

and, finally, in sudden death shortly after the introduction of food into the stomach. We shall next endeavour to ascertain the colour in Congestion.

II. *Colour of Mucous Membranes from passive Congestion.*

The materials for elucidating the laws and phenomena of passive congestion, are exceedingly imperfect and scanty. According to one writer,[*] congestion is the effect of torpor of habit, connected with an abstraction of stimulus, and is for the most part local. It is seldom accompanied with febrile irritation till it acts as an extraneous stimulus. Febrile motions may sometimes be the product of congestions: congestions, depositions, or evacuations are uniformly the product of febrile motions; that is, of irregular action. Dr. Armstrong has also written, indeed diffusely, on what he calls the congestive typhus fever,[†] but the cases which he has given in illustration of his views, would seem rather to belong to diseases of irritation, than to passive congestion of the organs affected. He has also made some capital omissions in not giving us the laws of congestion; in not saying a word about the state of the mucous coat of the stomach and bowels; and in confining his attention almost exclusively to the liver, spleen, and brain.

The congestion of red blood in any part of the body, is commonly produced by an obstruction of one or more of the large venous trunks, which return the blood to the heart. A ligature on the arm for the purpose of bleeding has this effect; garters worn too tightly, or indeed any other articles of dress which interfere with the return of blood produce the same; lymphatic or aneurismal tumours situated near the junction of the extremities with the trunk of the body, also produce a congestion of blood in the parts beyond them, by

[*] Jackson on Fever, 1803, p. 197.

[†] Armstrong on Fever, p 68, 97.

pressing on the adjoining veins.   Position will do the same, as throwing the head downwards and forwards in certain individuals who are corpulent and have short necks.   Permitting a column of blood to remain too long on a part, sometimes has this effect, as in standing or walking, which in certain persons is followed by a great accumulation of blood in the legs and feet.   The general character, however, of all these cases of congestion is, that the congestion disappears the moment the cause that produced it, is removed.   It very rarely happens that the capillaries and the larger veins are more than simply distended under such circumstances, and they quickly contract to their healthy diameters.   It however occurs occasionally in pregnant women, near the term, to have some of the fine blood vessels of the legs ruptured, in which case there follows an extravasation of blood in small bluish spots about half an inch in diameter; and which, being true ecchymoses, present the same variations of colour, and are removed by the same process as the latter when caused by bleeding.

It is practicable to produce a congestion of the whole venous system, by obstructing the general circulation.   If such obstruction be continued till the death of the individual, the phenomena of congestion are exhibited in swollen face, bulging eyes, blue lips, tumefied and red tongue, with purple or red blotches on various parts of the surface of the body, but especially about the head, neck, and trunk.   The most usual causes of such obstructions to the general circulation, are asphyxia, from hanging, drowning, or irrespirable gases. The mucous membrane of the lungs wanting in this case the usual stimulus of atmospheric air, refuses passage to the blood from the ramifications of the pulmonary artery into those of the veins, and a complete arrest is thus put upon the general circulation.   The lung becomes the seat of a congestion or engorgement in its capillary system, and all the mucous membranes of the body suffer in the same way.

17

Bichat's experiments,* are quite conclusive on this point. He says that in an animal in whose trachea a stop-cock has been fixed, if you draw out a portion of intestine and split it open, then close the stop-cock; in four or five minutes afterwards, a dark brown colour will succeed to the red, which previously characterised the mucous surface of the gut; and the same change of colour will occur in a granulating surface under similar circumstances.

The lividity of the surface of the body, and of its mucous membranes, may be made to come and go at pleasure, by interrupting or restoring the freedom of respiration. The arrest of the capillary circulation is, however, not to be considered as a mechanical phenomenon, but a physiological one; for the animalization of the blood being somewhat affected or altered from the want of respiration, the sensibility of the capillary system is not properly excited by it, and therefore this system refuses to propel the blood. The blood in this respect may be compared to extraneous fluids, which, if they be injected into living blood vessels, are found not to run so minutely as they do some time after death, when the vessels get into a passive state.† Parallel phenomena are common, and are well exhibited in the actions and sensibilities of many parts of the body. For example, the trachea, which is so large, yet closes immediately against the introduction of fluids which are unfit for respiration, as proved by Goodwin's experiments. The urethra in a state of sexual excitement will transmit the semen, but not the urine; the lacteals readily absorb the nutritious part of the chyle, but refuse the remainder, notwithstanding the equal fluidity of both. A moment's reflection will satisfy us that such powers of discrimination are indispensable to the operations of the system, for without them, the several fine tubes of the human body, vascular, absorbent, and secretory, would be continu-

* Bichat, Anat. Gen. vol i. p. 188.   † Anat. Gen. vol. ii. p 25.

ally mixing their fluids in a manner inconsistent with life and its objects.

It is not improbable that several species of purpura, as the urticans, the senilis, and the hæmorrhagica, all of which seem to be an arrest of the red blood in patches in the true skin, or rete mucosum, have, in their pathology, a close connexion with the purple spots from asphyxia—that is to say, that there is a want of reciprocal sympathy between the red blood, and the capillaries of the part, and therefore it is arrested in its passage through the latter. These spots may be distinguished from a common ecchymosis, by their boundaries being well defined, and also by their deep, varying colour, which being sometimes lighter, and sometimes darker alternately, show that the blood forming them, though arrested, is yet under the influence of animalization. The colour alternating is, however, not an invariable feature of this disease. I have lately met with a case of purpura hæmorrhagica at the Alms House following an inflammation in the cellular substance on the front of the knee, and extending over the anterior semi-diameter of the leg from the knee to the foot; where there were no alternations of colour, and the disease disappeared like a common ecchymosis. I have subsequently seen it a prelude to mortification in the leg of a patient, Anthony Hartman, aged 25, in the same institution. The patch which it formed, surrounded almost the whole leg about its middle, in a band of five or six inches.

In the more common cases of congestion, as the accumulation of blood is removed immediately upon the cause being withdrawn; so the organ of the body, which has been the seat of it, is quickly restored to its usual functions, and the disturbance which they have experienced, readily disappears. If, however, the congestion be permitted to remain an undue length of time, the preponderance of the fluids will cause the congested part to inflame and even to mortify, as in strangulated hernia.

The following dissection of a patient, who died in the

Alms House, will serve to illustrate the state of the stomach and bowels in congestion from a slow process of asphyxia, and to fill up partially the very wide gap in this part of physiology and pathology.

Observation 5th.—Congestion of Gastro-intestinal Mucous Coat.

Wm. Thomson, æt. 37, admitted June 8th, 1827, with abscess around cricoid cartilage, died June 10th.

Previous History.—While in France, some years since, had secondary syphilis, and other constitutional affections,— was salivated for a length of time—recovered—came to this country; where he has continued since in the capacity of coachman. Has drank freely for some time. About four months since, had common catarrh, the result of which was some difficulty in deglutition and respiration, and tremor in the throat.

Symptoms.—When admitted, there was a flattened, immoveable tumour in front of the thyroid cartilage, about two inches in diameter, half an inch thick—inspiration difficult in the extreme, amounting almost to suffocation— expectoration purulent—deglutition exceedingly painful— countenance anxious and distorted.

The tumour was removed by the knife on the day of admission, at four o'clock, P. M. I found it lying on the whole front part of the thyroid cartilage, between it and the sterno-hyoid muscles. The wound was filled with lint, and then covered with a compress of the same, maintained by a roller: in ten or fifteen minutes afterwards, it began to bleed rather freely. I then removed the dressings, turned the clot of blood out of it, sponged, and not finding any bleeding vessel, I directed it to be left undressed, with a light cloth thrown over it. This answered to arrest the bleeding until midnight, when it again bled half a pint, and then stopped. The tumour was of the hard encephaloid kind.

having, however, a small purulent softening in front; it seemed as if it might have come from a lymphatic gland; but its flattened shape was adverse to this idea: neither had it a distinct capsule.

He spent the night but slightly relieved by the operation; pulse rather full and tense—expectoration and deglutition less painful and difficult: the former thick, white, purulent, and consistent.—Ordered venesection ℥viij. R. Tart. Ant. gr. ii.—Aq. puræ, ℥viij. M. A table spoonful every hour—took six doses, then stopped on account of nausea.

June 9th.—Respiration very laborious—expectoration as yesterday—will not consent to tracheotomy, which I now proposed to him.   On the tenth, died at ten o'clock, A. M.

Autopsy, six hours after death.   An entire removal of the tumour over the thyroid cartilage—its bed thickly covered with coagulating lymph—thyroid gland healthy—superior laryngeal nerves not affected.—No marks of capillary congestion on the surface of the body.—Lungs healthy in structure, some old pleuritic adhesions on left side—no particular congestion, save at their posterior part; perhaps less blood than natural found on cutting into them—miliary deposites of coagulating lymph on the surface of both lungs.

In Pericardium about ℥iij. of straw-coloured fluid.

Abdomen.—System of vena portarum, filled with blood; even in the fine intestinal branches, which were very conspicuous under peritoneum, so as to give a light purple colour to the whole of the small intestinal canal: in places it was interspersed with mahogany-coloured patches of two inches diameter.   Colon externally was of a white pearl colour, contracted to three-eighths of an inch in diameter, and contained natural, hard fæces.   There were no fæces in small intestines, only flatus.

Along the whole anterior margin of the liver, a little above its edge, there was a white, hard cicatrix of old condensed coagulating lymph; mixed at intervals with hepatic structure, by penetrating, at various places, from three to six lines into it.   This terminated near the right end of the great lobe, by a depression, as if an abscess had once existed there.   On cutting into the liver, near the cicatrix, many small miliary tubercles were found there; but they were not observed at more remote places.

Gall-bladder filled with healthy bile.

Spleen healthy, but completely surrounded by old adhe· sions.

Stomach, common size; of a pearl colour on peritoneal surface.   Internal or mucous coat covered with mucus, tinged with bile—corrugated—light pink colour, generally—summit of rugæ, from accumulation in capillaries, appeared like red streaks, at the distance of six feet, from being covered with minute dots of red of the size of a needle point.   No large patches of ecchymosis or red blotches, so conspicuous in inflammation.

Intestines.—Mucous coat covered with similar small dots or points of red.   Internal membrane of colon slightly tinged with red dots.   Besides the hardened fæces in the commencement of this viscus, there were some small pieces of it along its course.

Œsophagus natural; internal coat white pearl colour, and the venous ramuscules filled with blood; but the dots not conspicuous.

Throat.—Along the upper margin of the glottis, as formed by the doubling of its mucous membrane, from the tip of the arytenoid, to the side of the epiglottis cartilage, a tumour existed on each side, formed of serum and coagulable lymph, about the size of small nutmegs, so loose as to hang over the glottis, and to be drawn over the rima glottidis in every act of inspiration.   *These tumours produced his extreme difficulty of breathing, and final suffocation.*

Cricoid cartilage, at posterior part, both externally and internally, separated from its perichondrium; whose surface was in the condition of a fistulous sore.

Aryteno-cricoid articulation, detached by the extension

of the latter disease.   A sinus formed communicating between the fistula and the right ventricle of the larynx.   Posterior part of cricoid cartilage reduced to a thin edge above:
its diseased surface rough, and resembling a carious bone;
lining membrane of trachea and bronchia, natural.

Head.—Skull-cap bled freely when torn up.   Veins of
dura mater and pia mater much congested.   Tunica arachnoidea, raised up from pia mater, by a serous effusion in the
interstices, between convolutions.

Mass of cerebrum, congested with blood.

Ventricles contained $\tilde{3}$ss. serum.   Serum, on basis of
brain, under tunica arachnoidea: arteries of base, filled with
blood.   *Pons varolii*, congested.   Fourth ventricle contained serous effusions.   Texture of the cerebrum and cerebellum, natural.

To sum up what has been said, it appears then—

1st. That mere congestion is not an active condition of the
part affected.   When active, inflammation exists.

2d. That congestion most frequently is the result of mechanical impediment to the venous circulation.

3d. That the other cases in which it occurs, are where
there is a want of reciprocal sympathy between the blood
and the blood vessels in the capillary system; in consequence
of which, the latter refuses passage to the red blood.

III. *Of the red Inflammation of Mucous Membranes.*

Red inflammation has for its symptoms, heat, pain, redness, and swelling; all of which are very obvious when it
attacks a portion of the external surface of the body.   It
differs from congestion, in the latter causing an accumulation of blood in all the capillaries of an organ in which the
blood is arrested; while inflammation is most frequently limited to a single tissue, and exhibits redness in it alone, or
at least, principally; as, for example, in mucous coats during

their inflammation, in muscular during theirs, in peritoneal during theirs, &c. This, however, must depend upon the intensity of the inflammation also; for where it is very considerable, adjacent coats will be affected.

Congestion is regular in its progress, and begins without constitutional symptoms; whereas, inflammation begins with a chill, has exacerbations and remissions, and a course of augmentation, of stasis and of decline. They both may terminate by delitescence or a disappearance of the accumulated blood, or by resolution when particles of red blood are infiltrated; but inflammation also terminates in suppuration, in scirrhus, in hepatization, and softening of a part.

The traces of acute inflammation are in many cases very fugitive, and entirely disappear upon death; because the local irritation which attracted the blood and accumulated it, having ceased, the blood abandons that part and retires towards the centre of the circulation. We can seldom tell by the appearances twenty-four hours after death, the quantity of blood which has penetrated an inflamed membrane, as the peritoneum, the pleura, the cellular and mucous membrane, the skin, &c. The eruption of measles, and the redness of sore throat disappear on the death of the patient. We are not, however, to infer from these circumstances, that the mere afflux of the blood to a part constitutes inflammation: on the contrary, it is attended with a dilated condition of the vessels independent of this afflux; for if death occur during the height of measles, the eruptions may be made to reappear by injecting the vessels.

Bichat[*] has very properly observed, that in inflammation we should distinguish between acute and chronic affections, for, though the blood readily vanishes from the former, yet it will remain in the latter, because it has combined with the diseased organ. Hence, induration, suppuration, and vitiated secretions are satisfactory signs of inflammation of a part.

* Anat Gen vol. ii. p 22

The increased irritability of a part is the cause of its inflammation, and of the afflux of fluids to it.   Frequently
this increased irritability depends upon the sudden diminution of irritability in other parts of the body, by depressing applications.   Thus, cold suddenly applied to the surface, by depressing the irritability there, causes an accumulation of it with inflammation in some one of the internal
organs, as the lungs or bowels.   Undue stimulation of an
organ or part, will produce an augmentation of its irritability amounting to inflammation.   The natural increase of
irritability of organs at particular periods of life sometimes
mounts up to inflammation, as that of the uterus at puberty
manifested by menorrhagia, amenorrhœa, &c.—the extreme
tenderness of the breast at the beginning of lactation—the
tenderness of the testicles during a state of sexual excitement.

It is principally in the capillary system, that the phenomena of inflammation occur, and that the varying degrees
of organic sensibility determine corresponding movements
in the circulating fluids, accumulating them at one spot, and
expelling them from another.   Inflammation is therefore
exactly the inverse of what Boerhaave believed; for, according to him, the blood pushed from behind by the heart into
an organ caused its irritation or inflammation; whereas it is
the irritation which attracts the blood.

Irritation has all the gradations from the light, fugitive,
and varying blush of virgin diffidence, to that rapid and tumultuous afflux of fluids to an organ which, in a few hours,
produces its dissolution.   In slight irritations there is no fever; but when they are more intense, there is an increased
heat of the body, and an accelerated circulation throughout
it.   Fever in such cases is merely a general symptomatic
affection, arising from the sympathy which connects the
heart to all other parts; and has nothing of the specific affection in it, but merely manifests the grade of the irritation.
Thus, a fever from a syphilitic bubo is the same as a fever

18

from measles, from small-pox, or even from a mechanical injury.*

When the irritation of a part goes beyond certain bounds, the sensibility is exhausted, and death ensues.† The vital condition having abandoned the solids, the fluids get quickly into a state of putrefaction: this state is the gangrene of writers, and is well depicted in strangulation of an intestine, or in mortifications which frequently occur in the legs of drunkards. Bichat‡ goes so far as to say, that when the organic sensibility of the part begins to diminish, the blood which has been attracted by the inflammation may even then tend to putrefaction, but always the want of tone in the solid precedes it.

There are many proofs of inflammation being seated in the capillary system, and of the circulation of the latter being in some measure independent of the general circulation. 1. The partial erythemas of the skin. 2. In slight incisions or scratches, the skin will bleed very little at first; but as soon as the irritation has determined a flow of blood to the part, the hæmorrhage is sometimes troublesome, as in shaving. 3. The secondary bleeding from operations is sometimes very profuse from this cause. 4. Another, and a very strong proof of the power of the capillary circulation to go on without the impulsion from the heart, is that if a limb be made turgid with blood by the application of a tourniquet, as in common amputation; when it is cut off, though it be completely withdrawn from the influence of the heart, yet the capillaries empty themselves, and the limb becomes as pallid as under any other circumstances of death. Though I feel satisfied of the capillary circulation

* Bichat says (Anat. Gen vol. ii. p. 30,) he believes, that if one examined attentively, local affections and general fevers, he would find invariably the species of fever to correspond in its nature with the species of local affection This sentiment can scarcely be adopted by a proselyte to the modern doctrines of pathology

† Anat Gen vol ii p 29   ‡ Ibid.

being different from the circulation in larger vessels, in not depending wholly on the heart, yet it is to be understood that I do not withdraw it entirely from this agency, for there are many strong proofs of its subordinancy.   In the inflammation of transparent parts, for example, of the skin under the finger nail, where vascularity is very perceptible, every pulsation of the arteries of the upper extremity is attended for the moment by an increase of the vascularity of the part inflamed, and a deeper suffusion of it.

From the several observations now made, it is clear that the blood upon reaching the capillaries moves through them by their peculiar tone, and not exclusively by the action of the heart.   But, as many causes alter this tone or sensibility, causing it to increase or diminish, the motions of the blood in the capillaries will undergo corresponding varieties, and frequently become irregular.   A slight irritation will cause it to advance, to recede, to turn to the right or to the left.   By the experiments of Haller, Spallanzani, and of others, often repeated and entirely well attested, it appears that the blood under ordinary circumstances moves straight forward from the arteries into the veins; but upon the application of an irritant, its movement becomes irregular, and inclines in every variety of direction, backwards as well as forwards.   These movements of the globules of blood are very distinct in the transparent parts of animals having cold but red blood; they are seen with more difficulty in the warm-blooded, even in parts of the same transparency.   As Bichat remarks, it is hence easy to see that all the phenomena of inflammations, of eruptions, of tumours, &c., are founded especially upon this susceptibility of the blood in the capillary system, to be borne into an infinity of different directions, according to the places where it is called by the irritation.*

Fevers can only exist in animals who have a regular

* Anat. Gen. vol. ii. p. 39

round of circulation, whose fluids move in mass. In zoophytes and animals whose circulation is entirely capillary,
we only see such phenomena as belong to the capillary system, as tumours, adhesions, &c. Vegetables, for the same
reason, have only the diseases of the capillary system.[*]

The irregularities in the capillary circulation are always
partial; for if the blood move more slowly or go backwards
in one place, it will proceed more speedily in another, so as
to maintain the general circulation. If it were otherwise,
life must cease, for it would be incompatible with it for all
the capillary circulation to be arrested, or to go backwards
at once. Hence arises a law of organism always strongly
exemplified in disease, that if the vital forces augment their
energy at one place, they diminish it in another. There
appears indeed to be only a certain quantity allotted to each
individual; and though it may be accumulated at certain
points, so as to present a disproportionate sum in different
parts of the body, yet it never can be augmented or diminished in mass by disease. This principle is the foundation
of all correct physiology and pathology, and is in fact, a
matter of daily observation. We learn from this why it is
that general bleeding is frequently inefficient in local inflammation, for so long as local irritation continues, whereby blood
is attracted, (not driven) to a part, the mass of blood may be
diminished one quarter, and yet the inflammation will continue; whereas, in an animal having no irritated point in
his system, you may double the quantity of blood by trans-
fusion, and yet not produce local inflammation.[†]

Every operation of nature manifests an economical or exact application of means, to effect an object: there is nothing
superfluous. We therefore see that during the waking
state, the vital energies and the currents of blood, are principally directed towards the senses and organs of animal
life, or those of relation, as the muscles, &c., and that during

sleep, the vital energies are applied to molecular nutrition, and the repairs and general restoration of equilibrium in the system. Infants sleep more than adults for the reason that their molecular nutrition or growth is more imperiously required. Deprive any one of sleep, and he soon becomes haggard and emaciated. There is a continued alternation in each individual, in the actions of the system, and in the currents of blood, depending upon the waking, and upon the sleeping states; one set of organs requiring the blood more at one time, and another set at another. It is impossible for an undue excitation, and an undue rush of blood to occur upon all points of the body at one and the same time, or in other words, for there to be a general disease. A general disease or inflammation would be as little consistent with nature, as a general rise in the waters of the ocean, which we know to be always lowered at one place when they are raised by the wind or other causes iro another. Such an inference would be a solecism in pathology for the reason that disease implies a loss of equilibrium in the actions of the body, by one or more parts having an unnatural preponderance. The general actions of life may all be increased at the same time, as one increases the weights upon each end of a pair of scales, and yet preserves an equilibrium; but so soon as we take from one or add to the other, the equality is destroyed.

It is perhaps owing to molecular nutrition being stronger at night, that the symptoms of inflammation, (which at least in its milder forms bears some analogy,) are increased at this time.

The general augmentation or acceleration of the actions of the body in exercise, as running, jumping, and so on, differs from disease in this respect, that there is no concentration of irritability in any one organ, and a consequent afflux of blood; but, on the contrary, the equilibrium of the system is maintained, notwithstanding the apparent haste and momentum of its actions.

The causes which produce inflammation of the mucous coat of the stomach and bowels are numerous, and in many individuals there is an idiosyncrasy which inclines them to it, from very slight causes. Persons who are exposed to the changes of the atmosphere by sleeping out of doors, as in military life, present frequent examples of it; bad aliment or an excessive indulgence in what is good, also disposes to it. Poisons of all kinds may produce it, also moral affections, as melancholy, rage, &c. As my principal object, however, is to point out the anatomical characters which are left after death by gastro-enterites, I must confine myself to such remarks as are pertinent to them.

In acute inflammation of the mucous membrane of the stomach, when the patient dies in the early stage of the disease, the blood vessels which ramify through the stomach, are enlarged and distended with blood. The membrane itself is covered by a coat of mucus, which is sometimes limpid like the white of an egg, but on other occasions, thick and purulent, like that from the nose. The mucus adheres frequently very strongly to the stomach, and is now and then so tenacious and consistent from the admixture of coagulating lymph with it, as to resemble a false membrane. When the coat of mucus is scraped and washed away, the mucous membrane itself being brought into view, is found most frequently in the greater part of its extent of a deep red, approaching on some occasions, a crimson red, on others, a purple or black. These colours are owing to the injection of a prodigious number of capillary vessels in the mucous coat; and, in addition to them, we find the inflamed part of the stomach interspersed with bands and patches of red, of the colour of coagulated blood, being a species of ecchymosis, in which the blood has escaped beneath, and in the substance of the mucous membrane. The mucous membrane at these places is somewhat softer than natural, and sometimes appears swollen; may be readily detached from the cellular coat with the end of a scalpel, and is in the condition of a bouillie. In cutting through all the coats of the stomach, and looking at the incised edge, it will be seen that where the general and diffused redness exists, the colour is only superficial; but at the ecchymosed spots, not only the whole thickness of the mucous coat is concerned, but even the corresponding part of the muscular, is more highly coloured than in common. In some cases where the gastritis has been occasioned by caustics, there are eschars of the mucous membrane, some of which are detached and leave the muscular, or even the peritoneal coat, bare from the depth of the impression made. It is said that such eschars become more distinct some hours after the stomach has been exposed to the air. [*]

In some cases of acute inflammation, where the symptoms have been those of army dysentery, or of typhus fever, the stomach and bowels are occasionally found a little thicker than usual, and of a yellowish brown or red colour on their peritoneal surface, and in their thickness; the fœtor from them, on opening the abdomen, is much greater than usual, and the peculiar smell of the halitus from the peritoneum is overcome by it.

The hues of an inflamed mucous membrane, vary according to the period of the disease. Thus it is stated by Drs. Physick and Cathrall,[†] that the appearance of the inflammation of yellow fever is affected by the date of the affection. "In two persons who died of this disease on the fifth day, the villous membrane of the stomach, especially about its smaller end, was found highly inflamed, and this inflammation extended through the pylorus into the duodenum some way." The inflammation was exactly similar to that produced by arsenic.

"In another person, who died on the eighth day of the disease, several spots of extravasation were discovered between the membranes, particularly about the smaller end of the

---

[*] Dict. des Sc. Med T. 17
[†] Rush's Inquiries, vol iii. p. 172 Philadelphia, 1809.

stomach, the inflammation of which had considerably abated. Pus was seen in the beginning of the duodenum, and the villous membrane at this part was thickened."

"In two other persons, who died at a more advanced period of the disease, the stomach appeared spotted in many places with extravasations, and the inflammation disappeared." It and the intestines contained a black liquor so acrid as to produce inflammation and swelling on the operator's hands, which continued for some days.

"The stomach of those who died early in this disease was always contracted; but in those who died at a more advanced period, where extravasations appeared, it was distended with air." The external surface of the stomach was healthy, but from its veins being distended with blood they had a dark appearance.

In the dissections performed by Dr. Physick in the year 1798–99,* the inside of the stomach in some cases resembled the black vomit precisely in colour. In most of these cases no black matter was found in the cavity of the stomach, but the blackness depended upon this fluid being retained in the vessels of the inflamed mucous membrane. The doctor remarks that he never observed any putridity attending it, and that the colour was very distinguishable from the dark purple of gangrene. In some stomachs the blackness was universal; in others, in spots only; there being some spots in a state of high inflammation, and giving the inside of the stomach a chequered appearance. These spots, in one instance, resembled one another precisely in shape, and in all other respects, excepting colour, in which they differed, one being black and the other red.

Dr. Physick's opinion on these subjects was, that this black matter, commonly called the black vomit, from its being ejected by vomiting, was a secretion from the inflamed vessels of the stomach, and one of the most common modes by which violent inflammation of the stomach has a disposition to terminate. "For in some cases where the vomiting of black matter had been considerable in quantity, or continued for several days, the inflammation was found very faint indeed; and in some the inside of the stomach appeared as if covered over with a vast number of small glands, like mucous follicles, crowded together."[*]

When chronic inflammation has assailed the mucous coat of the stomach, this membrane is frequently found thrown into numerous folds. Sometimes it is thickened, of a denser texture than natural, and reddish, with irregular white patches. On other occasions, the whole of it is red, with purple spots, as in acute gastritis; sometimes the whole of it is of a purple, approaching to claret colour. When the disease has been produced by poisons of a force insufficient to cause immediate death, small ulcers are found near the pylorus, and along the greater curvature of the stomach.[†]

In some observations that I have made on the stomachs of intemperate persons at the Alms House, I have found the mucous coat thickened and dense, without any remarkable contraction of the stomach, yet thrown into numerous, thick, elevated rugæ, and the summits of those rugæ, so reddened by numerous capillary vessels injected with blood, that at the distance of a few feet they appeared, when the distinction of the individual capillaries was lost in the distance, like red streaks. This, which is probably one of the pathognomonic signs of a recent debauch in an old drunkard, is frequently mistaken for congestion, from an arrest of blood in the agonies of dissolution.

The red blotches, which form the leading anatomical character of acute mucous inflammation in malignant fevers, may be readily produced by chemical irritants.

* Medical Repository, New York, vol. v. p. 129
† Dict. des Sc. Med. T. 17, page 379

Experiment 6th.—A full-grown white rabbit, fed three hours before on cabbage leaves, was fixed in a frame, and the abdomen opened, by a cut from the sternum to the pubes. The stomach was drawn out; it was found filled with the food, (which exhibited the appearance of having been boiled,) and had an hour-glass contraction in its middle, separating it into two sacs with a small orifice between them.   The stomach was opened all along its greater curvature, and the food turned out; the whole mucous coat was of a scarlet-lake colour.   This colour became deep crimson-lake, and the stomach more suffused with blood on wiping or rubbing the mucous coat with the hand.   To one part I applied the glass stopper of a bottle, wet with a saturated solution of corrosive sublimate in sp. vin. rect. which had the effect in three or four minutes of deepening the colour of that part still more.

The colon was in greater part filled with soft fæces. The small intestines, on being cut into, exhibited the mucous coat of a light-lake, approaching vermilion, which colour remained after death.

In this experiment, an ounce and a half of blood was lost from the cut vessels.   I had proceeded to open the trachea, and had fixed a pipe into it for the purpose of trying the effect upon the blood, of shutting off the air from the lungs, when the animal died after a faint struggle.

In five minutes after, the stomach was cut out, and put under a stream of water to wash it well.   The lake colour still remained in the whole mucous coat from the residence of red blood in the capillary system.   At the place where the corrosive sublimate was applied, *there were irregular, oblong, red blotches of two or three lines broad.* The mucous coat had indeed this variety of hue in other places also, but not so deep. In one part, there was a line of petechial spots, half an inch or three quarters in length, from half a line to a line in diameter, each resembling in colour the red blotches.

Observation 6th.—Acute Gastritis and Peritonitis.

Harriet Derrickson, an African, aged twenty-six years, was received near the term of pregnancy into the Alms House, July 13th, 1827, after a recent confinement in prison. On the preceding day she had got wet, which produced a pain in the right hypochondrium—she was relieved by immediate bleeding.

July 13th.—Her pulse was rapid and febrile, and skin rather above natural heat; but the symptoms were generally mild, and not alarming. She was ordered a dose of Epsom salts, and barley water for common drink.

July 14th.—Eye slightly sallow, tongue inclined to dryness, with dark fur at base, costiveness, skin of common temperature and moist, pulse rather tense and rapid. In the afternoon there was a violent pain over the whole head, which was rendered still more severe upon her stooping. Vertigo; thirst, lost of appetite; pains in the limbs. A dose of Seidlitz powders, and cold applications to her head were prescribed.

July 15th.—Tongue unchanged, thirsty still, skin hot, violent pain in the right side, eyes yellow, breathing hurried, pulse rapid, not strong. Treatment continued, with the addition of cups to the right hypochondrium.

July 16th.—She miscarried of a dead child to-day, at 6 A. M. with the loss of very little blood, but her strength was almost exhausted. Her skin continued hot and dry, her tongue dry; stupidity. The symptoms continued to increase during the day; twenty leeches were applied to the temples, and forty to the epigastrium. At 4 P.M. a saline mixture which she had taken in the morning, brought away some natural evacuations, but the skin continued excessively hot, the pulse rapid, without tension, and compressible; the tongue still furred with red apex and edges, the sense of pain in the head had diminished much, but there was great tenderness of the epigastric and hypochondriac regions. A blister was applied to her side, sinapisms to her ankles, and fifteen drops of spirit of turpentine were directed every hour.

July 17*th.*—Almost entire insensibility, eyes of a golden colour, pulse very feeble, soreness of flesh, restlessness and moaning, spirit of turpentine increased in the afternoon to ʒij. every hour.   She died at 6½ P. M.

This case was not treated by myself—the notes of it so far, were communicated by Dr. Ashmead.

Autopsy, eighteen hours after death, by Drs. Hodge, Ashmead, and myself.   We found the internal face of the uterus lined with red blood, which had blended with its ragged surface; clots of blood were in the uterine orifices of the uterine veins, and could be readily picked out.   There had been no undue hæmorrhage or lochial discharge.   The capillaries of the peritoneum, especially at the lower part of the abdomen, were distended with blood, and produced, here and there, rose-coloured patches.   The peritoneal covering of the uterus seemed to have exceeded other parts in the intenseness of its disease, and had beneath it several patches of from six to twelve lines each of ecchymosed blood.

The stomach presented a degree of inflammation, over its whole mucous coat, not often surpassed even in yellow fever.   Some inches square of its middle were almost in a state of sphacelation from the congestion and extravasation of red blood.   Small clots of black blood were found among the contents of the stomach, but there was no black vomit. (See Pl. I. fig. 5.)

The following case, with the appropriate drawing will serve to illustrate the appearance of the mucous membrane of the stomach, after an inflammation of two or three weeks.

Observation 7*th.*—*Chronic Gastritis.*

Women's Surgical Ward, Alms House.—Mary M'Graw, aged 28, moderately corpulent, common stature, lymphatic temperament, habits of intemperance, was admitted May 10th, 1827, for a fracture of the neck of the acromion scapulæ, destruction of the acromio-clavicular articulation, and an extensive laceration and injury to the shoulder joint, manifested by the extreme facility with which it could be thrown out of place and restored again. The account she gave was, that two years ago she fell into a ditch, upon which occasion she produced the injury mentioned, and also broke the os humeri about the lower end of the bicipital groove. The os humeri was cured of its fracture, by the attention of a surgeon, but the shoulder remained in the state described. She afterwards continued to do her ordinary work, till last January, when she began to suffer violent pain in the affected shoulder, and subsequently lost the use of her arm.

Without very sanguine hopes of the success of the treatment, I yet determined, as there was not much probability of the individual being made more helpless by the operation, to try the effects of a seton in producing a reunion of the broken acromion and of the acromio-clavicular articulation. The patient agreed to the proposal, and May 29th was fixed for its execution; but owing to her being feverish and unwell on that day, it was postponed to the next prescribing day.

June 1st.—The patient seeming sufficiently well, I passed a seton through the acromio-clavicular articulation, and another through the fractured neck of the acromion. The patient being exposed in returning through the yard to her ward, was seized directly afterwards with a chill, which lasted half an hour, and was succeeded by fever. The same night, or the succeeding, was attended with a storm of wind and rain. An unruly patient, in the same ward, threw up the window at the head of M'Graw's bed, while she was asleep, and left it open.

June 2d.—Chill at 10 A. M. followed by fever, headache, bad taste. Venesection $\tilde{3}$vii. R. Sulph. Magnes. $\tilde{3}$ss.—Carb. Magnes. $\mathfrak{Z}$ss. M. Ft. Haustus.

June 3d.—Renewal of symptoms of preceding day. Seidlitz powder, R. Sal. nit. ℥ij., ant. tart. gr. i., aq. ℥viii. A table spoonful every hour during fever. This mixture was discontinued after a few doses, from its producing too much nausea.

June 4th.—Pain in the epigastrium. Skin cool, pulse natural, tongue slightly furred, bad taste, restlessness. Shoulder manifests inflammation, and discharges pus from the setons. Desault's bandage applied. The symptoms continue with but little variety till the 10th. A mild febrifuge treatment was followed.

June 10th.—Pulse full, head-ache, face flushed, bilious vomiting, great tenderness in epigastrium—forty leeches to epigastrium—sodaic powder.

June 12th.—Tenderness of epigastrium diminished much, but vomiting continues at intervals. Skin cold and clammy, countenance distressed, bowels too loose. No sleep last night. Large discharge from shoulder. Lime water and milk. Cretaceous mixture.

June 14th.—Skin hot and dry. Tongue dry and furred. Stomach still out of order. Some tenderness in epigastrium. Blister to epigastrium. Ptisan of sal. nitri.

June 15th.—Stomach still irritable, tongue brown, alvine evacuations green. Tenderness in epigastrium. Fifteen leeches to epigastric region. Calomel half a grain every two hours.

June 16th.—Symptoms the same. Discontinue calomel. Saline mixture.

June 18th.—Severe chill, which lasted several hours, skin cold and clammy, frothing at mouth, extremities cold, countenance cadaverous. Hot bricks to feet and trunk. Hot lemonade.

June 19th.—Sinking still. Skin polished, pulse small and feeble, tongue dry and brown, extremities cold, especially the arms. Extreme pain in epigastrium on pressure; alvine discharges sometimes green and sometimes yellow.

Blister to abdomen. Volatile julep $\bar{3}$ss. every two hours. Wine panada. Garlic poultice to soles of feet.

June 20th.—Symptoms continue. Treatment continued.

June 21st.—Died.

Autopsy.—Abdomen. The peritoneal surface of this cavity and of its viscera, universally of a clear white pearl colour, and destitute of adhesion.

Stomach. Moderately distended with flatus, and contained the last articles of medicine and of nourishment. Its mucous coat for the most part of a white colour, and destitute of injected vessels; yet in the cardiac half, particularly the cul de sac, many of the large veins were occupied with blood, and led to blotches of blood now almost removed, but which were yet sufficiently obvious when the part was held between the eye and a window. Mucous coat in left half so softened that it could be readily scraped away with the finger.

Intestines healthy, light coloured, and diaphanous, excepting the duodenum, the internal coat of which was much injected, hardened, thickened, and with much less appearance of valvulæ conniventes than usual.

Liver of a brownish yellow colour, as in intemperate persons, somewhat indurated, and had on its upper surface a hydatid the size of a nutmeg.

Spleen natural, but larger than usual.

Pancreas white, and much indurated.

Uterus and its appendages, healthy.

The shoulder joint had been completely ruined by the original accident, its capsular ligament being torn up all around, and scarce a vestige of it left. The long head of biceps broken, insertion of supra spinatus detached, and head of bone next to deltoides could be thrown about in any direction. The articular cartilages of both bones had been absorbed, and the head of the humerus flattened. A new cavity on the posterior edge of the old glenoid had begun to be formed.

Acromion broken at neck—acromio-clavicular articulation destroyed; either the end of the clavicle, or an ossified inter-articular cartilage was in the place of the latter joint.

The seton in passing through the acromio-clavicular articulation, had been introduced into the cavity made by the lacerated state of the capsule of the shoulder joint.

This case, in which there was unequivocally marked gastric irritation, proves, that when an acute inflammation of the stomach has persisted for some days, though it terminates in death, no very great redness of the internal membrane may be manifest, and consequently that it is impossible to estimate the state of irritation of an organ during life, solely by the quantity of blood left in it after death. Dying seems to have the effect of concentrating more and more towards the heart, the vital powers, and the fluids, or in other words, withdrawing them from the circumference to the centre; in the same way that a prudent general, on finding his outposts too much extended for the size of his army, will contract them more and more, as his force diminishes by battle and disease. See Pl. I. fig. 6.

The highest grades of irritation are not always attended by pain nor vomiting. The state of inflammation is so exalted, that its effects approximate those of the most deleterious poisons which cause sudden death without local pain, fever, or any very sensible derangement of the functions, except mere weakness and a sense of illness. The following instance will illustrate this:—

Observation 8th.—Acute Gastritis.

Henry Turner, a black man, aged fifty-five, assistant in the apothecaries' shop, at the Alms House, after an apparently slight indisposition of a few days, which seemed to require rest rather than any thing else, while sitting up in his bed, suddenly expired almost without a struggle, May 4th,

1827. On dissection, twenty-four hours afterwards, the stomach was found of middle size, thick and dense, its mucous coat thrown into numerous, well-marked, elevated rugæ, and almost universally of a deep arterial red. The red globules of blood were extravasated in numerous spots and blotches in the thickness of the mucous coat, and along the summits of the rugæ. I declared unhesitatingly that the disease was an exasperated inflammation of the stomach; but owing to the want of an assignable cause for it, as well as the want of appropriate symptoms during life, the opinion was not very readily acquiesced in. In a few days afterwards it was ascertained through Mr. Marks, the apothecary at the Alms House, that Turner had been taking private draughts from a bottle of Hoffman's Anodyne; at least, the quantity missing, could be accounted for in no other way.

Observation 9th.—Chronic Peritonitis and Gastro-enteritis.

Alms House, July 26th, 1827. Examination twelve hours after death.

John Neaman, aged seventy-seven, has been for two years a resident of this house. For the last nine weeks he suffered want of appetite, a sense of fulness over the abdomen, and pain in that region, but not so severe as to make him complain, or disquiet him much. Has had no diarrhœa, no vomiting, and no fever which called the attention of persons around. Eight days ago the little food which he was in the habit of taking, produced such a sense of fulness and distress that he determined to take no more, or at least the smallest possible quantity: since then he has taken a little bread, and now and then a spoonful of milk. His complaints being obscure, there has been no medical

20

treatment within those eight days, and scarcely any before. At a distant time, which is not precisely remembered, some tincture of bark was administered by one of the young men of the house. He died seemingly from exhaustion.

Exterior habit. Skin pallid as usual after death. Marasmus not exceeding that common at his time of life.

Abdomen. Peritoneum rough, with universal small miliary bodies, resembling tubercles; thickened somewhat by a coating of coagulating lymph, continuous with the tubercles. Peritoneum, on abdominal muscles, and also on diaphragm, interspersed with patches of red blood; small coagula of blood adhering to its interior in many places—and abundant points of the same, as if from ruptured vessels; its cavity contained about three quarts of fluid, half serum and half blood, blended; with coagula of blood floating in this mixture Mesentery studded at distant intervals with these small points of blood.

Stomach. Exterior or peritoneal aspect, pallid and healthy. Internal condition; contained no food, but a little mucus tinged with bile; cardiac termination of mucous coat of œsophagus of a deep red, from distinctly injected vessels; the whole mucous coat interspersed at somewhat distant intervals with small black spots of extravasated blood, from half a line to one line in diameter. For three inches around the pyloric orifice, these spots were more abundant and larger.

Small intestine. Mucous coat healthy, but the peritoneal coat of the colour of lamp-black in many parts, and more or less of a sooty hue in its whole length.

Large intestine. Exterior or peritoneal face, healthy, but dull from the disorganization beneath it. Mucous coat covered with black patches of blood extravasated in its thickness and beneath it; it resembled very much the spotted appearance of some of the sea shells, and contained a small quantity of hardened fæces. Small miliary bodies, like those on the peritoneum, abounded in it; but I could not distinguish whether they were mucous glands, or such tubercles as existed on the peritoneum

Liver. Small and flabby.

Spleen. Natural.

Thorax. Lungs healthy, a slight manifestation at very distant intervals on the pleura, of the same sort of action that prevailed in peritoneum—but no effusion, except of serum in a small quantity, which might have occurred after death.

Head not examined.   See Pl 1st, figs. 7, 8, 9.

The following are examples that redness is not found invariably in those exalted irritations of the stomach producing immediate death.

Observation 10th, Jan. 28th, 1827.—*Gastric Irritation.*

The daughter, aged eight months, of Mrs. A. D. without previous indisposition, and while playing in apparently excellent health on the lap of her aunt, was taken with a sudden spasm, and died instantly.   This occurred after a hearty draught of cow's milk, on which the child was accustomed to feed.

The day following I made an examination, twenty-four hours after death, with Dr. James, the family physician, and the following appearances were presented:—

Head. The flat bones much tinged with congested blood. The veins of the pia mater turgid.   Serum under tunica arachnoidea; a drachm of serum in the right ventricle of the brain.

Thorax. Every thing natural.

Abdomen. About one gill of a cheese-like coagulum of milk in the stomach.   The serous part had been continually running out of the mouth and nostrils since the death of the child, so as to require the constant use of cloths to soak it up; the quantity, therefore, could not be rigidly estimated, but probably did not fall short of two gills. *The mucous coat of the stomach was not vascular, but of a pearl colour.*

All the mesenteric glands were very much enlarged, but had nothing of a scrofulous consistence or texture

The child, owing to the ill-health of the mother, had been weaned at the age of one month, and brought up on cow's milk. That the coagulum formed from the latter was indigestible perhaps from the quantity, is proved by the fact, that pieces of it tinged slightly with bile, were found in the lower part of the jejunum. It is pretty clear in this case, that the undue quantity of coagulum in the stomach was the cause of death.

Observation 11th, March 29th, 1826.—*Gastric Irritation.*

Yesterday the infant daughter, aged ten months, of Mr. W. H. was seized, in a short time after eating half a table-spoonful of rice pudding, with convulsions. The insensibility was complete, and the spasm universal; respiration was carried on with the greatest difficulty, irregularity, and interruption. This was at half past four o'clock, P. M. Happening to pass the house, almost at that instant, my assistance was requested; in a few minutes, Drs. Hodge and Griffith arrived.

A warm bath was immediately resorted to. Three grains of tartar emetic were dissolved in a wine-glassful of water, and administered by the tea-spoonful, every five or ten minutes. The attempt to raise a vein in the arm being ineffectual, I opened on the right side of the head, three superficial veins, and on the left side two, along with a branch of the temporal artery. From these several openings, about three and a half ounces of blood were drawn. About three-fourths of an hour were thus consumed, when the convulsions ceased. As the infant was teething, the gums were then cut with a lancet.

The child was an unusually fine one; had to the moment of illness enjoyed most excellent health, and had, indeed, been out on a visit to its friends that very morning. The indication seemed, therefore, sufficiently marked, that the rice pudding, along with a prune which had been eaten in the morning, was the cause of the convulsions; and that these matters, if possible, should be expelled from the sto-mach.

As, notwithstanding the cessation of the convulsions, the insensibility and difficult respiration still remained with-out much mitigation, about twenty-five grains of pulv. ipe-cac. in three tea-spoonfuls of brandy, were administered in divided doses, at small intervals of time. This not pro-ducing the desired effect, a tea-spoonful of powdered mus-tard was given by portions; which also failing, twelve grains of sulphate of zinc were next given in divisions. This also failing, we next resorted to tickling the fauces with the finger, and to the introduction of a feather down the œsophagus, almost to the cardiac orifice of the stomach, some five or six times: still there was no vomiting induced. These several trials occupied until eight P. M., when the child revived very much, and was able to sit up.

It should also be mentioned that sinapisms had been, during our efforts, applied to the soles of the feet and to the epigastrium; and that two or three injections of spirit of turpentine had been administered, with the effect of purging as often.

About ten o'clock, P. M. the infant seemed to recognise persons, smiled on being addressed in a soothing, playful manner, and afforded a prospect of recovery. At half past twelve o'clock at night, after a slight convulsion, it died.

Autopsy, seventeen hours after death, the weather being moderate, and no putrefaction.

Head. Vessels of pia mater so congested with blood as to be almost apoplectic. Brain congested also.

Abdomen. Stomach flaccid and of the middle size; contained the rice pudding undigested, with a small part of the skin of a prune; its mucous membrane of a light pink colour. The mesenteric glands were enlarged and numerous: the child had been fed occasionally on cow's milk.

Dr. Physick informed me that he had saved a child, affected in a similar way, from eating a piece of pear. During the prevalence of the convulsions, the child not being able to swallow, a large quantity of tart. emetic and ipecacuanha was injected, by a syringe, into the stomach, through a catheter introduced down the throat; the piece of pear was thrown up by vomiting, and the child saved. He also told me that a Mr. L. once lay in a stupor for several hours, from swallowing some article of food extremely difficult to digest. He also was relieved by its expulsion.

Observation 12th.—*Mollescence of the Stomach.*

In the summer of 1825, I dissected, for Dr. Otto, an infant child, (about two years old,) of Mrs S. S who was unwell for a week, without there being any well marked symptoms of the nature of its disease. I found the left extremity of the stomach disorganized in all its coats; having been reduced to a light mahogany coloured and pulpy state, about the consistence of a piece of glue soaked in cold water for twenty-four hours. Having no suspicion, at the moment, of such a state of the organ, I lacerated it, inadvertently, while only using a common force in drawing it upwards for examination. There was no undue redness in the mucous coat.

The brain of this child was large and somewhat congested, but not to a remarkable degree.

Observation 13th.—*Mollescence of the Stomach.*

Dr. La R. of this city,' lost a child, in 1826, about four weeks old, in whom I found the stomach in a similar state of dissolution or softening. There had been, however, much pain in his infant, and flatulent tension of the abdomen.

Observation 14th, Mollescence of Stomach, Jan. 5th, 1829.

Charles C., aged three years and four months, a well-grown, florid, and healthy child, began seven weeks ago to show marks of indisposition, by a loss of complexion and flesh, a disposition to inaction, and some fœtor of his breath. These symptoms, with but little alteration, went on till I was called in, Dec. 26th, 1828. The treatment, in the mean time, had been with such remedies as the family thought well of, who considered the affection to be worms. Two bottles of Swaim's Vermifuge were among the articles given.

December 26.—When I first saw the infant, the symptoms were a wax-like, cadaverous complexion, inaction and langour; appetite good, abdomen somewhat tumid, bowels regular, pulse voluminous and frequent. No signs of cerebral or pectoral affection. Prescribed bark tea, made of Cort. Peruv. ℥i. Aquæ pur. 1lb., to be taken often during the day: vegetable diet; salt bath.

This treatment was continued for two days with but little or no advantage. In this time he lost his appetite, and was seized with flying pains in the limbs and different parts of the body, which we supposed to be rheumatic.

December 29th.—He was purged with calomel and rheubarb.

December 30th.—Nitre ℨi. ant. tart. gr. i. aq. ℥viii. A dessert spoonful every two hours

December 31.—Do. do. A dose of Sulphate of magnesia.

January 1st.—Do. do A fomentation in a blanket was directed, which relieved the pain in the limbs, &c.

January 2d.—Took at night Dover's powder, which produced some sleep.

January 3*d.*—Seized with symptoms of congested or pe-ripneumonic lung, manifested by high, laborious breathing; the pulse being full and frequent, with occasional cough. This continued till January 4th, when he died at 1 P. M.

Autopsy twenty-seven hours after death:—weather very cold.　Present Dr Randolph.

Exterior aspect.　No putrefaction—colour like bleached wax universally.

Abdomen.　Peritoneum healthy.

Mesenteric glands somewhat enlarged.

Liver somewhat enlarged, and of a healthy colour.

Spleen healthy.

Stomach.　Contained about one pint of gas, and some mu-cus with articles, as gum water, swallowed not long before death.　The mucous membrane of the left half was of the colour of lamp oil, and reduced in consistence to that of a cold, thick jelly.　For a space next the spleen of two inches in diameter, the mollescence of all the coats was so complete that they tore through in lifting up the stomach for exami-nation; and, upon further trial, they seemed to present col-lectively about the consistence of cold calf's-foot jelly—not admitting of any handling, from their being so completely altered.　Contained a lumbricus worm six inches long, and dead.

The small intestines seemed generally healthy, the duode-num was stained with bile, the gall bladder being turgid with it.

Large Intestine.—Mucous coat in left half of a very light slate colour, in right half the mucous follicles were nume-rous and very perceptible, and were black like the follicles on the face and nose when they collect dirt.　The parietes of the ascending colon were thin.　Two years ago he had cholera infantum.

The kidneys were very hard and almost white.　He had a fashion of pulling at the prepuce, and had some uneasiness occasionally in passing his urine.　I found a red calculous deposite in the urine the day before his death. The bladder was healthy, with the exception of some few spots of ecchymosed blood, in its mucous membrane.

Thorax —Heart large   The right auricle and ventricle filled and distended by a polypous concretion entirely destitute of red blood.   A similar concretion was in the left auricle, but not so much of it; and also a little in the left ventricle. These concretions were traced for a considerable distance into the vascular trunks, adjoining the cavities, respectively. There was not even enough red blood in the heart, to stain the surface of the fibrinous concretions; indeed, there seemed an almost universal destitution of red globules.

Were not these concretions forming for several days before death, for the heart was evidently much distended by them, indeed almost blocked up?

There was a peripneumonic congestion of blood in the posterior half of each lung, especially the inferior lobe, marked by the solidity and want of elasticity of the lung; and also slightly by the colour, but less so than usual from the defect of red globules in the blood.

The head and spine were not examined.

These observations upon the stomachs of children, illustrate sufficiently the fact, that the most extreme irritations of the stomach may exist during life, and may even be fatal, but yet not be manifested after death, by unusual redness of the tissues affected.   It would be indeed unphilosophical, and inconsistent with pathological observations on other parts; to expect from the stomach an invariable manifestation of disease, by redness and injection of its mucous surface after death.   Let the redness of the skin in erysipelas be ever so strong during life, it frequently disappears wholly, by the retreat of the blood from the capillaries upon death. Measles are similar in this respect, and the fact already mentioned is very worthy of attention, that if a fine injection be thrown into a subject who has died at the height of the eruption, the vessels originally dilated by the irritation, manifest themselves by the greater quantity of injecting matter they receive; or, in other words, the eruption may be renewed after death, as I have satisfactorily ascertained by experiment.   If any conjecture can be hazarded on these points, we are disposed to believe that during the process of death, the vitality of parts in a state of inflammation is frequently so far diminished, that they no longer have the power of attracting the fluids in undue quantity to them; consequently, their redness disappears.

Acute inflammation of mucous tissues generally only thickens inconsiderably, the part affected. It is attended by an increased secretion of mucus, of serum, of fibrino-mucous matter, and even an exhalation of red blood, from the blood vessels being so extremely superficial. We see continually these phenomena going on in inflammation of the Schneiderian membrane and in colitis.

It has been seen that if an acute inflammation of the gastro-intestinal mucous membrane does not kill in its early stages, the injection with red blood is frequently by no means so great as it would have been in the case of an earlier death, and the changes which I have generally observed are as follow·—The stomach and bowels assume a dirty yellow, or liquorice colour; the stomach presents, internally, small blotches of red at intervals, and frequently small filaments of coagulated blood are found adhering to the mucous coat of the stomach, seemingly at the orifices of the vessels from which they were discharged. The veins of the bowels are either partially or generally filled with blood. The intestinal mucus is abundant, adheres closely, and is tinged yellow by the bile. The mucous membrane of the stomach is easily peeled or scraped off by the finger nail. The brain in this state most frequently exhibits marks of congestion, and with some inflammation of its meninges. The eyes and skin are yellow. In the skin there are not unfrequently blotches of red blood, resembling purpura.

Yellow Fever.—In my notes of dissections, performed on four yellow fever patients, in the year 1820, I find the following remarks. In a female patient, aged forty, whose period of the disease I did not learn; the stomach contained a gill of black vomit, was of a natural thickness and texture, and presented over its whole mucous coat in different regions, patches or blotches of extravasated blood. In a seaman belonging to the brig Martha, who had been sick at least nine or ten days, the stomach also contained black vomit, and was beset with small red points, and spots of ecchymosed blood. In a third patient, a man aged forty, who complained slightly in the morning of one day, and was dead the next at seven o'clock, A. M., I found the stomach extensively ecchymosed in its mucous coat, and its veins distended with blood; the black vomit was in great abundance in the stomach and intestines   In the fourth patient, a girl aged fourteen, who died on the fourth day of the disease, the mucous coat of the stomach and small intestine did not present the appearance of ecchymosis, but merely a minute arborescence of its veins.

Observation 15th.—Acute Gastritis.

During the month of July of the year 1826, I lost a patient, Jno. Henderson, aged about sixty, from a violent remittent fever of nearly eight days' duration, attended with great prostration of strength, tenderness in the epigastrium, irritability of stomach, high fever with coma and occasional delirium. A saffron-coloured skin and black tongue attended the last days of his disease.   I examined him in the presence of Drs. Hodge and La Roche; the peritoneal surface of the abdomen and of its viscera we found healthy, but the mucous coat of the stomach presented in its cardiac portion a large motley patch of ecchymosed blood, as big as the palm of my hand; it also presented smaller patches of ecchymosis in other regions. His symptoms were, with the exception of black vomit, of such intensity, that his death would, in times of yellow fever, have been ascribed to that disease.

The same patched appearance sometimes is extended into the intestinal canal.

Observation 16th.—May 30, 1827 —Gastritis.

I dissected Edward Bloom, aged thirty-eight, a patient in the Alms House. After a debauched course of life, of some continuance, he was brought into the syphilitic ward, for a sloughing ulcer of penis, with mortification of the adjoining skin: without any well marked sympathies, except a general prostration of his intellectual and physical pow-ers, he died in five or six days after his admission. Though there were no prominent gastric symptoms, as extreme irritability of stomach, tenderness in the epigastrium, &c.; we yet found the left end of the stomach, the jejunum, and the ascending colon in a patched ecchymosed state, with here and there mahogany coloured spots along the intestinal tube, arising from the collection of blood. The yellowish, semiputrescent tinge which the intestines under such circumstances are apt to have, was also present.

Observation 17th.—Acute Gastritis supervening upon a chronic one arising from intemperence, and attended with Arachnitis of the Cerebrum. (Plate 2nd, figs. 1st and 2nd.)

Nov. 22nd, 1827.—W. C. aged forty-three, innkeeper, has used alcoholic drinks in excess for the last eight or ten years, and become much enfeebled from them. The last summer he had a severe dysentery which lasted for several weeks.

Habitude.—Not much emaciated, skin pallid and temperate.

1

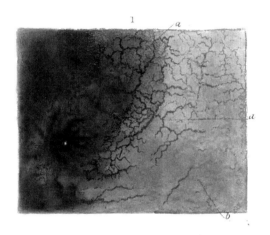

2

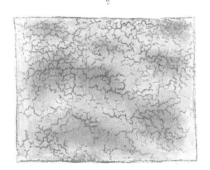

Drawn from nature & Eng'd by J.Drayton

Countenance.—Dull and unmeaning.

Intellectual Functions.—Disposed to taciturnity, and dull in apprehension.

Sensitive Apparatus.—Hearing dull.

Respiration.—Natural.

Circulation.—Natural.

Locomotive Apparatus.—Very much enfeebled, scarcely able to walk.

Digestive Apparatus.—No appetite.

He did not complain of pain in any particular part. I ordered valerian tea.

Nov. 25th.—I visited him again, and found him with hallucinations; he observed that though the figures were before his eyes, yet he knew them to be deceptive. He complained also of pain in the epigastrium, and suffered from a retention of urine. The muscles of the abdomen were rigid, and drawn towards the spine. He had spent several nights without sleeping. Ordered a pill of opium two grains, camphor one grain; to be repeated every three hours, till sleep be procured. Four of these pills produced the desired effect, and he slept soundly the following night.

The next day forty leeches were applied to the epigastrium, with much advantage in diminishing the pain there: and two days afterwards a blister was put upon the same region.

December 1st. His speech became suspended; great tenderness occurred in the abdomen, and the most excruciating pain was felt in the lower extremities upon their being moved, either by an assistant or by himself. His tongue became covered with a thick, yellow coat, and his strength exceedingly prostrated. Vol. alkali was administered in a julap to the amount of five grains every two hours. He took several doses of it, and the next day I found that the moisture of the tongue had disappeared, and the yellow coat had dried up into a dark brown one.

In the further progress of his treatment, up to the day of his death, a mild cathartic was administered on three or four occasions, also a decoction of serpentaria and bark at intervals. It was attempted twice to leech him on the head, but the leeches refused to bite. He was then cupped on the temples: half a dozen cups were also applied on each side of the spine, and mustard poultices were applied to the ankles.

His nourishment was wine whey, arrow root, and such light articles as he could be induced to swallow.

From the period of his first retention of urine to the day of his death, the bladder continued paralytic and required the daily introduction of the catheter, which brought away a dark, fœtid, ammoniacal urine. For several days before death, he lost all voluntary motion in the lower extremities, notwithstanding the continuance of their extreme sensibility.

He sunk away gradually and died without a struggle.

Autopsy December 7th, twelve hours after death.

Head. Very strong adhesion of dura mater to bone. Several drachms of serum lost in attempting to remove the latter, which were supposed to come from the tunica arachnoidea. The latter turbid, and raised in vesications.

Blood vessels of pia mater and of cerebrum very turgid. The latter, on being cut into, bled freely, and much serum exuded from it. Cerebrum soft; adhesion between the thalami unusually strong. A cluster of transparent vesicles on each side of the plexus choroides. Blood vessels of the velvum interpositum very turgid.

Spinal marrow—veins on surface of very turgid;—very great vascular fulness internally, giving a red pink colour along the roots of the anterior fasciculi of nerves, where they came from within the medulla spinalis. Spinal marrow not so vascular along the roots of posterior fasciculi, but still having a superabundance of blood.

Thorax. Ancient universal pleuritic adhesion on both sides. Lungs healthy. Heart healthy; its blood not coagulated.

Abdomen. No peritoneal disease.

Stomach small, universally inflamed; and of a deep pink colour, not coming from extravasation, as in fever; but from the immense number of its veins which run along the surface of the internal coat, and their fulness. At many places, their capillaries were so numerous, as to look, at a little distance, like small spots of extravasation, which, however, with the aid of a microscope, were found to be congeries of very fine vessels. Near the cardiac orifice there was a round patch two or two and a half inches diameter, consisting of thickly interwoven veins, containing black blood, and looking as if they were varicose: they were on the internal surface of the mucous membrane. In the pyloric region were two reddish slate-coloured patches, the indications of a chronic irritation there, and about twenty-four lines in diameter. Pylorus thickened.

No gas scarcely in bowels—Mucous coat of duodenum and of jejunum inflamed to almost the same red colour with the stomach; ileum and colon of a lively pink colour internally. No ulceration of intestines. Colon contained some well elaborated fæces. Liver of common size, colour degenerated into a drab, hard vascularity diminished, acini consisting in little hard scirrhus like grains. The secretion of bile seemed to have been suspended, for the gall bladder contained only a little black-coloured mucus.

Pancreas healthy. Spleen healthy. Kidneys healthy. Mucous coat of bladder inflamed; being injected with a network of veins, large and small, which were particularly abundant about the neck.

This patient had a mortification from pressure on sacrum. On cutting into it, as it was in the early stage, the blood was identified with the cellular substance and skin, so that it all looked like a bad bruize about the size of a dollar.

Observation 18*th.* *November* 26*th,* 1828.—*Chronic Gastro-enteritis, with tubercular condition of Mesenteric Glands.*

Mr. M. aged fifty, about six years ago, perceived a slight enlargement in his right testicle. It continued to increase, and finally became a confirmed scirrhus, and was extirpated by a surgeon at the end of three years. It did not re-

turn. Before this operation, he was seized with symptoms
of dyspepsia, that lasted with extreme severity until the
day of his death, which occurred yesterday morning. To-
day an examination of him was made, about 34 hours after
death, assisted by Dr. Randolph, his attending physician.

Exterior aspect. Considerable emaciation, several of the
superficial veins of the abdomen very serpentine, and enlarged, being distended by gas. Some putrefaction in the
muscles of the abdomen. A hard and prominent knot felt
along the spine, in the abdomen.

Abdomen. Peritoneum generally healthy, but in the hypogastric region, its sub-peritoneal tissue was interspersed
with several dark spots, a line or so in diameter.

Stomach. Mucous coat of a dark red colour, and highly
injected; and its veins in that varicose state, indicative of
chronic inflammation, such as is drawn in last case.* Neither this coat, nor the others of the stomach were thickened
in a perceptible degree, and there was not an obvious change
in its consistence. The small intestines were in very much
the same state with the stomach, and the commencement of
the large also. The rectum was tinged of a brownish colour, as in chronic phlegmasiæ of mucous membranes; but
not more injected than usual. There were no hardened
fæces in the large intestine, but a lamina of fæces adhered
to its sides.

The whole of the mesenteric and lumbar glands, were
enlarged, and formed into a scirrhus or tubercular mass; and
probably the majority of them softened into that puruloid
state which follows tubercle. This was the second time that
I had seen scirrhous abdominal lymphatic glands, follow
scirrhous testicle.

Liver, spleen, and pancreas not sensibly deranged. Contents of gall bladder principally mucus.

Thorax. About 3 gills of bloody serum in each pleura.

* Fig 1

Lungs collapsed but little; the inferior two thirds of each were in that congested peripneumomic hepatized state, which according to Mr. Laennec, sometimes occurs a few days before death, and resembles the hæmorrhagic state of active peripneumony.   A very large quantity of serum was discharged from both of them, when they were cut into, and a few small crude tubercular masses existed.   The superior third of the lungs was in a healthy state.

The heart was healthy, but enlarged: the pericardium contained about an ounce of serum.

Brain not examined.

From the liability of persons to confound the redness of the stomach, indicative of its inflammation during life, with the redness depending upon an obstruction to the circulation during the agonies of death, a principal object of the preceding pages has been to point out their difference, and to establish the important fact of gastric inflammation, in most of those cases where the redness is observed.   It is now proved that the redness arising from simple congestion, like the redness from injection, is uniformly diffused, whereas the redness from inflammation is generally partial and in patches, sometimes in the mucous membrane of the cardiac extremity of the stomach, and sometimes in that of the pyloric extremity.

Simple obstruction to the current of blood during the agonies of death, could never produce such appearances; for if it could, we ought to meet with them invariably.   On the contrary, where an obstruction does occur, which I am disposed to believe is very uncommon in natural death, whether this obstruction arises from the liver or from the lungs, the arrest of blood should be manifested by a uniform tinge of red in the organs concerned, and not by patches here and there.   Such marks of obstruction should also be more frequently seen and better developed, in cases of enlarged, in-

22

durated liver, in consumption, in dropsy of the thorax, and in all cases of obstruction of the lungs.

In concluding these observations, I should do injustice to an artist of uncommon merit and ingenuity, were I to with-hold the marked expression of my sense of the invaluable services rendered by Mr. Drayton, in promptly and faith-fully executing the drawings of the parts represented in the plate, and in subsequently executing the engravings. I have also to acknowledge the characteristic liberality of the pub-lishers, in freely allowing me the advantage of an unre-strained use of his talents.

PLATE III

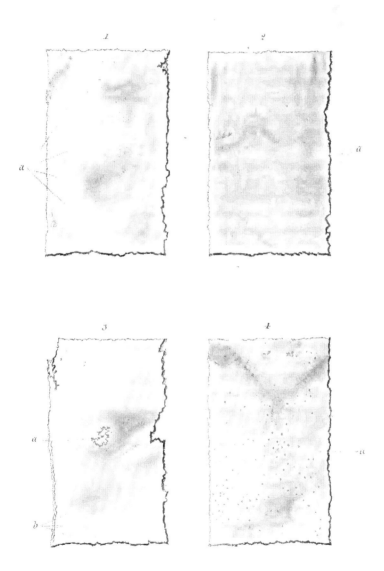

CHAPTER XI.

ON THE FOLLICULAR INFLAMMATION OF THE GASTRO-INTESTINAL MUCOUS COAT IN CHILDREN, AND ITS PROBABLE IDENTITY WITH CHOLERA INFANTUM.

SEVERAL dissections of children performed latterly, have inclined me to adopt the opinion that Cholera Infantum is in its essential anatomical features, an inflammation of the Muciparous Follicles of the gastro-intestinal mucous membrane. And that this affection, like hooping-cough and measles, may be considered as ingenerate to the human family. The present chapter will show the grounds upon which the theory rests. The subject is, however, so far open, that it still solicits inquiry and further observations; and whether my own opinions be confirmed by them or refuted will be equally acceptable; as I can have no farther desire, than a suitable exposition of the truth. Among the difficulties of a rigid conclusion at the present time may be ranked the few reports of dissections in cholera infantum; for it is lamentably true, that a disease so entirely American as this affection is, and which, from its annual recurrence and extensive prevalence, presents its facts so continually to the physicians of this country; yet stands in need of many developments to fix it upon a sure and perfect pathological foundation

In the city of Philadelphia alone, the number of deaths under two years of age from cholera infantum, is on an average two hundred annually; on some occasions it has amounted to two hundred and thirty, and is seldom less than one hundred and seventy. Its ravages are witnessed along a space of three thousand miles, from Quebec to New Orleans, and as a general rule may be considered to increase proportionably to their approximation to the equator. I have no doubt that a bill of mortality for the United States alone, on this single disease, would exhibit thousands of victims to it annually. It is then a remarkable fact, that from such an immense store of information, there is not one dissection a year reported to the medical public. Indeed, so completely have the pathological characters of the disease been neglected, that in hastily looking over several of the most popular American journals for the last twenty years, I have found but one dissection reported in detail.*

I have no doubt that many dissections have been performed in the mean time, indeed, they are alluded to in a general way; and possibly there may be much valuable information suppressed by the reserve of its owners; but if either, or both of these cases exist, they have remained in an obscurity, scarcely exceeding the precincts of a port folio, or the limited circulation of a medical coterie.

The indications of the existence of this affection, are so familiar to parents and physicians, and have been so well described by the eminent medical writers and practitioners of the United States,† that it will not be necessary to enter into a detail of symptoms, with a view of illustrating still more satisfactorily the subject of this inquiry. It may be

* See Coxe's Medical Museum, vol iii page 94, Philadelphia, 1807, case of Cholera Infantum, &c , by James Stewart, M D.

† See Medical Inquiries and Observations by Benjamin Rush, M. D. Professor, &c. in the University of Pennsylvania, vol. ii p 361. New England Journal of Medicine and Surgery, vol i James Jackson, M D Professor of Theory and Practice of Physic in Harvard University, Remarks on the Morbid Effects of Dentition. A Treatise on the Medical and Physical Treatment of Children, by William P. Dewees, M D Adjunct Professor in the University of Pennsylvania, Philadelphia, 1826. Nathaniel Chapman, M. D. Professor in the University of Pennsylvania, Manuscript Lectures The Medical Works of Edward Miller, M. D. Professor. New York, 1814.

stated in a summary way, that the affection prevails in the summer among children of two years and under; and that the morbid phenomena resolve themselves into a strongly marked change of the alvine evacuations, which cease to be natural and well-elaborated fæces, but consist in articles of aliment discharged in very much the same state in which they were swallowed, in an unusual quantity of the mucus of the bowels, frequently tinged green in places by bile, and holding, if the child have been fed on milk, (or small masses of food) the pieces of curd or food in clusters, resembling, in the mode of their connexion, the spawn of frogs. In serum in large quantities, coming either from the exhalents of the intestines, or from the muciparous glands, and augmented perhaps by the watery drinks of the patient,— and in bloody stools, which are also spoken of by writers, but are comparatively unfrequent.

Dr. Jackson* has expressed, in a very summary and striking way, as a leading indication, that the natural stools are retained, and such as are passed are derived principally from the chylopoietic viscera themselves; and that the proper fæcal smell is wanting in cholera infantum as in dysentery, being sour or putrid, or like water in which putrid meat has been washed. He also says, that some *red* portions are discharged as in true dysentery. I regret that he has here applied the name of a colour in such a way as to leave us in doubt of the substance to which it refers.

Other morbid phenomena are found in the frequency of those alvine discharges, which occur from three to twenty times in the course of twenty-four hours; in the want of appetite, irritability of the stomach, and vomiting; in extreme thirst; in an uneasiness, ever tempting to a change of posture; in fretfulness and quick perceptions; in frequent pulse; in fever of a remittent form disposed to evening exacerbations; in extreme emaciation and languor as the disease advances; and in delirium, coma, or hydrocephalus, in its last stages. This

* Loc. cit

affection, when it leads to a fatal termination, runs its course
generally in from a fortnight to six weeks. Dr. Rush[*] reports a case where death ensued in twenty-four hours. The
restoration to health may in like way be accomplished at
any time of the disease, and there are few or no symptoms so
aggravated but children have recovered from them. Among
those of the most fatal kind, are stools with pink-coloured
margin;[†] live worms crawling from the throat, and small
transparent vesicles on the chest.[‡]

The practitioners of the United States are as generally
agreed on the anatomical characters of this affection after
death, as they are on the symptoms indicating it. In common cases, the brain presents no other pathological state than
that of congestion of red blood: occasionally, however, the
disease becomes complicated with hydrocephalus, (chronic
inflammation of the arachnoidea.) The viscera of the thorax are in a sound state. In the abdomen the liver is generally enlarged: sometimes so much so, as to occupy two-
thirds of the cavity of the abdomen: it is also more firm
and solid than natural; but the derangement of structure, if
any exist, cannot be seen or appreciated. The gall-bladder
is sometimes found distended either with bile or colourless
mucus; on other occasions, it is flaccid with the same kind
of contents. The structure of the spleen and pancreas continues natural.

It is evidently in the mucous coat of the alimentary canal
that the true anatomical characters are found; the peritoneum
being generally entirely sound. In the stomach and small
intestines, especially the duodenum, red, inflamed patches,
inclining to a purple, have been observed. In the large intestines, according to Dr. Jackson and Dr. Dewees, it is rare
to discover marks of disease: in this, however, I do not agree
with them. The contents of the intestines are feculent matter in hard lumps, involved in a hard adhesive mucus, and

[*] Loc cit.   [†] Chapman, loc. cit.   [‡] Dewees, loc cit.

coloured either yellow or green by the bile. These feculent substances are sometimes in considerable quantity, but it is uncommon to find undigested matter; because the patient, in the latter stage of life, refuses all nourishment which is not in a liquid form. Dr. Dewees states that coagulable lymph is in some instances spread on the surface of the small intestines, or found in detached pieces; and, in many parts, their coats are thickened, so as to reduce considerably their calibre.

In some rare cases the intestines are filled with flatus, and distended much by it. In the majority of instances, however, the intestines are contracted, which is manifested during life by the collapse and diminution of the abdomen, and the wrinkling of its parietes.

Without entering into a further detail of the received anatomical characters of cholera infantum, it may be stated that they are considered to consist in an inflammation of the mucous coat of the stomach and small intestines, rarely if ever followed by ulcerations,* and that rare as ulceration is, it is more frequent in the large than in the small intestines.

From the foregoing exposition of symptoms and of pathological changes, it is evident that the authorities who treat of this disease, fix it in the mucous coat of the alimentary canal; and, so far as my experience goes, they have been entirely correct, and happy in giving this location to it. I have, however, some reason to believe, as the subsequent cases will tend to show, that this affection is rather a follicular than an erythemoid inflammation; that it is rather a disease of the innumerable mucous glands or follicles extended from one end to the other of the alimentary canal, than a common vascular or erythemoid irritation. With the view of presenting the grounds upon which this notion rests, the attention of the reader is called to the following dissections, with the plates illustrating them.

---

* New England Journal. ut supra, p 118, vol 1

CASE I.—*Follicular Inflammation of Intestinal Canal, the symptoms being those of Cholera Infantum.*

June 30th, 1828, *Autopsy eighteen hours after death.*— Present Drs. Dewees and Edward Jenner Coxe, attending physicians.

The infant daughter of Mr. F. aged about twenty months, has had for the last three weeks the usual symptoms of cholera infantum, manifested by eight or ten green-coloured discharges with mucus, in the twenty-four hours, but there has been no sickness of stomach. The complaint was attended with whooping-cough, but no other complication which was apparent. During the progress of her malady she did not seem to be very ill, but last evening she died very unexpectedly to her family and physicians.

Autopsy.—Abdomen: peritoneal surface of viscera healthy: liver of a light yellow colour: gall-bladder distended with bile: spleen healthy.

Mucous membrane as follows: that of the stomach of a sienna colour, and of a consistence which permitted it to be scraped off very readily with the finger nail. On the small intestines it was generally of the same colour, but interspersed at distant intervals with patches of injected blood-vessels, but no extravasation.* The clusters of muciparous glands or follicles were very distinct to the naked eye, and had their orifices also enlarged and tumid. The same condition of the muciparous follicles prevailed in the large intestines from one end to the other; but they were larger and more tumid, and gave to the mucous coat somewhat the appearance of having been sparingly sprinkled with fine white sand. In both small and large intestines the mucus seemed less consistent than usual.

The upper part of the small intestines contained yellow

---

* The colour of the intestines may be understood from fig. 4. plate 1st, though the latter belongs to a different subject

bile, almost pure, excepting some mixture of mucus. In the large intestines, the contents were also bilious, but greenish, like the discharges which had prevailed. There was a small blue spot on the large intestine, the colour somewhat like that of chronic inflammation.

The weather being sultry and oppressive, we did not extend the examination further. I carried, however, the whole of the large and a portion of the small intestine away, macerated it so as to remove the blood, and then suspended it in spirits of wine. This process has made the anatomical characters of the follicular affection much more distinct, by removing the tinge and mucus; and by floating the affected tissue, its folds and processes are kept extended and separated, and thereby give more prominence to the glands or follicles. Thousands of them, the ulceration of which was previously imperceptible, are now seen very clearly to be in this state. The maceration and suspension in a fluid, has moreover brought into view, on the jejunum, several common erythemoid ulcerations about two lines in diameter, and which escaped my observation entirely during the dissection. They are so different in size and appearance from the ulceration and tumefaction of the follicular system of the intestine, that they could not be mistaken for them, and the contrast in the drawing must be very evident. See plate III fig. 3d. a.

An observation worthy of consideration in this case, is, that yellow bile was in the jejunum, but green in the colon. The inquiry resulting from it, is what produced this change of colour? We know, that frequently in cholera, the alvine discharges are in a state of fermentation, and are sour. Is this condition confined to the colon? If so, the rationale is, that the bile retains its natural character in the small intestines, but becomes green in the large, from meeting there with acescent matters made so by fermentation. See Plate III. fig. 4, for a representation of a section of the colon, and fig. 3, for a portion of jejunum. The preparations are in the Anatomical Museum.

Q

CASE II.—*Follicular Inflammation of Intestinal Canal, the Symptoms being those of Cholera Infantum.*

September 3*d*, 1828.—A coloured female child, aged eighteen weeks, has been ill at least a fortnight, and probably more, from cholera infantum; the date, however, could not be ascertained precisely from the mother, owing to her imperfect intelligence and ill health. Within a few days, the mother has taken refuge in the infirmary of the Alms House, bringing with her the infant alluded to; and a twin of the same age, having an affection of the same kind and date. The subject of the present observation died last evening, and this afternoon I made the examination, in presence of the resident students of the house: thermometer 77°. The child, during its illness, had convulsions, which are by no means an uncommon symptom in the last stages of cholera. The attending physician, to whose care the infant had been confided, Dr. John K. Mitchell, was absent.

Autopsy.—Exterior aspect: no percepticle putrefaction; considerable emaciation.

Abdomen.—Stomach empty, contracted; mucous coat, of a light sienna colour, almost white, and destitute of blood-vessels, excepting a very few; the rugæ well marked, laid for the most part in longitudinal rows, and so elevated that they were in contact. The mucous coat was also so soft that it could be scraped away easily, in the form of a pulp, with the finger nail.

The small intestines likewise of a light sienna colour on their mucous coat, and empty, excepting a little mucus, which was here and there greenish. The large intestines presented the same colour as the small, and were destitute of fæces; in place of the latter, the two inferior thirds of the colon were occupied, to the extent of a slight distention, with

pure pus of a cream colour, proper consistence, as well elaborated as I ever saw, and destitute of any excepting a very
faint odour. The muciparous follicles of the colon were
all enlarged, so as to represent small grains of white sand
sprinkled over the mucous membrane, and about the size of
millet seed; there was in each a little depression of a darker
colour than the rest of the gland, which, from its position at
the apex, was taken for the orifice of the gland. The muciparous glands of the small intestines were also tumid and irritated, but could not be so well distinguished at the time of
examination, as they were by the subsequent management.
In a few of the follicles, ulceration had begun to show itself,
in both small and great intestines, only to an inconsiderable
extent, but maceration in this case also being resorted to,
both the tumefaction of the glands and their ulceration were
made more distinct by it, for the reasons stated in case 1st.

The liver was healthy, but its colour was lighter than
usual, and somewhat variegated by a yellowish ground, being interspersed with its natural brown. The gall-bladder
was distended with inspissated green bile.

The other viscera of the abdomen were healthy, as well
as the peritoneal coat. The thorax and head were not examined by myself. The preparation of the colon is deposited in the Anatomical Museum. See Plate III. fig. 2d.

After what has been stated in these two cases, on the
consistence of the mucous coat of the stomach, it becomes
a very interesting object of inquiry, whether this was a normal or a morbid state of its texture. I am as yet deficient
in those facts from personal observation, which would enable me to assign some standard of consistence to the mucous coat of the stomach under two years of age   I have,
however, no doubt that it is much softer at that period of
life than it is in the adult, and the probability is, that from
being so soft as to be readily scraped off with the finger nail
in the early months of existence, it then increases successively and gradually in its consistence as it advances in age,

until it finally becomes a membrane of sufficient tenacity to permit very readily its being fully dissected up with a scalpel. The subject is, however, quite open to inquirers, especially in this country; and sound conclusions upon it made by multiplied observations, would confer a great benefit upon the profession.

CASE III.—*Follicular Inflammation of Intestines with Cholera Infantum.*

September 7th, 1828.—The twin child alluded to in the preceding case, after having languished under the same disease with similar symptoms, died, and was examined today.

The mucous coat of the stomach was in a natural state. The duodenum contained healthy bile, and the other small intestines abounded in fæcal matter, of a light yellow colour. There was also fæcal matter in the cœcum, of a light yellow, and chopped appearance, but none in any other portion of the large intestines.

The muciparous glands of the cœcum were very obviously enlarged, as also those of the sigmoid flexure of the colon, and of the rectum. A mucous inflammation was seen on the lower portion of the ileum, and there was a considerable injection of the rectum, apparently of an inflammatory kind.

The appearance of the liver was healthy.

The facts of the last case were communicated to me by Dr. Ashmead of the Alms House Infirmary, who has now for some years distinguished himself there by a devoted attention to its scientific and charitable objects, and by a ready co-operation in the inquiries of the prescribing physicians and surgeon.

CASE IV.—" Maria Boulefray, aged ten months, head

large, considerable embonpoint, pale complexion, skin soft and flaccid, died February 5th, 1824, after an illness of six days; during which she was somewhat comatose, had no fever, no pain, very frequent vomiting, incessant alvine discharges; rejected pap, (bouillie,) and the breast of her mother.   The stools were first yellow; they then became white, frothy, inodorous, of a glairy consistence, slightly ropy, and without tenacity.   The body was opened ten hours after death.

Head—Serosity effused in the cranium; cerebral convolutions almost effaced; substance of the brain infirm; arachnoid membrane injected, middle and lateral ventricles distended by a considerable quantity of serosity.

The larnyx and chest in a sound state.

Abdomen not distended; peritoneum dry, and without effusion into its cavity.   Exteriorly the intestinal convolutions were white, and only a few small blood vessels, not much divided, were seen to creep under the serous coat

The stomach being empty, was in a middle state between dilatation and contraction.   The mucous membrane was of a natural thickness, sufficiently adherent to the subjacent membrane, of a milky whiteness, and was moistened by a proper quantity of clear, ropy mucus.   The villosities were very distinct on the great curvature, and scarcely perceptible elsewhere, the cardia and the pylorus had nothing remarkable, *but all the extent of the mucous surface was covered with a prodigious number of white granulations, the size of a millet seed*, indiscriminately scattered over the gastric surface, which presented no marks of inflammation.

The antrum pylori, (espace pylori-valvulaire,) was sound and covered *with small glands,* like the stomach.   A similar follicular developement had occurred in the duodenum; the valvulæ conniventes did not yet overlap, as in the adult; there were glands on the summits of these valves, as well as in their intervals.   From the beginning of the jeju-

num to the middle of the ileum, the internal membrane retaining a white satin colour, sufficiently villous, and of an
ordinary thickness, was covered with *granulations of an
appearance and size similar to those of the duodenum.*
From the inferior third of the ileum to the valve of Bauhin,
there was a white, frothy, fluid, tinged yellow, without a
particular odour, having almost the liquidity of water, and
filling the entire cavity of the intestinal tube.   Besides
the granulations generally scattered upon this part of the
intestine, there were groups of follicles united in small
masses, and in elliptical plates which all occupied the curvature of the intestine.   They were bordered by a winding,
colourless line, their surface was rough, and surmounted by
glands, similar to those which existed alone in the environs
of the plates; mucous folds extended from one gland to another.   The plates generally were four lines wide, and half
an inch long.   In the ileo cœcal region they were very near
one another.   The different glands which existed alone on
the mucous surface, offered for the most part at their summit,
a grayish point, indicating their excretory orifice.

   In the whole length of the large intestine, down to the
rectum, and even the anus, *these glands were found in
abundance.*   The colon contained frothy, yellow matter,
similar to that of the small intestines.

   The mouth, the pharynx, and the œsophagus presented a
similar developement of follicles.

   The intestinal mucous membrane was detached with difficulty; but at the end of eight days of maceration in water, a large shred could be peeled off.   The plates and the
granulations came off with it, being as it were, incrusted
in it."

   M. Billard,[*] from whom this observation is translated,
continues his remarks in stating that we may conclude that
there was here an unnatural developement of the mucipa-

   * De la Membrane Muqueuse Gastro-intestinale. p. 422, Paris, 1825

rous glands, from their being much more numerous than they are in the healthy state. It may also be remarked that the membrane was not inflamed, that the intestinal tube contained a prodigious quantity of liquid matters almost aqueous, and which seemed to constitute what is called the mucous flux; and that in fine, the young patient, though dead in a short time, had not presented very evident febrile symptoms.

It is evident to the American reader, that if this case of M. Billard, had occurred in this country, it would have been registered, and was, in fact, cholera infantum. But the paucity of his observations prevented him from recognising in it the anatomical characters of this disease: for he says the follicles probably are not developed by inflammation, because the membrane upon the surface of which they manifest themselves, offers none of the characters of inflammation laid down in a former part of his work. The difficulty with M. B., however, comes from his not making a sufficient allowance for the difference between the erythemoid or common vascular inflammation, and the follicular irritation of the intestinal tube. In the observations by myself, the indications of erythemoid inflammation have also generally been either absent or defective.

Strange as the assertion or rather suggestion may appear, I am inclined to the opinion, that if this follicular inflammation be the primary or essential affection in cholera infantum, cases may, and indeed do occur, where the diarrhœa is wanting, and where perhaps the most striking symptom are convulsions, no doubt arising from the sympathetic irritation of the brain. The following case, at least, where the anatomical characters after death were the same as in the cholera infantum, will go to show how far this notion is supported by facts.

CASE V.—*Follicular Inflammation of the Colon with Convulsions.*

Examination about twenty-four hours after death.—Present Dr. Hays, attending physician, and Mr. Theodore Dewees, student of medicine.

Miss P. aged two years, for about three weeks had been disposed to constipation, requiring the use of cathartics frequently. She was attended by Dr. Dewees, who informs us that her stools had been white with an absence of bile. Eight hours before her death she was suddenly seized with convulsions which lasted to the end of life.

Autopsy. Jan. 9th, 1828.—Exterior aspect, nothing unusual.

Head.—Brain and membranes natural.

Thorax.—Lungs natural; half an ounce of straw-coloured, transparent serum in the right pleura.

Abdomen.—Peritoneum healthy; liver hard and of a yellowish hue; stomach of usual thickness; its mucous membrane could be scraped off with the finger nail, and was of a pearl or sienna colour, interspersed every few lines with small specks of blood of a light pink colour, and not larger than the head of a very small pin. The mucous membrane was also smeared all over with a coat of tenacious mucus, and at the left end of the stomach was of a light gamboge colour, which I attributed to discoloration from the bile.

The intestines were distended with flatus and of a light pearl colour. Nothing pathological could be detected in the small ones, but in the large, all the muciparous follicles from one end to the other seemed to be affected. These follicles were converted into small cysts of the transparency and size of the itch vesicle, and on being punctured with a needle and pressed, readily gave out their transparent fluid. Their orifices could be seen very readily with the assistance of a lens, and appeared to be closed generally, but some were opened and slightly ulcerated; neither could a distinction of colour be observed between these orifices and the remainder of the gland. See Plate III. fig. 1. (This is also deposited in the Anat. Museum.)

Case VI.—*Enlarged muciparous Glands of Colon, without Diarrhœa; with congested Brain, and Peripneumonia from Measles.*

April 29, 1829.—An infant boy, aged six months, was taken six weeks ago with violent cough, and symptoms resembling pleurisy, they were attended by squinting, which finally went off entirely. There was no diarrhœa at any period of the complaint, except what was produced by certain cathartic medicines. He died last night.

This afternoon I examined him in the presence of Dr Dewees, the attending physician, and Dr. Hays.

Autopsy. Head.—A considerable effusion of serum beneath the tunica arachnoidea, all over the brain; the lateral ventricles contained each about one drachm of serum. The whole amount of the sub-arachnoid effusion, when collected, was about two ounces. The brain was of the consistence common to this period of infancy, and congested highly with blood; the white part of it had a light pink colour, from the quantity of blood in it

Query. Is the effusion of serum beneath the arachnoid, indicative of an irritation of this membrane, or of the pia mater? I am disposed to believe the latter, for membranes, when in a state of irritation, secrete from their free surfaces, and not from the adherent ones: the secretion of the arachnoidea would, therefore, be between it and the dura mater, and not between it and the pia mater. Pure hydrocephalus is, a secretion from the arachnoidea, covering the ventricles;

24

and sub-arachnoid secretion must be from the pia mater, as in mania a potu, &c.

Thorax.   Lungs white, like those of a veal, and spongy; did not collapse on opening the thorax.   Filamentous adhesions between the convex surface of the right, and the parietes of the thorax.   The whole inferior lobe of the left lung of a cherry colour, carnified and hard; having a purulent tubereulous infiltration throughout; the air cells being completely obstructed.

The trachea was filled with pus, which could be traced into the lungs.   There was no enlargement of the muciparous glands of the trachea, or undue injection of its lining membrane, or that of the bronchia.

There was a recent adhesion of the fissure between the two left lobes, with vascular injection, and redness of the surfaces which adhered.   The irritation of the lower lobe seeming to have been continued to the upper, on the surface of the fissure.

No effusion of serum in thorax on either side.   Heart healthy.

Abdomen.   Viscera generally healthy, but extremely pallid and transparent, probably from the small quantity of blood in the system.

The muciparous glands of the colon were, from one end to the other of this intestine, enlarged to about the size of the head of the smallest pin in common use: there was no ulceration perceptible in them or in the coat of the intestine.

Were these glands in a state of irritation or not, as there had been no diarrhea or abdominal symptoms?

I have now adduced a sufficiency of evidence to excite inquiry, and perhaps to lead to the conclusion, that cholera infantum is pathologically a follicular inflammation of the intestinal tube, attended with increased peristaltic motion in most cases, but not in all; and in its extreme stages, exciting various sympathies of the different organs of the body.

In its anatomical characters, it has a very strong resemblance with the vesicular diseases of the skin, and in its extreme stages it seems to progress from the interior to the exterior of the body; by showing itself in the mouth by inflammation of the mucous follicles there (aphthæ;) and on the skin by an irritation of its follicular system, the appearance of which has been compared by Dr. Dewees to the vesicles which would be produced by an immense number of minute drops of scalding water.*

The disease seldom becomes fatal until the sympathies with other organs are well established, and the indications of their irritation be strongly marked by disordered circulation, incessant vomiting, coma and convulsions; all of which show the lesion of the organs presiding over the great functions of circulation, digestion, sensitiveness, and myotility. It is under the advanced stages of cholera that the meningeal inflammation of the brain, (hydrocephalus,) is evolved; the sympathetic affection being converted from one of mere irritation of the arachnoidea, into a pathological change of structure followed by effusion.

Follicular inflammation of the intestines sometimes appears in the eleventh year; the following case will prove it.

Case VII.—*Follicular Intestinal Inflammation.*

May 17th, 1824.—Louis Joui, aged eleven years, of an infirm constitution, but having a certain degree of embonpoint, being thrown from his horse, his skull was fractured, and he died the next day, in the hospital. It could not be ascertained whether he was labouring under a diarrhea at the time, or not.

Autopsy, eighteen hours after death.—The fracture of the skull was found extended to the base, and there was

* Op. Cit p. 398.

much effusion.   The lungs were sound, with some ancient adhesions of the thorax.

Abdomen—Peritoneum sound, the intestines thin and transparent.   The mucous membrane of the stomach was of a rose colour, wrinkled, and covered with a thick layer of mucosity.   By scraping it, a number of red points became visible, and it contained some bread and the skins of stewed apples.

The antrum pylori was long, yellowish, and marked with a great number of small, grayish spots.   The mucous villosities were well marked there; the duodenum, and the remainder of the small intestinal tube, were the seat, in places, of a very fine ramiform injection.   In the interior third of the ileum, was a cluster of twelve lumbrici worms.   The large intestine was healthy, and contained a great quantity of fluid matter, which was yellow, frothy, and moderately odorous; at the end of the colon, the fæces had a consistence sufficiently firm.

In the whole extent of the intestinal mucous membrane, was a great number of muciparous glands.   They were extremely numerous on the duodenum, and occupied both the valves and their intervals.   They all had the size of the head of a pin, and exhibited, very visibly, their excretory orifice.   In the jejunum they were more rare; but they reappeared in great numbers on the ileum, and united themselves in little masses, and by plates.   The cœcum was covered with those glands; at the end of the transverse colon they became more rare, and none existed in the sigmoid flexure, nor in the rectum."*

M. Billard goes on to remark that the state of this intestinal tube is entirely analogous to most of those opened by Rœderer, and Wagler.†

* Billard, op cit. p 420
† De Morb. Mucos. Paris, 1810.   I regret not having been able to obtain this book in the United States   It alludes to an epidemic which prevailed in Gœttingen, the violence of which seems to have exploded on the intestinal canal, according to the allusions which I have seen concerning it.

There was evidently here an abundant mucous flux; a re-markable whiteness of the mucous membrane, and a marked development of the muciparous glands. Nevertheless, this infant did not die from the affection; it appears even that he was not incommoded by it during life, so far as to require repose and care, inasmuch as he received, while working, the wound which caused his death in so short a time.

There are certain diseases considered as contagious, one of the remarkable peculiarities of which is, that when once individuals have gone through them, the charm is dissolved, and they are for ever afterwards innoxious. Another cir-cumstance worthy of remark is, that these diseases have their primary seat in the follicular system, as for example the small-pox and the chicken-pox. They appear occasion-ally under such doubtful causes, that the opinion may be rea-sonably entertained of their spontaneous production, in the localities where they appear from time to time. Have we not then mistaken too freely this peculiarity of disposition in the organism to fall into certain morbid conditions, for distant sources of contagion; for a power in disease as an essential existence to propagate itself, like plants or animals, by its seeds as they are ridiculously called? May not cho-lera infantum, as a follicular disease of the intestines, be the inevitable lot of every individual of the human family, but under circumstances of various severity, being mild, scarce-ly perceptible in some; and in others aggravated by the season of the year, by the local circumstances of the in-dividual, and by his early infancy? May not, in fact, the whole follicular system of the body be successively under the necessity, in most individuals, of undergoing inflamma-tion, the symptoms of which will of course vary, according to the functions of the part in which the follicles are placed, and give rise apparently to diseases having no external ana-logies? As, for example, in the inherent follicular inflam-mations of the skin, we have what is called small-pox, from its vesicular or bladder-like appearance;—in the inherent in-

flammations of the follicles of the intestines, we have what
is called a cholera or flux of children, because the bowels
are continually expelling their contents, being too irritable in
most cases to retain them; and is it not perfectly consistent
with the laws of induction; that when a similar innate inflammation attacks the follicles of the trachea and lungs,
we shall of course have symptoms suited to the organs assailed? In fact, what is whooping-cough but an ingenerate
inflammation of the mucous follicles of the air passages,
manifested by the immense transparent mucous discharges,
which are sometimes brought up by the tea-cupful after a fit
of spasmodic coughing? May not then the theory of contagion rest upon the explanatory fact, that till the ingenerate
diseases of the follicular system have been gone through,
the individual is liable to have them excited by such individuals as are labouring under a similar affection.

CHAPTER XII.

DISSECTIONS, ILLUSTRATING THE PATHOLOGY OF THE
ABDOMEN.

ACUTE PERITONITIS.

John L., aged twenty-four, of rather a strong frame, submitted to an extirpation of the testicle, by Dr. Randolph,
in consequence of a chronic enlargement of it of a scirrhous
character. The operation was performed September 5th,
1827, and *the testicle weighed at the time three pounds
two ounces.* Its original glandular structure had entirely
disappeared, and left this enormous body constituted by an
immense congeries of small cysts, of yellowish serum, adhering together by an indurated scirrhous substance of various
thickness in different parts of the testicle. The preparation
is now in the Anatomical Museum, having been presented
to it by Dr. Randolph.

In a few days after the operation, the patient was seized
with symptoms of acute peritonitis, and died, Sept. 13th.
He was examined seventeen hours after death, when the following appearances were presented:

Thorax—Great accumulation of blood in the lungs, especially the right one.   Heart healthy; white coagulum in
right auricle and in right ventricle.

Abdomen—Universal peritoneal inflammation of intestines marked by the redness and extreme congestion of the
vessels. The convolutions of the small intestines adhered
together by a recent secretion of coagulating lymph, which
formed upon several of them, on the surface next to the abdominal muscles a complete layer. The omentum was in-

jected highly, and adhered slightly to the front of the intestines.   Mahogany patches of blood vessels were distributed over the intestines.

The superior portion of the jejunum was dilated by flatus
to one and a half inches in diameter: its lower half, and
the ileum were of a common size.   Left lumbar portion of
colon constricted by contraction of its muscular coat, so as
to obliterate its cavity.   The other portions of the large intestine were of the usual size, and contained hardened well
elaborated fæces in lumps, and adhering all along to its surface.

The *mucous coat* of the stomach was yellowish, soft, and
with many small spots about half a line in diameter, scattered over its surface: that of the small intestinal canal was
injected fully with distinct blood vessels, and spotted from
one end to the other with tubercles at various distances
apart, supposed to be the muciparous glands.   These tubercles were from half a line to two lines in diameter; and as
they approached the ileo-colic valve became more and more
ulcerated.   The largest of the ulcers were twelve or fifteen
lines in diameter, with thick indurated injected edges, as in
the ulcerations of the intestines in the last stages of pulmonary consumption.   The ileum, for the last five inches of it,
was one continued sheet of ulcerations to the ileo-colic valve.
The adjoining part of the colon was highly injected for seven or eight inches, but presented no distinct ulcerations:
the remainder of the mucous coat of the colon was healthy.

The mesenteric glands were all enlarged, indurated, and
some of them injected.   A tumour the size of the fist was
on a level with the right kidney, in front of its vessels.   It
consisted in a congeries of cysts, and indurated gelatinous
matter; resembled very much in structure the testicle
which had been extirpated, and was precisely in the course
of its lymphatics; we supposed it to be a degenerated lymphatic gland affected by the carcinomatous condition of the
testicle.

The liver healthy, but congested with red blood, and seemed to have had an old peritoneal inflammation, a little above its anterior edge.—Spleen healthy.

Head not examined.

Acute Peritonitis, from Inflammation of the Urinary Bladder.

A patient aged about fifty, and having a stone in the bladder, had a paroxysm of inflammation brought on by the introduction of instruments into the latter. He was seized with violent symptoms almost immediately afterwards; such as extreme tenderness of the abdomen, flatulent distention of it, and a diffused blush of red over its skin. During his illness he vomited some stercoraceous matter. Death followed in fifty-eight hours after the beginning of the attack.

Autopsy twenty-two hours after death.

Universal peritoneal inflammation, marked by the effusion of coagulating lymph from the entire surface of the peritoneum,—by the full injection of the capillary blood vessels of the latter,—and by purulent secretion. The convolutions of the intestines, were all coherent by the recent effusion of lymph.

The stomach and intestines were much distended by gas, and exhibited also a high grade of inflammation on their mucous coat, marked by an abundant punctated redness. The parietes of the intestines were somewhat thickened, and the stomach contained a bilious stercoraceous matter.

The scrotum and the extremity of the penis were of a dark purple, from the settling of blood by ecchymosis. Along the course of the lining membrane of the urethra, there were many small blotches of extravasated blood

Within the pelvis the whole cellular membrane around the bladder and rectum was in a state of suppuration, which extended beneath the peritoneum, almost to the umbilicus.

25

The cellular membrane connecting the peritoneum to the bladder, was in a dark gangrenous suppurated state.

The bladder was thickened and closely contracted upon a stone nearly the size of a goose egg. The internal coat was also in a state of suppuration, and presented the dark slate colour common to chronic inflammations of the mucous membranes. There were two openings from the cavity of the bladder, to the purulent collections beneath its peritoneal coat.

Ascites and Hydrothorax.

Mr. B. æt. 38, being under the professional charge of Dr. Dewees, suffered for eighteen months with dyspepsia, followed within the last six months by dropsy, of the abdomen. Having died under these symptoms, he was examined eighteen hours after death, (April 12th, 1829.)

Exterior Aspect.—Considerable infiltration of lower extremities and posterior parts of the trunk of the body, with settling of blood in integuments of the latter.

Thorax.—Universal peripheral adhesion of right lung, which, upon inquiry, could not be traced to any known sickness at a former period. Left pleura contained about fourteen ounces of straw-coloured transparent serum. The parenchyma of both lungs perfectly sound. Heart itself sound: pericardium contained two ounces straw-coloured serum—root of aorta somewhat dilated, wrinkled, and presented the beginning of an aneurismal change of texture.

Abdomen.—One gallon of serum in peritoneum, with shreds of coagulating lymph floating in it. The peritoneum itself transparent and smooth, but considerable numbers of the sub-serous capillary vessels were seen every where beneath it. The omentum was tucked up into the epigastric region, and from it a round cord of vessels proceeded through the cavity of the abdomen to the sigmoid flexure of the colon, where it terminated in one of the appendiculæ epiploicæ.

This cord was free, except at its extremities, where it adhered; it ran almost vertically down in front of the small intestines, was the thickness of half a line, and we supposed
had arisen primitively from an adhesion between the omentum and the sigmoid flexure; which adhesion had elongated
by the retraction of the former, to about ten inches in length.

The stomach was distended.   Its mucous coat had but little mucus on it, was slightly thickened and felt hardened
when brushed with the hand; had a shining smooth surface
destitute of the villous appearance, and resembled more an old
mucous membrane, which, by exposure to the air is becoming almost like skin.   It was of a sienna colour, with
no vascular injection, except here and there in the left half
some clusters of a light punctated redness.

The intestines were much distended with flatus.   The
mucous surface of the duodenum had the unequal granular
appearance of chronic duodenitis.   The whole length of the
jejunum was infiltrated to nearly three lines in thickness;
the water being in its cellular coat, and the valves almost
obliterated by it.   The ileum was not so.   The colon had
a light blue or slate colour in its whole length.   No ulceration any where in the intestinal canal.

The liver was only two thirds of its common size, and
had a collapsed or shrivelled appearance.   On its convexity
were six or eight marks like cicatrices, which were traced
into the substance of the liver eight, ten, or twelve lines, and
seemed to be the remains of former abscesses, which had been
healed and cicatrized for a long time.   Among these cicatrices several tubercles of four or five lines in diameter, were
found.   The bile was yellow, but thin.

Spleen healthy.

Kidneys enlarged; secerning part of a very light yellow,
and softened, so that it tore easily; tubuli uriniferi of common colour.

The semi-lunar ganglion of the sympathetic nerve on each
side was hardened and surrounded by a compact matting of

cellular substance; but I could not perceive any departure from the natural colour.

Head not examined.

Ascites and Tubercles of Liver.

Mr. T——, innkeeper, 40 years of age, of intemperate habits, injured himself about six months ago in the right iliac region by a fall, which he always considered as the beginning of his illness: ascites followed, which terminated his existence. I examined him thirteen hours after death, Nov. 25th, 1827, assisted by his attending physician Dr. Emerson, and some others.

Exterior Aspect.—Skin very yellow, abdomen extremely distended, slight œdema in feet and ankles.

Head.—Scalp bled very freely on being cut. Arachnoidea raised up from the upper convexities of hemispheres of cerebrum, by a layer of serum. Glandulæ Pacchioni very numerous; and not far from them there were some specks of condensed substance, as if from inflammation in the arachnoidea. With this exception, membranes healthy. Brain and cerebellum of a very healthy consistence; about a drachm of water in each lateral ventricle: there was no disorganization of former. Many small veins turgid with blood in encephalon; but from the horizontal position of the body, we supposed the blood might have been confined there, by the pressure of the ascites on the vena cava ascendens.

Thorax.—Heart large and flabby; an ossification twice the size of a wheat grain, between the corners of the semi-lunar valves of the aorta. A small ossification on mitral valve, but not large enough to derange its functions. There had never been intermittent or irregular pulse within the knowledge of his physician:—lungs, right one sound, no water in pleura; left one had a universal adhesion to pleura costalis, from an old pleurisy, but in other respects it was sound.

Abdomen.—Liver smaller than usual, of a chocolate colour, very hard, diminished vascularity, knotted on the surface, and presenting a complete hard tuberculous degeneration; but nothing like suppuration. Gall bladder contained a very dark green bile, principally mucus, much of which had been discharged by stool a day or two before death.

The spleen was in a sufficiently healthy state. Stomach distended with gas, and had adhering to its inner surface broad patches of the same kind of fluid bile, as the gall bladder contained. The patient had much sickness of stomach a day or two before his death, which accounted for its being there. The mucous coat of the stomach was thickened, of a lively red colour all over, which upon near examination, was found to consist of numerous spots of extravasated blood, from half a line to a line in diameter; but there were no large patches or blotches, such as attend fevers. It was in fact the stomach of a man accustomed to an undue use of alcoholic drinks.

The intestines, though not healthy, had not a change of colour or condition, so decided as to admit of description.

Kidneys healthy. About three gallons of straw-coloured transparent serum were in the peritoneum, and had strings of coagulating lymph floating in it.

Stricture of Œsophagus.

W., aged fifty, an inhabitant of Georgetown, D. C., came to Philadelphia to obtain the professional advice of Dr. Physick. He has for seven months suffered from extreme difficulty in swallowing his food. This difficulty increased so much, a few days before his death, as to render deglutition entirely impracticable, and he died from absolute inanition.

Autopsy, March 14th, 1828, eighteen hours after death.

The œsophagus was obstructed for two inches, about the middle of the trachea, by a scirrhous tumour on its whole circumference, which reduced its calibre to less than the size of a writing quill. The muscular fibres around it were ulcerated, and in a state of chronic inflammation, which seemed to render them incapable of acting in the transmission of food downwards to the stomach. The tumour itself was also ulcerated, and of a soft consistence. The stomach was distended with flatus, and contained about a pint of watery fluid, with thick flocculent mucus floating in it. The mucous coat was smeared with this thick mucus, which adhered to it; its consistence not being sensibly altered, nor its thickness. It presented, very generally, patches and spots of a deep punctated redness, arising from the residence of red blood in the ends of the fine vessels, as is often seen in drunkards. This is one of the indications of mucous inflammation, and as the individual died from starvation, arose probably from it alone; as there was no evidence of his being intemperate, and it was impossible for him to have been so for some time previous to death. The black bronchial glands were much enlarged and schirrous, and a spherical ossification six lines in diameter, was found on the front surface of the left lung. The lungs themselves, and the other viscera of the thorax and abdomen were healthy.

Fever.

It occasionally happens, after symptoms of considerable intensity, that the derangement of organs is not found upon examination, of a kind so marked as to give a satisfactory solution of the cause of death. The following autopsy is of that description. I experience now much less difficulty than I did formerly, in ascertaining the mode of deranged organism; but yet pathological anatomy is not sufficiently advanced, to throw light upon every case of death.

Master D., aged three years and six months, died after thirteen days' indisposition, attended with high fever, but no well marked local affection. His illness was supposed to arise from eating heartily of oyster pie.

Autopsy, twenty-one hours after death, Nov. 27, 1827, assisted by Drs. Dewees and Griffith, the attending physicians. Exterior aspect of body nothing remarkable, face tranquil.

Head.—Membranes of brain, natural.—Brain voluminous, with many blood-vessels traversing its substance, a small quantity of serum under arachnoidea of upper portion of hemisphere, and about one drachm in each ventricle. The fornix very hard and well developed. Periphery of cerebrum rather softer than usual. Pons varolii hard. Cerebellum natural, with only a slight congestion. The state of the brain generally, might be considered as indicative of an afflux of blood to it, though there was no strongly marked inflammation.

Thorax.—Heart natural. Lungs natural. Pleura, on right side contained about two ounces of transparent fluid, but it was not injected; left, contained about two or three drachms, but its capillary blood vessels were injected; there was no thickening of it, or false membrane on either side, or any other mark of an effusion of coagulating lymph.

Abdomen.—Peritoneum healthy universally. Stomach distended with gas, and for the most part of a healthy aspect, but on the right side of the cardiac orifice there was an irregular patch of inflammation, about two inches in diameter, made up partly of injected blood vessels, partly of extravasated blood, and partly of stellated spots. It was of a red rose colour. The consistence of mucous coat natural, and there were no wrinkles in it.

Small intestines of a healthy aspect on their mucous coat. The jejunum was very much distended with gas, but the ileum was much contracted in the greater part of its length, with partial distentions here and there of gas; duodenum healthy. Mesenteric glands enlarged, but no disorganization of them. Large intestine spasmodically contracted in almost the whole extent, with the exception of its right side; mucous coat of a very light pink colour, and covered with a thick layer of mucus. A thin layer of fæces in it. Liver healthy, but very red, and filled with blood. Spleen healthy. Kidneys healthy.

Scirrhus of the Stomach.

The following is the narrative of a case, which I dissected a few years ago. It is rendered highly interesting by the extent to which the disease had proceeded, and by the manner in which the symptoms during life indicated it. The attending physician, Dr. Otto, politely addressed to me its history in the following letter.

Philadelphia, August 28th, 1824.

My dear Sir,

I was called to attend the late Mr. D., the middle of January, and continued my services for nearly five months. He had been previously visited a considerable time by a medical friend of mine. I was informed, that for more than ten years he had regularly given himself an enema in the evening, as his bowels were never naturally moved. He had been gradually declining in strength and appearance for more than two years, about which period his stomach began to manifest disease. When I first saw him, he had a slow irregular fever, and it continued occasionally during my attendance, especially the latter part of it. Sometimes it seemed to be increased or renewed by causes not connected with his disease, as exposure to cold. He manifested the usual symptoms of dyspepsia. His diet was regulated, but as his complaint increased, there were very few articles he could take with impunity. As the stomach is often capricious in this disorder, occasionally digesting the most improbable things, he was ultimately permitted to eat whatever he had a strong desire for—the whole round of food was resorted to for his support. His appetite declined, and his powers of digestion gradually lessened. His stomach refused what had been formerly acceptable to it, so that it was difficult ultimately to find any thing that would long remain on it. At first he

seldom vomited; but during the latter part of my attendance, he rarely passed two days without discharging the
contents of his stomach, and then he thought that every
thing he had taken since he last vomited, came up.   The
gradual accumulation oppressed him, and he felt uneasy
until it was discharged.   Great care was taken not to over-
load it.   He often complained of acidity and uneasiness in
the stomach, but never, to my recollection, of pain.   His case
appeared to me to be purely dyspeptic.   His strength gradually failed, but he was sometimes stronger than at others;
and when I ceased to attend him, he was able to walk abroad,
if the distance was short, and to ride many miles.

Yours truly,

Dr. Horner.   .   J. C. Otto.

Autopsy.—The mucous membrane of the stomach in the
left half of this organ was healthy.   But the whole remaining portion of it was in a scirrhous state.   From the beginning of this disorganization to the pylorus, the mucous membrane increased gradually until it became half an inch thick.
It was of a semi-transparent gristly appearance, and the internal surface of it like a honey comb.   The muscular stra-
tum of the corresponding part of the stomach was increased
to one quarter of an inch in thickness.   A sort of tuberculous degeneration seemed to have occurred under the peritoneum of the corresponding region of the stomach.

Scirrhus of Colon and Rectum.

March 8th, 1829.—Autopsy, twenty-four hours after
death.

Mr. ——, aged 35, under the professional charge of Dr.
Meiggs, was affected eighteen months ago with dyspepsia,
from an intemperate course of life.   The symptoms subsided
after a few months of treatment, and was succeeded by pain

26

and uneasiness in the rectum; which, upon examination, was
found to be in a scirrhous state.   Towards the conclusion of
his life, a diarrhea came on which nothing could arrest; and
he was reduced to an extreme state of marasmus, in which
he died.

Abdomen.—The front parietes drawn so far in, as to be
in contact with the spine.

Peritoneum healthy; liver, spleen, and stomach, healthy.
Small intestines:—duodenum healthy—upper part of jejunum
presented several large ulcerations about twelve lines in diameter, the lower part of the ileum did the same.   In both
cases the ulcerations amounted in depth to a perforation of
the intestine, excepting its peritoneal coat.   At several of
these places the intestine was constricted.

Large Intestine.—The rectum in its whole length had
its mucous coat thickened three lines, indurated and ulcerated; with a high vascular chronic injection, and with a
slate colour.   The head of the colon, for five inches, was in
a similar state; and the ileo-colic valve was constricted and
ulcerated, as well as the contiguous parts of the ileum.   The
mucous coat of the sigmoid flexure of the colon was thickened, highly injected, and looked granulated.   The remaining portion of the mucous coat in the left half, presented the
slate colour so indicative of chronic inflammation, in mucous
tissues.

I examined, in this case, the semi-lunar ganglia of the
splanchnic nerves, and found them healthy, as well as the
contiguous branches of the solar plexus.

Thorax.—Heart healthy, except some white plates on its
surface, which are common in chronic affections of other organs.

Left lung tuberculous in its upper lobe, excepting the peripheral part, some of the tubercles softened and presenting
excavations; had an adhesion at its upper part.   Right lung
generally healthy, but presenting several insulated tubercles
in a cheesy state, but not suppurated.

Exsiccation of Colon.

A gentleman of a full habit of body; whose clerical office should have secured him from the fascinations of intemperance, died in 1824, under the charge of Doct. S. Jackson, in a state of mania a potu. On examination, we found the following diseased appearances.

The liver was diminished in size, white, deficient in the usual degree of vascularity, and harder than natural. The stomach, the small intestines, and the large intestines presented the stellated condition which occurs frequently in gastric affections, from blood being extravasated in the course of the extreme or capillary vessels. The head of the colon was enormously distended, perhaps to the amount of four or five inches in diameter with flatus, and contained a layer of dried and hardened fæces adhering to it. This portion of the gut was so dry as to be almost crisp, like a bladder which has been suspended for some time in the air.

The brain had the blood vessels of the pia mater congested, and had suffered from the effusion of about four ounces of serum into its ventricles, and on the surface of the pia mater.

Cholica Pictonum.

May 16th, 1829.—Autopsy twenty hours after death. Present Dr. Edward J. Coxe, attending physician.

Cornelius Hopkins, a black man aged about 38, stature full, worked for thirty days in a white lead factory belonging to Mr. Roberts, Druggist, in Second Street. About ten days ago he began to complain of colic pains, for which he drank plentifully of chamomile tea. He continued to work till the 12th instant, when he became too ill to proceed longer in it. The next day he employed Dr. Coxe, who found him labouring under inexpressible anguish in the abdomen; obstinate constipation, with frequent and violent

nausea and vomiting. He was bled to the amount of forty
ounces at once, and took calomel and opium, which were rejected. He then took calomel, opium, and sacch. saturn. on
one occasion, and three doses of Epsom salts subsequently;
fomentations of cold water applied to the abdomen afforded
great relief from pain. On the 14th his bowels opened, and
he discharged, in frequent stools, large quantities of a black
watery fæcal matter, highly offensive. His stomach continued so irritable, as not to retain any thing except for a few
moments. On the fifteenth, in the morning, his pain eeased;
but the stomach and bowels continuing disordered, he died
in the afternoon.

This day at 12 M. we examined him, and found as follows:

The abdominal muscles were drawn inwards towards the
spine; and the parietes of the abdomen, when struck, indicated the presence of a smaller quantity of gas than usual,
in the hollow viscera.

Liver healthy, but of a yellowish tinge, the pori biliarii
were occupied with bile, and had their parietes dyed by it.
Gall bladder empty and contracted, containing only a few
drops of bile.

Spleen healthy and about three inches in length. Pancreas healthy.

The stomach contained a pint of gas, the mucous coat
was covered with a layer of viscid mucus, coloured yellow
by bile. On removing this lamina, only a slight vascular
injection was seen; a patch an inch in diameter, of small
ecchymosed spots existed near the lesser curvature. There
were here and there, at distant intervals, other small dots of
blood; but the general complexion of the mucous coat was
of a dingy or yellowish white, like old ivory. The mucous
coat was generally so soft, that it could be torn off by
scraping with the thumb nail, and then came away in a pulpy state, instead of in strips. In the left extremity it was so
soft as to suffer abrasion from much slighter causes than
scratching with the nail.

The duodenum and jejunum were internally of a yellow colour, from being stained by their contents, which were bile and mucus mixed. The ileum was occupied by a small quantity of green purulent matter, formed of, probably, the same substances; the colour of the bile having been altered, perhaps, by some acid fomentation or secretion there. The contents of the colon, which were merely enough to smear its surface, were the same as those of the jejunum.

The great intestine was collapsed, and in the highest possible state of irritation on its internal coat; which was of the colour of coagulated venous blood, from the quantity of blood deposited in the substance of this coat. This appearance was produced as follows.—At the base of each of the rugæ, or small folds of the mucous coat, there had been a deposite of serum in the cellular coat; which thickened it, and caused the folds to project in the form of pendulous tumours into the cavity of the gut These tumours were blackened on the surface by the quantity of blood infiltrated as aforesaid, in the substance of the mucous coat covering them. The gut had thus the appearance of a beginning mortification, as in the highest forms of dysentery. This condition of purple tumours prevailed almost universally at the caput coli, forming nearly the entire surface there, and for some inches upwards: it then decreased gradually in the transverse colon, and vanished in the sigmoid flexure.

The muciparous glands of the colon studded its whole surface where this violent hæmorrhagic irritation prevailed, and were very conspicuous in the intestines between the purple tumours: they were for the most part only two or three lines or less from one another, and projected into the cavity of the gut; their size was about half a line, as it is in cholera infantum. I did not perceive any ulceration in them; the disease being, perhaps, in too early a stage for that. They were also conspicuous in the inferior six inches of the ileum.

Perhaps the best general description which could be given

of the condition of the internal coat of the large intestine would be to represent it as having its whole surface in the region indicated, covered with tumours, resembling very accurately in colour and configuration those of the bleeding piles, which, it is generally known, have a broad base, and are of dark purple colour.

The peritoneal surface of all the abdominal viscera had a yellow tinge from the bile. The kidneys and bladder were healthy.

The semi-lunar ganglion of the sympathetic was white, firm, and healthy.

The viscera of the thorax were healthy, excepting some slight old pleuritic adhesions.

Foreign matters discharged at the Umbilicus.

July, 18*th*, 1824.—A girl aged sixteen, the daughter of a farmer, near Reading, had suffered for some time violent pains in the stomach, and cramps in the legs; and had never menstruated. A few months ago she began to discharge at the umbilicus, pieces of aliment consisting in boiled beef, ham, white of eggs cooked, bits of tendon. These matters were discharged at intervals, having been passed through a fistulous orifice, which formed when the first attack commenced. Commonly this orifice is too small to admit a probe; but when any of the above articles are to be discharged, the orifice ulcerates and enlarges itself sufficiently for the purpose. A bleeding to the amount of half an ounce, occurs in two or three days afterwards, and then the orifice is reduced to its usual size.

No fæces have ever made their appearance at this orifice, and the pieces discharged have not the appearance of mastication or solution by digestion.

I have not myself seen the patient, but the circumstances were narrated to me by a medical attendant, who brought with him five ounces of these materials, with the view of obtaining my opinion in the case, as several very ridiculous notions had been propagated about it.

It is difficult to afford a satisfactory solution of these phenomena; yet one may hazard a conjecture, that, at an early period of life, perhaps during infancy, the individual, being fed on these articles, they were for the want of mastication, passed undigested from the stomach into the intestinal canal, and lodged permanently in some of the cells of the colon. That becoming surrounded by a cyst, an effort is now making to discharge them from the cyst, by ulceration through the umbilicus.

About the same time, I examined for Dr. Samuel Tucker, a female, in Third Street, who had previously discharged gall stones at the umbilicus, on several occasions. The channel, however, whatever it might have been originally, had left no traces which were evident, either by adhesion or fistulous communication.

Inflammatory Intus-susception of Intestines.

The daughter of Mr. Jno. N., aged two years, on Monday afternoon, the 30th of December, 1823, fell down the kitchen stairs four steps. The servant girl hearing her cries, came speedily down to her aid; the way being dark, she passed over the child without seeing her, but is not conscious of having touched her. The child, after recovering from the agitation of her fall, resumed her play, ate supper, and went to bed apparently in good health. At 12 o'clock at night, she became unwell and restless. A dose of calomel was given, which produced a stool on Wednesday morning, and another on Thursday evening. She began now, as far as she was able, to complain of pain in the front of the right iliac region near the hypogastric. Dr. Otto being sent for, gave cathartics, bled, leeched the abdomen; and blistered her head,

in the course of Wednesday, and Thursday, from an apprehension of hydrocephalus.

Dr. Physick was consulted on January 3d. The symptoms were constipation since Thursday evening; medicine
and aliment rejected from the stomach, swelling in the right
side, and fracture of a rib. It appeared to him to be a contusion of the canal, and obstruction of it: he advised to desist
from any thing, and leave it to nature.

The child died on Saturday morning, at 4 o'clock. On examination in the afternoon of that day, an intus-susception of
the intestinum ileum was found. It was about three inches
long, and almost in a state of gangrene. The intestine,
above, much distended with wind, but below, contracted to
eight lines in diameter, and empty. No ecchymosis of parietes of abdomen, or other mark of injury about it. *Query*.
Was the disease produced by the fall, or was it a mere coincidence?

*A Case of Hernia, attended with Death, from the Sac
having been lacerated at its Orifice, so as to form a
loop hole which produced Strangulation of the Intestine, by the escape of the latter through it.*

John C., aged forty, of a good habit of body, (pump
maker, in Fitzwater street,) had suffered for five years, from
inguinal rupture on the left side, owing to violence. Had
neglected the use of a truss all that time. On Monday, at
6 P M., January 30th, 1826, was taken with symptoms of
strangulation.

I saw him on Tuesday afternoon, in company with his
physician, Dr. Neill. In the mean time, 6 ounces of castor
oil, the warm bath, bleeding to the amount of 40 ounces,
had been all fruitlessly resorted to. I found a protrusion,
at the internal ring, apparently of intestine, reaching in the
scrotum down to the testicle. By a proper position, I suc-

ceeded after a while in replacing the protuded bowel; the local pain in the groin was thereby relieved, but no stools followed. Injections were then administered. The night was spent somewhat restlessly, and without stools.

February 1st, at 10 o'clock A. M., the rupture had returned, tension of the abdomen very great; vomiting. A tobacco suppository, introduced into rectum. At 4 P. M. no relief, protrusion still existing, I then operated as follows:

Beginning the incision an inch from the upper angle of the external ring, towards the spine of the ileum, it was continued through the skin to the lower end of the tumour; a corresponding incision, was made through the subjacent adeps. The tunica vaginalis communis being thus exposed, was divided, with the assistance of the forceps, to the same extent: a single fasciculus only of the cremaster was visible. The hernial sac next came into view, which, being punctured below, was, with the aid of the director and blunt pointed bistoury, divided to the external ring. A couple of drachms of dark coloured scrum was contained within the sac. The protruded portion was a mass of omentum, the size of four fingers; by passing the finger up to the internal ring, a bit of intestine seemed to be engaged in it, which was replaced without difficulty. The omentum, though its blood vessels were turgid, was not mortified, and by a slight dilatation of the external ring, I succeeded in returning it.

On passing my fore finger into the abdomen, through the neck of the sac, on the iliac side of the latter, a process was felt, corresponding with the semi-lunar process of peritoneum, from the side of the bladder to the umbilicus.

I therefore concluded, with the fullest assurance of certainty in the indication, that the disease was ventro inguinal hernia; and supposed that the symptoms of strangulation would now be entirely relieved. The epigastric artery could not be felt, as the tension of the abdomen was extreme. In order to prevent a repetition of the hernial protrusion, a truss was applied, after dressing the wound as usual.

At 9 oclock, P. M., the symptoms continued to progress: stercoraceous vomiting; a small discharge, two ounces, of stercoraceous matter through rectum.   An enema of water lb. iss. Epsom salts 3 ounces, administered. February 2d, the symptoms still progressing, the patient died about 11 A. M.

February 3d. Post mortem examination.—The upper part of the jejunum was distended with flatus and thin fæces, to such a degree, that it looked like the colon. A loop eighteen inches in length, of the lower end of the jejunum, was found bridled, strangulated, and mortified, in a ring of five-eighths of an inch in diameter.   This ring belonged to a process of peritoneum, that came from the internal abdominal ring; and was found drawn two or three inches above the latter, towards the lumbar region.

The strangulated intestine was therefore fairly in the cavity of the abdomen.   In front of this process of peritoneum, was the abdominal orifice of the neck of the hernial sac, through which the omentum had descended.   The hernia being on the left side, the formerly prolapsed omentum, now reposed in the left iliac region.

The failure of the operation, arose from the annular stricture of the intestine, which was drawn so high up into the abdomen, that the finger not being able to reach it, no suspicion was entertained of its existence; all the symptoms being referred to the strangulated omentum.   Again, such was the confusion in the position of the intestines, from their swollen state, that even when the abdomen was fairly laid open, in the post mort. examination, it required several minutes of close examination, by sliding the intestines through the fingers, before it became clear what was the real nature of the malady.   It would therefore have been impossible for the single finger, introduced into the abdomen during life, to have detected the actual condition of the parts, even if it could have reached the point of strangulation.

The ring which produced the stricture I supposed was originally the orifice of the hernial sac; which sac became permanent by the intestine getting into it, and remaining there. It is also probable that the intestine, in the progress of time, or suddenly from some cause, drew the neck of the sac into the left lumbar region. That while this state was existing, some violence applied to the stretched neck of the sac, caused it to tear in front. That through this laceration the omentum descended into the scrotum, and the hernial sac contained in it. That previously to this step, the intestinal loop at its lower part, had escaped through the lacerated orifice, and by that means encircled itself inextricably. There was no appearance of the laceration having been a recent affair; no jagged edges: on the contrary, the latter were rounded, indicating a duration of several weeks at least. At the period of operation, there were then two places of strangulation, the annular portion of peritoneum for the bowel, and the internal abdominal ring for the abdomen. The latter was relieved, the first not.

The process of peritoneum, belonging to the annular stricture, deluded me into a belief of the disease; that is, the omental protrusion, having been ventro inguinal, while in fact it was inguinal.

Inguinal Hernia.—A case of successive Strangulation of the greater part of the small Intestinal Canal.

Joseph Clarke, aged about 55 years, was admitted into the Alms House on Saturday, January 7th, 1825, between one and two o'clock P. M. He then had an enormous hernial tumour hanging between his thighs, almost as far as the knees, and extremely painful. He was very restless,—the countenance expressed a great deal of anxiety, accompanied with irritability of stomach and inclination to vomit; great thirst with distinct but rather feeble pulse and cool skin. The swelling was tense and hard, but occasioned little or no pain on handling. There was much tenderness over the abdomen, which was increased on pressure. The patient stated he had been afflicted with the complaint about twenty years;

that it frequently descended, but was easily reduced; that it
was much larger at the present time than it ever had been,
and his sufferings much greater. He said it came down
about two o'clock the same morning, attended with intolerable pain. He confessed he was addicted to drink spirituous
liquors freely, and had been intoxicated the preceding day
and night. A very gentle attempt was made to return the
contents of the tumour; but being of no avail, a large and
stimulating enema was administered. Between four and five
o'clock the injection had operated several times copiously,
and the swelling was found considerably relaxed: in other
respects the patient the same. An attempt was made at re-
duction by the taxis; in a few minutes a portion of the contents passed up with the usual guggling noise: by degrees,
more and more was gradually replaced. The patient was
now attacked with vomiting, and discharged large quantities of water from the stomach, which he had drank from
time to time. When about two thirds of the contents of the
sac had been returned in the cavity of the abdomen, the patient was unexpectedly seized with a slight convulsion, and,
to our surprise, expired almost instantly. By the contraction of the abdominal muscles during the fit, the intestines
were again forced down into the sac. It may be observed
that the abdominal ring appeared to be so large and free as
to admit two or three fingers. The patient was perfectly
sensible till the convulsion came on, and went to the close
stool a few minutes before he expired.

Dissection.—The different fasciæ were unusually distinct
and extremely well marked; the fibres of the cremaster muscle were apparently absorbed, as no traces of them could
be discovered: the vessels composing the spermatic cord
were found lying on the outer side of the sac. On dividing
the peritoneal sac, a large quantity of bloody serum escaped,
and numerous folds amounting, to nearly one half of the entire length of the small intestine protruded; one portion of
them was of a dark brown or chocolate colour: the remain-

der of a bright scarlet, resembling the most successful artificial injection, and, on minute inspection, had very much
the appearance of ecchymosis succeeding to an injury inflicted on the surface of the body. The greater portion of
the small intestines in the cavity of the abdomen was also
engorged, but diminished in intensity of colour in proportion
as they receded from the herniac sac. The same kind of
bloody effusion was found in the cavity of the intestine as
observed in the sac. No part of the intestine was mortified.

Inguinal Hernia with a double Sac.

A white male subject, aged sixty, was examined by me,
Dec. 10th, 1827. He had on both sides inguinal rupture.
On the right, the head of colon and end of ileum, were in
the sac; the cavity of the latter was completely obliterated
by an old universal adhesion between the gut and the sac. In
attempting to open the latter from below, I unavoidably cut
into the cœcum. The appendiculæ vermiformis adhered
vertically to the anterior parietes of the sac, and in slitting
up the latter it was inadvertently cut. On the left side the
sac was empty, but *double, by one sac protruding into
another, like a double night-cap.* On the outer face of the
spermatic chord, there was a series of large lumps of fat,
which, when examined through the skin, gave the sensation
of an omental protrusion.

In another subject in whom there was a large scrotal hernia as well as in this: on a careful examination, I could not
perceive any thickening in the sac. My impression is, that
the peritoneum simply slides, in such cases, from one point
to another, as in distentions of the bladder and uterus.

Enlarged and suppurated Ovarium.

This case is explained by the following letter from the
physician Dr. O. H. Taylor, who attended: the preparation
is deposited in the Anatomical Museum.

" On the 26th of January, I was called to visit A. Brown, aged 35 years, who had for the last four or five years been suffering (as was supposed) from gradually increasing dropsical symptoms. The previous history of the case, as detailed by the patient, was somewhat singular. She had been under the direction of some respectable physicians of this city, by whom she had been treated for ascites. During the treatment, recourse was had to paracentesis abdominis, which was attended with a discharge of merely a small quantity of blood and serum. She was subsequently placed in the Hospital, and there underwent the same operation, with a similar result. From these circumstances, it was considered as a case of encysted dropsy, and treated accordingly.

" At the time of my first visit, she was labouring under a harsh cough, accompanied with mucous expectoration, together with great dyspnœa, particularly on motion. Much difficulty was experienced in lying in the recumbent posture; so much so, as to render it necessary to prop her up in bed. The pulse was weak and somewhat irregular, and she complained much of flatulency and constipation. Her abdomen was unusually large, presenting the appearance of a person labouring under ascitis: there was also some œdema of the lower extremities. Fluctuation was very indistinct.

" In this urgent state, I ventured to encourage some hope of relief by the use of purgatives of gamboge and super-tartrite of potash· inasmuch as the state of the bowels indicated their employment as an incipient treatment. From the operation of the first purgative, she was soon able to lie in a horizontal position, and to walk across the room. The purgatives were continued for a day or two longer, apparently with much advantage. Diuretics were exhibited for a few days, and a copious diuresis was the consequence.

" On the 31st of January, the patient was submitted to the care of my friend Dr. Wiltbank, who deemed it proper

from the then existing symptoms, to administer tonic remedies, which were persisted in until her death; which unexpectedly took place on the 3rd of February.   From the
interesting history of the case, we were particularly desirous of making a post mortem examination, which was accordingly proposed and submitted to.   We commenced the
dissection by making a longitudinal incision along the whole
course of the linea alba.   In the first place, the anterior
part of the abdomen presented an unusual degree of thickness, at least two inches: although the skin and adipose substance appeared very thin.   Upon continuing the dissection still farther, we were considerably surprised at the
ejection of a large stream of genuine pus.   The unexpected
and sudden discharge of this immense quantity of purulent
matter, induced us to apply for aid from some more experienced persons; in consequence of which, Drs. Horner
and Hodge were called upon, and politely gave their services.

"The whole of the pus being discharged, which reached
to the almost incredible amount of four gallons, we proceeded to the examination of the tumour containing it.
This was ascertained to be an immense hollow tumour, filling the whole abdomen, and protruding the intestines, liver, &c. very high within the cavity of the ribs.   On being separated from its adhesions to the surrounding parts,
the tumour was discovered to be the right ovarium.   The
vascularity of the tumour was remarkable, arteries and
veins, as might have been conjectured, running in every
direction.   Its weight upon examination, after being emptied of its contents, was seventeen pounds.   After having
made an examination of the ovarium, our attention was
next directed to the state of the uterus, which, contrary to
our expectation, presented a perfectly natural and healthy
appearance; the other contents of the abdomen were found,
with the exception of some adhesions and thickening of
the coats of the intestines. in a natural state.''

Extra-uterine Fœtus.

In June 1823, I was called to execute for Drs. Physick and James, the dissection of Mrs. B., under the following circumstances. On a former occasion, she had borne a fine healthy child. This was followed by another pregnancy, in which the symptoms of gestation had nothing unusual, and at the expiration of nine months, she was seized with the pains of parturition. The practitioner who attended her, states that membranes presented, waters were discharged, and an organized mass resembling the placenta was expelled, but no fœtus.

The symptoms of parturition then went off, and her health recruited much, but a large tumour was left in the lower part of the abdomen on the right side, giving indistinctly, the feel of a head. By alternate pressure on the sides of the abdomen, it could be made to move sensibly. After a while her health began to decline, she was seized with vomiting and diarrhœa, and finally died about twelve months after this pseudo-parturition.

Autopsy.—A cyst was found in the pelvis and hypogastric region, containing a fœtus of about the size of one of six months. The head of the fœtus was in the pelvis, between the rectum and the uterus; the buttocks were in the right side of the hypogastric region; the umbilical cord was about six inches long, detached at its placental extremity, and very small. The placenta itself was about three inches in diameter, and consisted in a thin growth of detached flocculent masses, which sprang from the parietes of the sac. They resembled very much the filamentous flocculent masses into which a common placenta is reduced by maceration, but were not near so thick or abundant. This condition may indeed have been produced by the species of maceration, to which the structure was exposed by a duration of twelve months. I could find but one umbilical artery running to these remains of a placenta.

The cyst, seemed to have been formed originally on the posterior face of the broad ligament of the uterus; and extended itself along the posterior surface of the uterus itself, and of the rectum; the latter being forced much to the left side of the pelvis The cyst appeared to have ascended subsequently, and had adhered to the anterior parietes of the abdomen, to the contiguous convolutions of small intestines, to the transverse colon, and to the omentum.   There was a fistulous communication between the lower part of the cyst and the rectum.

The fœtus was in a semi-putrescent state, and horribly offensive; this condition, having been generated perhaps by the admission of air to it, through the fistulous opening of the rectum.   The more prominent parts of the fœtus, as the vertex, the spine, the great trochanters, and some other portions were denuded down to the bones, by a process of ulceration, or absorption perhaps from the parietes of the sac.

The uterus presented no where the mark of a cicatrix, which deficiency with the vestiges of placenta in the sac, would oppose the idea of the fœtus having escaped, by rupture of the parietes of the uterus, at the time of parturition, into the abdomen.   The neck of the uterus was two inches long, and its cavity straighter than usual.

Lumbar Abscess attended with Artificial Anus in the Groin.

James Culberton, a carter, aged twenty-four years, of a very strong and athletic constitution, in consequence of some injury or strain received in the prosecution of his business in August, 1814, felt a severe pain arise in the lumbar and iliac regions, which was followed with fever and the common symptoms of inflammation.

Bleeding, purging, and other means usually resorted to on such occasions were adopted, without any other effect than that of alleviating in some measure the intensity of the attack. From the inadequacy of the remedies to produce discussion, suppuration took place; the matter formed, passed out under Poupart's ligament, and produced a prominent and fluctuating tumour, a little below it. This tumour was opened with a lancet, and a considerable quantity of pus discharged. With little subsequent attention the wound got well, and the energies of the patient's constitution seemed to have restored him, in a short time, to his ordinary state of health.

In the middle of the next winter, from being exposed to a snow storm, he caught cold;—the place in the groin which had been occupied by the tumour and in the vicinity of the incision became heated, painful, red, and tumefied;— suppuration followed, and a spontaneous opening was made, through which pus, mixed with feculent matter, was discharged. Doubts might have been entertained at this time in regard to the real nature of the feculent discharge: but the patient having eaten some rice shortly before, it so happened that a few grains of it passed undigested through the opening. This accident demonstrated that a connexion existed between the intestinal canal and the orifice in the thigh.

A number of perplexing considerations grew out of this circumstance: 1st, it was thought that a femoral hernia, lying under the tumour, might have been wounded by the plunge of the lancet; but upon a rigid scrutiny into the case, it appeared, that the patient had never in his life been affected with any of its symptoms; and a local examination of the part itself at the time, indicated nothing of the kind. It, however, was considered possible for it to have had a temporary existence, and to have been afterwards returned by the voluntary action of the bowels, assisted by the position of the patient. 2d. If the primitive inflammation in the lumbar and right iliac regions had invaded the intestinal canal, and by the process of adhesion to it and of ulceration into its cavity, established a communication, it was still a desideratum to ascertain what portion of the bowels was thus affected

In ten days this orifice healed, and continued so till April 1815, a period of three months   At the expiration of this time another inflammation about the orifice took place, followed by suppuration and ulceration, fæces were again discharged for ten days along with the pus; the parts then healed, and continued so till February, 1817.   During this interval his health became sufficiently good to induce the patient to consider himself exempt from the chance of similar attacks; but these hopes were destroyed about the middle of February, by a recurrence of the inflammation in the thigh, with discharge of fæces.

Between this date and the following August four fresh attacks supervened; after that he suffered from them every three or four weeks till December   It is now necessary to observe, that in the recent recurrences of the disease, the old orifice, which had been situated not far from the anterior superior spinous process of the ilium, remained cicatrized, and a new one formed nearer the pubes. Also that the inflammation which had been the precursor in every instance of the discharge of fæces, was not attended latterly with suppuration; but that the integuments affected by it, being protruded by the accumulation of fæces, burst and gave vent to them. The inflammation then subsided and the part healed.   It was therefore apparent that the fæces occasioned the inflammation in the groin   The inflammation had, during this time, extended itself into the contiguous parts; and amongst others, affected the inner side of the thigh, two thirds of the way down to the knee.

The sequel of the case, is as follows: In December, 1817, Dr. Gebbard the attending physician first saw it.   The patient was then labouring under a violent symptomatic fever; the most rigid antiphlogistic plan was pursued, such as bleeding, low diet, refrigerants, &c. By these means he was relieved from the constitutional affection.   The subsequent exhibition of bark seemed to strengthen him, and to diminish the intensity of succeeding paroxysms, which took place in

connexion with the bursting of fæces through his thigh, every two or three weeks till his death.

In February, 1820, he became anasarcous and continued so
until the middle of July; he was then seized with a sore
throat, which in its sensations of pain was extended along
the œsophagus into the stomach.   The sensibility of those
parts became so highly excited, that the swallowing of such
bland fluids as flax-seed tea, milk and water, &c. was excruciating.   Examination showed the pharynx and palate inflamed, but no swelling of the tonsils, gargles being ineffec-
tually exhibited, the application of a blister on the throat
relieved him.   The dropsical affection began to disappear simultaneously with the commencement of the sore throat;
and by the time the latter was cured, the former had subsided entirely.   A diarrhœa had attended the dropsical affection from its beginning—his health sunk apace under its
influence, notwithstanding the continuance of a good appetite.   The exhibition of medicines suppressed the discharge
per anum, but produced no effect on that through the artificial opening.   Wasted by this continual drain from the alimentary canal, he at length died on August 15th, 1820.

Autopsy.—The appearance of the abdominal viscera generally healthy. The psoas magnus and iliacus internus muscles,
which were considered to be the seat of the primary affection,
had lost entirely their muscular fibres, were diminished in size,
somewhat indurated, and converted into a ligamentous-like
mass.   The head of the colon, besides being bound down to
the right iliac region by the usual reflection of peritoneum,
had contracted an extensive adhesion to the contiguous muscles.
The peritoneum, at the part alluded to, seemed unaffected by
disease.   It is known, that the colon at its head, is covered
only in two thirds of its circumference, and that anteriorly,
by the peritoneum; the rest of this portion of the gut being in
contact with the iliacus internus muscle, and connected to it
in health by loose cellular substance.   The latter part of
this intestine had united itself to the iliacus muscle by a

preternatural adhesion, which was strong and so compact as to produce a continuity of substance with the muscle itself. At this place, about an inch and a half above the valve of the colon, two orifices existed through the parietes of the gut; each large enough to admit a finger; these orifices communicated with one fistula of the same size, in the centre of the iliacus internus. The fistula passed out of the abdomen, and continued in the centre of this muscle, till it had got beyond Poupart's ligament; it then became superficial, and terminated in the orifice of the groin alluded to.

A prosecution of the dissection exhibited another fistula arising from the lower termination of the first, and extending downwards six inches, parallel, or nearly so, with the femoral vessels. It was not known whether this fistula had arisen at the commencement of the disease, or from the aggravation of the local inflammation which took place about August, 1817. Its connexion with the other was subsequently demonstrated by the ability of the patient, to discharge fæces from the external orifice, by pressing along the course of the adductor muscles from below, upward. The femoral artery and vein were imbedded as far as the place where they perforate the tendon of the triceps adductor, in a ligamentous sheath, which, I presume, had been fabricated in order to protect them from the extension of the disease in their vicinity. The parietes of each fistula were so thick and perfect, that they might have been with ordinary facility dissected from the contiguous parts, and preserved in their membranous form. The vertebræ of the loins were in a healthy condition.

This case I believe to have been unusual, in regard to the communication established between the abscess, situated in the iliacus internus and psoas magnus muscle, and the cavity of the colon: and it may, perhaps, prove serviceable, by calling in similar cases the attention of the practitioner to the cause of a series of symptoms, which embarrassed exceedingly all the medical gentlemen who were consulted

about it.   It is also a good example of the species of lumbar abscess, which, in the language of Mr. Abernethy, pro-
ceeds from phlegmonoid inflammation in the part.   The circumstance is familiar to most surgeons, that there are two
species of lumbar abscess; the one preceded by pain, tumefaction, increased heat, throbbing and a hurried circulation
of blood through the loins, and a secretion of coagulating
lymph, by which the parts are united to each other, and the
boundaries of the abscess circumscribed, constituting by all
these symptoms common inflammation; the other species
belongs to chronic abscesses, in which collections of matter
take place without any evident act of inflammation.

In these latter, the surrounding parts remain in a great degree unaffected by the diseased action; the purulent discharge
commences from very small beginnings, increases gradually,
accumulates indefinitely, its boundaries are soft and unattended with thickening, affording but little impediment to
its gravitation, and the matter, therefore, passes from one
part to another, appearing sometimes in the groin, sometimes
just above the knee, and occasionally in the perinæum, giving
occasion by this change of place, to the distinction which Mr.
Hunter has made between abscess *in a part, and of a part.*

This last form of the disease, supposed to depend
on a scrofulous habit, has its peculiar mode of treatment,
which is very satisfactorily illustrated in Mr. Abernethy's
Surgical Observations, but the former, differing essentially
from it, and partaking largely of the attributes of common
inflammation, has its remedial indications accordingly.   The
case just recounted, seems to me from the primary symptoms, and from the alteration of structure in the parts affected, to have been one of phlegmonoid inflammation, and
would have been cured by the treatment, had not the diseased action extended itself through the parietes of the colon;
and by that means, produced a constant evacuation of fæces
into the cavity of the abscess, which eventuated in incurable
fistula and artificial anus.

CHAPTER XIII.

IRRITATIONS OF THE PULMONARY TISSUE.

THE lungs, in climates subject to frequent mutations of temperature and moisture, and in seasons presenting these varieties, are much disposed to the various forms of irritation, from an active pneumony to the slow process of a consumption. Hence we find them in a pathological state quite as often, as any other tissue of the body.

There are some appearances of the lungs which are merely cadavarous, being the effects either of the last struggles of life and the debility preceding them, or of the changes subsequent to death. As these appearances may be very readily mistaken by the inexperienced pathologist for disease, it is of some consequence to warn him of them, especially as they mimic very serious affections.

Whoever has examined with attention the lungs at the several periods of life, must have been much struck with the contrast of their appearance and condition, between infancy and old age. In the first, they are of a uniform pink colour, and retain it for some years. In the progress of life, as the individual advances to puberty, this pink is converted into a very light gray; which from that time forward becomes darker and darker, until it is changed into an iron gray. This change of colour is produced by a deposite of a black pigment, on the surface of the lungs beneath the pleura, and in the intertices between their lobules and cells. It penetrates throughout the thickness of the lung, and not unfrequently is deposited so superficially on its cells, that it is excreted and coughed up with the common mucus. It

is deposited also in the lymphatic glands, on the trachea
and bronchia; and makes them jet black. Its principal line
of deposite is along the intertices between the lobules, and
in their connecting cellular substance; hence the surface of
the lung is divided into mathematical figures of various
sizes and forms, lozenge shape, squares, triangles, and so
on.   The black discoloration now described, which has
nothing unhealthy or uncommon in it, is worthy of recollection, because it may be confounded with melanosis; a
cancerous tumour, resembling a black bronchial gland,.
sometimes found in the lung, but much more commonly
elsewhere;* and is distinguished with some difficulty from
it.   M. Laennec says that the most satisfactory mode of
distinguishing such tumours is, by rubbing the skin with
them, and permitting the part to dry. The colour from the
gland is more permanent than the other, and will remain
for some days in spite of the attempts to remove it.   Moreover, the bronchial gland contains a great quantity of car-
bon and hydrogen; principles which do not exist in mela-
noses, as they are composed almost entirely of albumen,
and of a peculiar unknown colouring principle.

In extreme old age, the pigment of the lung rather diminishes again, and another peculiarity is presented.   The
lung becomes attenuated in the parietes of its air cells, and
its whole volume of matter is so much less, that it is evidently much lighter.   The elasticity of its tissue being destroyed, it collapses completely under atmospheric pressure
on the opening of the thorax, and recedes so as not to occupy more than one third of the cavity of the pleura.   M.
Laennec† has happily compared this state of it to the difference between fine muslin and coarse. It appears, also,
that the calibre of the vessels is contracted in old age; that
they are more destitute of blood (ex-sangues) and feel much
more dry than at other periods of life.

* Laennec, De l'Auscultation, vol. ii. p. 32.
† Op cit. vol. ii. p. 282

Another purely cadavarous condition of the lung liable to be mistaken for disease; and of very common occurrence; is the bloody engorgement at its root, and in its posterior part. If individuals have died from a chronic affection where the marasmus is considerable, the diminution of the general mass of blood renders this engorgement inconsiderable, and rather of a light red, but yet it is sufficiently evident. On the contrary, if they have died in a full habit of body, the quantity of blood there accumulated and infiltrated into the substance of the lungs is so great: that the lungs have a deep violet colour, approaching here and there in spots to a blackness; which might and has been mistaken for mortification, and reported as such in courts of justice.[*] The blood thus collected, is in a half clotted state, and when putrefaction has commenced, the lung is easily squeezed into a dark pulpy mass· especially when the infiltration has commenced before death, and has been joined to that form of peripneumony, which· supervening where the agonies of dying have been somewhat protracted, manifests itself by distinct points of hepatization.[†]

In individuals who have died from dropsy, the posterior part of the lungs contains, frequently, a frothy serosity, slightly tinged with blood; and strongly resembles the first state of pneumony, or of œdema of the lung. It is to be distinguished from the two latter, by their being found in various situations of the lung; whereas the serous engorgement, like the bloody, is always in the most depending parts. In order to settle the question about the collection of blood, in the most depending part of the lung, being a cadavarous condition merely, Bichat directed patients to be fixed in different positions immediately after death, and he always found the blood of the lungs subsiding to the lowest point; but as the common position of dead bodies is

[*] Laennee, Op. Cit. vol i. p. 282   [†] Id. 479.

on their back, this usage determines the usual congestion and infiltration of the lungs, at their back part. The
same experiment has been repeated by Laennec,* with
similar results; and to them he has added the observation,
that the sanguineous or serous engorgement of the back
of the lungs, often commences some hours before death:
which accounts for the oppression of respiration in the dying, even when they have not been afflicted with disease of
the lungs, during the progress of their malady.

Bichat's explanation of this is,† that as the lungs alone
receive all the blood of the body: when their strength diminishes, the blood stagnates there, and accumulates in
such a way, that according to the state of their strength in
the last moments, whatever may have been the malady,
they are more or less heavy, more or less filled with fluids.

Having thus pointed out the more common cadavarous
appearances of the lungs, with the view of drawing the
distinction between them and the alterations which are really pathological, I proceed to speak of the latter. The chief
of them are hypertrophy, atrophy, emphysema, œdema,
pneumony, and phthisis. of these, the two last are by far
the most common.

Hypertrophy of the Lungs

Is manifested by an augmentation of their volume, and an
increase in the consistency of their tissue. It is very seldom exhibited by both lungs at once, but is more commonly seen on one side only; in cases where accident or disease of some duration, as empyema, has produced a collapsed
and permanent atrophy of the lung on the other side. The
lung here takes on an increase of vitality and energy, as well
as of volume, in order to execute its double task. Under
this view the condition can scarcely be regarded as a disease,

---

* Laennec, vol 1. p 284   † Anat. Gen. vol II p. 65.

and is similar to what occurs under corresponding circumstances in other double organs, as the kidneys, the testicles, and the mammæ, when one has been destroyed.

It would appear indeed from the report of M. Laennec,[*] that any cause rendering one lung useless for a few months, will be productive of an increased organic development of the other lung. He met with it in one case where empyema had prevailed for six months only, being caused by a softened tuberculous mass rupturing its way into the pleura, and producing inflammation there. It is the result also of hydro-thorax, of the collapse of the chest following severe pleurisies and extensive pulmonary excavations; and of that condition of the pleura called pneumo-thorax, which is a collection of gas of some kind in it.

It is more than probable, though extremely difficult to prove by inspection, owing to the minuteness of the object; that each air cell in hypertrophy of the lung is enlarged, and its parietes thickened. The texture of the lung becomes more firm and elastic, and it, instead of subsiding on the opening of the thorax, remains more stationary than usual; and, in some cases, escapes upon the removal of the sternum, as if it had been confined in a cavity too small for it. The mediastinum, in these cases, is generally pushed from the middle line of the thorax over towards the side of the collapsed lung, and the heart consequently also. In a subject brought to our dissecting-rooms many years ago, (about 1818,) where empyema prevailed on one side, the thorax was unusually prominent and rounded upon the other side, owing to this unusual evolution of the sound lung.

Atrophy of the Lung.

In ordinary cases of general emaciation of the body, the lung is one of those organs whose size and condition are not

[*] Id. vol. i. p. 285.

sensibly affected; its atrophy, therefore, is more immediately
the result of causes acting locally upon the lung itself, as
pressure from without as just stated, from effusions of different kinds into the cavity of the pleura; and the developement of diseased masses within its substance.

In several of these cases of atrophy of the lung, which I
have examined after death, the lung was pushed to the back
of the thorax, was lying in a state of perfect collapse along
the sides of the dorsal vertebræ, and reduced to a thin flat
cake, having a hard fleshy feel.   Confined to this restrained
position for some time, it loses its permeability and power
of expansion, so that in inspirations, only a very small quantity of air is introduced into it.   Another great obstacle to
its dilatation, probably the most important and effectual one
is, that the coating of coagulable lymph with which it is
covered, becomes converted into a strong organized membrane of a somewhat fibrous structure, which will not yield
to the expansive tendency of the lung.   This factitious membrane which covers the lung, also modifies very sensibly the
shape of the thorax.   For, when the absorption of the effused
fluid begins, as the dilatation of the lung does not keep pace
with it, the thorax is pressed in by the weight of the atmosphere acting on its surface; and it finally becomes flattened
on that side, or caved in, as is spoken in common language.
This depression of it is arrested at a certain point, and then
it remains stationary during the residue of life, the space between the lung and the ribs being filled up with pus. · This
constitutes a chronic form of empyema, which seems to be
perfectly consistent with general good health, and which, if
ascertained during life, it would be exceedingly improper to
interfere with by an operation; as no good could result, and
the constitution would be thrown into great disturbance, by a
new inflammation supervening on the pleura, from the admission of air.

In some cases it has happened that the pus of empyema
being entirely absorbed, the depression of the ribs, has

brought the factitious membrane on the lung, in contact
with that on the pleura covering the ribs; and an intimate
adhesion has followed, which has identified the two factitious
membranes and at the end of some months they have acquired the consistence and all the characters of a fibrous or
fibro cartilaginous production. *

The following dissection will illustrate what I may call a
dormant empyema, from its not awakening any symptoms
of an unpleasant kind in the system.   In May, 1822, I was
called upon to examine a boy aged fourteen at Mr. Hatt's
boarding-school in Market Street near Ninth, the leading
character of his last illness, had been pain in the abdomen
with fever.   His physicians were Drs. Chapman and Dewees.

We found nothing out of order, or in a diseased state in
the abdomen.   This is my note of the dissection, and, in
reflecting on it at the present day, I think it very probable from the symptoms, that there were some pathological
changes there; but I had not the light of information at that
time which enabled me to see them.   To our great surprise,
though there had been no indication of either an acute or
chronic thoracic disease, we yet found the left pleura filled
with well elaborated pus of a suitable colour and consistence;
and the corresponding lung reduced to a tubercle about the
size of the fist, with a small part collapsed and adhering along
the spine.

To account for this, it appeared upon inquiry, that this
young gentleman had a pleurisy in Paris two years before.
His general health had been subsequently re-established, and
he seemed like any other boy of the same age.   Though, at
the time of dissection, the state of the lung and of the pleura
seemed sufficient to account for death, and the difficulty was
the aberration of symptoms, yet I am now satisfied of the conclusion being erroneous.   I think it more probable that the
system had become accommodated to that state of the thorax,

* Laen. vol. ii. p. 121

and that if I had been a better pathologist, some more satisfactory cause of death would have been discovered.   I am
now fully convinced, that if an officious surgeon had opened
this pleura, to let out the pus; and had thrown in his detergent
washes, that a renewed inflammation, hectic fever, and
death would have followed from it.   The disease was evidently dormant and required no treatment.

The following case which occurred to me in the practice
of the Philadelphia Alms House, will illustrate the effect
upon the general health of a patient, when an opening is
made either artificially or naturally for the relief of the empyema.   It will also show, how careful a physician should
be in interfering with such collections of matter: unless the
patient be so distressed in his respiration, from the accumulation of pus; as to make its evacuation of primary importance
to the expansion of the opposite lung, so as to admit a sufficient volume of air.   In which case we substitute one evil
for another, a renewed inflammation, hectic fever and death
at a remote time; for that death which threatens to come instantly, without a mechanical relief, of the lung on the sound
side.

Philadelphia Alms House, May 4th, 1825.—Charles
Shaw, aged 28 years, was admitted a patient in this institution on the 25th of January, 1825, labouring under symptoms of pneumonic irritation, as cough, mucous expectoration,
difficult respiration, hectic fever, &c.   He stated, that some
months previously he was attacked by pleurisy, of unusual
violence, in the city of Lancaster, where he then resided;
which terminated by the formation of pus between the pleura pulmonalis and costalis.   On examination, a scirrhous
ulcer was discovered on the left side, about the sixth rib,
mid-way between the sternum and spine, through which a
small quantity of puriform matter was constantly issuing.
As the symptoms became daily more urgent and distress-

ing, and particularly the respiration, which was extremely
laborious; it was conjectured, that a large quantity of matter had formed in the left cavity of the thorax, and was prevented from escaping through the narrow and tortuous
opening, that with difficulty admitted a probe. Accordingly, about two weeks after the patient's admission, an opening was made in the direction of the sinus; and, as had been
anticipated, a quantity of puriform matter was discharged,
amounting to two pints at least. The respiration was immediately relieved, and in a little time his general health was
considerably improved. The wound was kept open by
means of a tent, which was occasionally removed to give
vent to the pus. After a while, however, the discharge
from the side became very much increased, with a return
of hectic accompanied with profuse night sweats, and great
emaciation: he was gradually exhausted, and expired on
the night of the third day of May. No local means were
resorted to, to arrest the discharge, till a few weeks before
his death, when stimulating injections were employed. At
this time, however, he was too much exhausted to derive
benefit from any kind of treatment.

On the dissection of Shaw, the left lung was found in a
collapsed state lying along side of the thoracic vertebræ,
and covered by a thick coat of coagulating lymph, or rather
by the same kind of membrane which lines an ancient fistula. This membrane was so strong, that no effort of the
lung at expansion could possibly have stretched it out. The
pleura costalis, was also in a state of chronic inflammation, and
much thickened. The left cavity of the thorax, was much
below its usual capaciousness, owing to the diminution of its
circumference, by the extreme depression of the ribs, and
the ascent of the diaphragm: it did not appear capable of
containing more than a quart of fluid, in addition to the collapsed lung.

From this case it would appear, that the natural cure of
empyema, where an opening exists for the discharge of pus

through the parietes of the thorax, is by a contraction of that side of the thorax from the circumference to the centre; and, as there is no tendency to heal it by granulations from the pleura, nature might, perhaps, finally obliterate the cavity by contracting it; but, unfortunately, the patient's health is generally exhausted, and he dies before this can be done.

In the case of Shaw the injections were of no use; neither could they possibly have 'been so, at any period of this disease; and their effect, being irritating, would of course increase a discharge already too profuse. A week before his death, I therefore ordered the injection to be discontinued, and also forbade that any means should be taken to get the pus out of the thorax, from a belief that the least irritating body applied to the pleura would be its own secretion. Notwithstanding this, not two gills of pus were found in the cavity after death.

While on the subject of empyema, I may state cursorily, that sometimes the tendency of the matter, from its excessive quantity, is to find its way outwardly through the parietes of the thorax, and it will be seen bulging out the intercostal spaces. I met with one case where it formed a large bag on the side, just over the lowest ribs; and, from the necessity of the patient for air, there could be no alternative for evacuating the matter by puncture.

In empyema and other effusions into the cavity of the thorax, where the quantity of fluid has been less considerable, and adhesions have occurred between the lungs and the sides; the primitive volume of the lung is never restored, although respiration be re-established in the most perfect manner.[*] This will account for the shortness of breath which persons thus circumstanced suffer, on undue exercise, or in ascending an eminence.

In addition to the collapse and atrophy of the lung, occasioned by pressure from a fluid in the pleura, tubercles de-

* Laennec, vol. i. p 287

veloping themselves in its tissue will produce the same degree of diminution in its respirable surface, by occupying the spaces of the air cells. In these cases, the air cells between the tubercles are frequently in a healthy state, and do not seem either compressed or pushed aside, but removed by a species of atrophy; and as the whole volume of the lung is not increased, but rather diminished, it is evident that the atrophy of the lung is equivalent to the aggregate quantity of the tubercles developed in its structure, which are sometimes very numerous, and of different sizes.

Emphysema of the Lungs.

Emphysema of the lungs is of two kinds, the one consists in the distention by air of the air cells of the lungs; and the other in a distention by air of the common cellular substance, holding the air cells and the lobules together. The characters of pulmonary emphysema have generally been taken from the last; but it appears from the observations of M. Laennec,[*] that the former is a very common condition with the asthmatic, though it has heretofore been supposed a rare complaint.

In emphysema of the air vesicles, they become much larger than usual, and much less uniform in their shape: some are the size of millet seed, and are by far the most numerous; others equal in volume a flax-seed; and others are of different gradations of size, up to that of a kidney bean. In the approximation to the latter size, it is probable, that several primitive cells have suffered a rupture of their partitions, and by that means concur to form a single large chamber; but, in some cases, they are evidently formed by the dilatation of a single one.

In the celebrated work of Dr. Baillie, on Morbid Anato-

* Laennec, vol. 1 p. 289.

my, there is an excellent representation of this pathological change in the air cells of a lung. According to the plate, they occupy the whole lung; are of very different and irregular shapes; and the largest of them do not seem to be more than two or three lines, in their greatest diameter. The structure thus altered, has according to the comparison of Dr. Baillie,* an analogy with the air cells of the lungs in amphibious animals.

In some cases, the cells near the surface of the lungs are so much enlarged, that they project beyond their general periphery, and have the appearance of a number of thin globular vesicles the size of cherry stones; and they adhere by a pedicle, which communicates with the adjoining branches of the bronchia and cells.

The branches of the bronchia and especially the smaller ones, are also sometimes dilated in lungs where emphysema exists. It is a very rare complaint.† I am not aware that a case of the kind ever presented itself to my notice. It is, however, easy to conceive of the same cause which produces distention of the cells, also producing an enlargement of the bronchia.

Emphysema may exist, partially or generally, in one or both lungs at the same time. Like hypertrophy, it increases the volume of the lung, and seems to make it too large for the thorax; so that, upon opening the latter, the lung escapes from it in part, instead of collapsing. When the lung is squeezed, the air escapes with more difficulty than in the healthy state, and its crepitation resembles more the slow passing of air from a bellows. If put into water, an emphysematous lung does not sink so deep as a sound one, and often seems to float on the surface, scarcely displacing any of the water.

While the cells of the lungs are in this state, the disease consists in a permanent and excessive distention of them.

* P. 43.   † Laennec. vol 1 p. 292

This, by increasing still more, or by occurring too rapidly, produces a rupture of their parietes, and an infiltration of air into the connecting cellular substance, as in common sub-cutaneous emphysema. In this state vesicles filled with air, which may be displaced by pushing, are seen on the surface of the lung, and vary in size from a line . to twelve or fifteen lines in diameter. When the infiltration of air occurs, however, at the union of several interlobular partitions, the air becomes fixed there, and cannot be transferred from place to place. * These several infiltrations of air from rup-tured cells are generally superficial; and do not extend them-selves much into the thickness of the lung, by following the sheaths of the bronchial branches, and of the pulmonary vessels; except in very rare cases.

It sometimes happens that a rupture of the air cells will occur in the depth of a lung; and a large globular accumu-lation of air is the consequence, which is manifested on the surface of the lung, by an irregular projection. This cavity contains generally a little clotted or decomposed blood, and the cells bordering it are in a collapsed state.

An emphysematous lung is less humid than a sound one, and is destitute commonly of the cadaverous engorgement about its root which was alluded to; unless it be complicated at the time of death, with peripneumony. When the affec-tion is confined to one lung, it becomes much larger than the other, and displaces the heart and mediastinum. In this case the thorax of the corresponding side is protruded, and more elevated, and when struck, it is also more sonorous than the other. When the affection is equal on both sides, the sound is equivalent, and is well heard every where; the whole thorax becomes of a cylindrical or globular shape, the sternum is held high up, and the intercostal spaces are enlarged. I have a patient, a young gentleman of twelve, who having had asthma from early infancy; the conforma-

* Laennec, vol i. p 291

tion of his thorax is precisely what is now stated, being evidently much modified by the disease.

The most usual cause of cellular emphysema of the lungs is that form of catarrh called dry,* from the trifling expectoration attending it; and which is marked by a tumefaction of the lining membrane of the fine bronchial branches, with an expectoration of pearl-coloured mucus. The dilatation of the air cells, according to the theory of M. Laennec,† is produced in the following manner: as the office of inspiration, owing to the greater force of its muscles, is executed with more vigour than that of expiration; it often happens that the air which has by inhalation, surmounted the obstruction of mucus, and the tumefaction of the bronchial ramifications; cannot find its way back again from the cells of the lungs, except partially; and renewed inspirations only add to its quantity, from the same cause   Again, as cold air is introduced, especially in winter, it expands in volume when it has got into the cells   These two causes then, a difficulty in the return of air, and its expansion by the heat of the lungs, produce a permanent and preternatural dilatation of their air vesicles, and the disease called emphysema is the consequence.

Emphysema may also arise from the exertion of the lungs, in playing upon wind instruments; or from any other violent exercise of respiration, making it necessary to hold the breath for a long time, with simultaneous efforts to expel it. Hence singing, screaming, hallooing, produce the same effect. Tumours of the thorax developed within its cavity tumefactions of the bronchial glands, or aneurisms of the aorta, also produce the same effect; and, it is stated by M. Laennec, not to be uncommon to find some cells dilated, where tubercles of a moderate volume prevail in the lungs.

The second form of emphysema, it has been stated, is called interlobular, from the air being extravasated from the

---

air cells by a rupture of their parietes, and insinuated into the partition of common cellular substance, holding the lobules together. These partitions, from the almost inappreciable thickness which they naturally have, are thus swollen out to a breadth of from one line to twelve; traverse in this state the surface of the lung, and penetrate some distance into its thickness. Such infiltrations of air, frequently follow the course of the pulmonary vessels, especially the superficial ones; and form bubbles resembling a chaplet, along them. Bubbles of air are also found beneath the pulmonary pleura; and when this interlobular emphysema occurs near the root of the lung, it passes on to the mediastinum, from there to the neck, and to the intermuscular and subcutaneous cellular tissue of the whole body. I once met with interlobular emphysema in an infant who had died from croup.

This affection, it is admitted, is the consequence of a rupture of air cells, yet the places of rupture cannot be seen; and it very rarely happens, that there is a dilatation of the air cells along with it. By inflating and drying a lung with this affection, and afterwards removing slices of it with a knife, the situation of the air becomes very apparent, as well as the perfect integrity of the air vesicles themselves, of the affected lobules.

The same causes which produce the vesicular emphysema also occasion the interlobular, as all violent exertions of the organs of respiration in the discharge of their natural functions; and it is also supposed that the air may be developed there also, as in other parts of the cellular substance of the body.* It is a remarkable fact, that the cases of coincidence in the vesicular and the interlobular emphysema, at the same time, in the same lung are so rare; this may arise from the induration and thickening of the pulmonary texture which takes place in the former.

* Laennec. vol 1 p 342

Œdema of the Lungs.

Œdema, in this case, is a serous infiltration which pervades the pulmonary tissue, and diminishes remarkably its permeability to the air. It is said* to be a very common disease, yet it is but little known, perhaps owing to the imperfect manner in which observations have been made upon it, by most pathologists. It is seldom a primary affection, but most commonly, one of the attendants of such chronic diseases as dropsies, and organic affections of the heart. It is also a consequence of severe peripneumony.

Its anatomical characters are as follow:—The colour of the lung becomes of a pale gray, or pale yellow; its vessels contain less blood than usual; and it does not collapse upon the opening of the thorax. It crepitates as in health; the finger will make a slight indentation into it, and from it when cut, there issues an abundant, transparent, and almost colourless serosity, with but little froth, except in recent cases. It is frequently blended with acute peripneumony, and is considered by M. Broussais as a grade of that affection.

Peripneumony.

This is an acute inflammation of the substance of the lungs. It is frequently uncombined with an inflammation of the pleura covering them; when combined with it, the disease is a pleuropneumony. Though the gradations of this affection are numerous, yet the more prominent stages of it are three: *suffocation*, (engorgement,) *hepatization*, and *purulent infiltration*.

1. Peripneumony, in the stage of suffocation, makes the lung heavier than usual, of a much greater firmness than na-

* Laen. vol. i. p. 349

tural, and of a livid or violet colour. Its crepitation on
pressure, though it still continues, is much diminished; and
it feels evidently like a body engorged with a liquid, and it
retains the impression of the fingers. When cut through, its
tissue internally is of the same dark red or livid hue with
the surface, and is found infiltrated with a bloody serosity
which flows freely, and is frothy and muddy. The spongy
texture of the lung is not entirely extinguished, with the exception of some few places, which have advanced to the second stage, or that of hepatization.

2. The term hepatization, expressive of the second stage
of peripneumony, is derived from the resemblance of it to
the liver, in compactness and weight. The lung in this state
presents internally a red colour, varying in places in the intensity of its shade, from a violet to a blood red. There
is a strong contrast between this and the bronchial ramifications, the blood vessels, the colouring matter of the lung,
and the interlobular partitions of cellular substance, which
are more distinct than usual, and frequently are free from inflammation.

Little or nothing escapes from the surface of incisions of
a lung thus situated; and, on scraping them, a little bloody
serosity may be forced out, with occasionally some white
puriform matter. The vesicular arrangement of the lung is
extinguished. A cut or lacerated surface exhibits in the place
of air cells, a granular arrangement consisting in small red
rounded masses, considered by M. Laennec,[*] as the vesicles
themselves transformed into solid grains, by the thickening
of their parietes and the stuffing (infarctus) of their cavities.

In pneumonic subjects of this grade, the lung does not collapse upon the opening of the thorax, owing to its universal
inflammation and its being completely destitute of air. It is
not, however, more voluminous than in the natural state,
neither is the corresponding side of the thorax, which, according to M. Laennec, establishes a great difference be-

[*] Laen. vol. 1. p. 337.

tween the signs of a pneumony and of a pleurisy. On this subject a very sharp controversy has arisen between M. Laennec and M. Broussais; the latter asserting that the lung is sometimes so tumefied as to have the marks of the ribs upon it: which is both denied by M. Laennec and declared by him to be impossible, from the ribs and intercostal muscles, being on exactly the same plane.

3. In the third degree of pneumony, that of purulent infiltration; the pulmonary tissue, besides the state last described, assumes a pale yellow colour, like straw. First of all are seen small yellow points of pus: these points afterwards coalesce, and the whole lung becomes of a citron colour. From the incisions which may be made into it, there issues a yellow opaque, viscid, purulent, fluid; by no means so disagreeable as the pus, from an external wound. The substance of the lung becomes much more soft and humid than in the red hepatization; the granular texture is effaced, and before the process is finished, the lung will resolve itself into a soft grume by pressure from the fingers.

The inferior parts of the lung are the most common location of pneumony; and when it invades the whole lung, it starts usually from these points. The various degrees which have been set forth may exist at the same time in the opposite lung, and in different places of the same one. The right lung is more subject to this affection, and indeed to all others than the left;* also, the lungs may be only partially affected and not generally, by the irritation being confined to a circumscribed spot.

Of Abscess of the Lungs.

This affection has been called vomica by the older writers in medicine, and till lately was considered as rather a common termination of pulmonary inflammations. The ob-

* Laen. vol 1. p. 406.

servations of M. Laennec and others, have now settled the question upon the ground, that instead of being common, it is one of the rarest pathological conditions. On several hundred peripneumonic subjects, M. Laennec has met only five or six times with purulent foci, and, in my own observations on probably more than fifteen hundred dead bodies of different kinds and ages, I remember to have seen it only twice, and then it was but small. The parietes of such abscesses are formed of the contiguous pulmonary substance infiltrated with pus, and in a state of semi-putrid softening, which decreases from the abscess outwardly in every direction.

It has been remarked,[*] in purulent collections, that the inflammation prevails in a part only of a lung, and not in the whole; it is supposed that the following rationale of the circumstance may be given. In universal inflammation, death occurs before the matter can collect into one or more foci; but nature and art together, can succeed against a partial inflammation for a longer time, and even cure it when it has gone into the state of suppuration; as done by M. Laennec,[†] in eighteen out of twenty cases.

There is but little doubt now, that the supposed frequency of vomica has arisen from the prevalence of tubercles, softened down and discharged by expectoration; but the anatomical characters of these are essentially different, as I shall show; and also the constitutional symptoms.

Gangrene of the lung is next in order; it also is an extremely rare affection. It may be either partial or general: in the latter case death follows in a very short time, preceded by extreme prostration, and intolerably fœtid, green expectoration. The lung diminishes in consistence, and is found of various shades of colour, from a light green to a dark one almost black, with a mixture of brown. Some

* Laen. vol i p 408.   † Id. p. 400

parts of the lung are so softened, as to be in the state of putrescence. I have seen it but seldom, and then it was partial. It does not seem to be so much the result of a highly active inflammation, as of a tendency to gangrene;* hence, the inflammatory changes around it are inconsiderable, and seem to be rather a consequence, than the cause of the gangrene.

* Laen. vol. i p. 443.

CHAPTER XIV.

IRRITATIONS OF THE PULMONARY TISSUE.

PHTHISIS PULMONALIS.

This affection is a slow disorganization of the pulmonary tissue, occasioned by the development in it, of a number of masses of matter, called *tubercles*. Similar masses are frequently found in the thickness of the alimentary canal, along its line of junction with the peritoneum, scattered over the surface of the latter, in the spleen, the liver, in the lymphatic glands, in the brain, and in other parts of the body. But it is principally, and most frequently in the pulmonary tissue that they exist, and go clearly through those stages of development and subsequent dissolution which characterize them.

A *Tubercle*, when examined chemically, seems to be co-agulated albumen, containing an excess of alkali, which is manifested by its turning green, vegetable blues. When plunged into boiling water, into an acid, or into strong spirits of wine; it, like all other animal textures containing much albumen, becomes opaque and more firm than it was previously. No pus can be detected in it, in its early stages. It is only in the later ones that the surrounding pulmonary texture, becomes evidently inflamed, and the tubercular masses softened; and that the expectorated matter consists in a mixture of the latter, with the purulent secretion of the adjoining parts. These facts may be ascertained by receiving the expectoration into a vessel filled with cold water, when the pus will be found precipitated to the bottom, and characterized by its globules, and pulverulence.*

The principal difference between tubercles is their relative state of aggregation. Some are found *disseminated* and perfectly distinct from one another; and in this state have been called by M. Laennec and Bayle miliary tuberculous granulations. In such cases they do not exceed the size of a millet seed, and may be recognised by their ovoidal shape and colourless transparency. Others are found collected into masses, or, in the technical language of anatomy, are *agglomerated.* And lastly, there exists what is called a *tuberculous infiltration.* In some subjects, we find exclusively one of these forms, and in others, all of them at once: so that whatever may be the mere mechanical condition and arrangement, the pathological one is identical in all. Notwithstanding this obvious inference, the subject has been very much complicated; by a most learned and excellent writer, Mr. Bayle,† making several distinct species; which he declares are of a nature entirely different, though he admits their occasional union in some subjects.

These species, in the phraseology of Mr. Bayle, are, 1. Tuberculous Phthisis, (agglomerated;) 2. Granular Phthisis, (disseminated;) 3. Phthisis with melanosis, (tubercules covered with the pigmentum nigrum of the lungs.) 4. Ulcerous Phthisis, (cavities from gangrene;) 5. Calculous Phthisis. 6 Cancerous Phthisis. The old fashion of infinitesimal differences in diseases has scarcely been more fully exemplified, in a modern book of celebrity, than in these six distinct pathological forms of phthisis pulmonalis. The first three are evidently of the same nature, to wit, that of tubercle; and the three last have scarcely any thing in common with phthisis, but that of being seated in the same organ.

* Gendrin, vol. ii. p 598.
† Bayle, Phthisis Pulm. p 21—24, Paris, 1810

According to the computation of Mr. Bayle, these various forms of phthisis observed, in nine hundred patients, the following proportions to one another:—

Tuberculous Phthisis,		-	-	-	624 ⎞
Granular,	do.	-	-	- -	183 ⎰ 879
Melanosis,	do. -	-	-	-	72 ⎱
Ulcerous,	do.	-	-	- -	14
Calculous,	do. -	-	-	-	4
Cancerous,	do.	-	-	-	3

Considering the three first to be all modes of what we call tubercle, it follows that this mode of chronic derangement in the structure of the lung, is about ninety-eight and a half per centum on the whole, of those forms called phthisis by Mr. Bayle.

When tubercles exist in the *disseminated* state, they consist in innumerable granuli dispersed throughout the lung: are from a scarcely perceptible magnitude to that of one or two lines in diameter, and are separated from one another by the intermediate air vesicles of the lung, seemingly in a healthy state. It is thus that we find them in the fœtus for the most part, or the very young infant, where they have been congenital. These granuli are semi-diaphanous; when cut, they shine, and are of the colour of ground glass, but much more lustrous. Some of them are contiguous immediately to the pulmonary tissue, others are enveloped by a distinct membrane or cyst separating it from them. * They adhere intimately to the pulmonary structure, and cannot be detached without tearing it. They have no apparent vascular organization, though they, no doubt, derive their growth from an interstitial circulation, as many parts of the body do even in a state of health. In this, however, there is some difference of opinion; for Mr. Bayle says that they are pierced by capillary blood vessels, and M. Laennec,†

* Laennec, vol 1. p 21   † Bayle, vol 1 535

that they grow by intussusception. I am disposed to believe that the latter is the case at first: but as they increase
in size, either by individual solitary growth, or by adhering
to the contiguous ones; it is likely that vessels will be found ,
penetrating their interstices to a limited extent, as in other
tumours.

In a short time after a tubercle is evolved, its centre
becomes a dark yellow point, from some change in its
organization; and the tubercle itself diminishes in transparency, and becomes of a milky colour. The tubercles in
this state are called *crude,* and it is probable that they frequently remain so for a considerable time, without a material change in their organization. There is then, so little
constitutional disturbance from them, and the physical symptoms of their existence are so equivocal, that they are frequently unsuspected.

Tubercles are evolved in the cellular substance of the
lungs, between the air cells and lobules; so that the two latter
are not obstructed, but rather compressed, and are slightly
indurated where they border on the tubercle.

As the proper pulmonary tissue is but little impaired in
this state, the function of respiration is duly performed,
with the exception of being somewhat hurried from exercise.

Agglomerated tubercles are formed from the disseminated ones coming into contact as they grow, and then coa-
lescing. The intervening portions of the lung become
more indurated, are infiltrated also with tuberculous matter, and become identified with the general mass of tubercle. By this mechanism, balls or masses of the latter
are found of all sizes, from that of a disseminated tubercle
to a hen's egg, and even much larger. The structure in its
arrangement may be compared to the particles of pudding
stone, with their intermediate cement; it being recollected
that the cement itself is finally assimilated to the tuberculous nature itself

As the agglomerated tubercles progress towards liquefaction and dissolution, the tuberculous infiltrations are made extensively into the adjoining pulmonary tissue. Frequently, however, these infiltrations occur, without the preliminary step of disseminated or agglomerated tubercles. Under whatever circumstances tuberculous infiltrations are made, the affected pulmonary tissue becomes more compact than usual, grayish, semi-transparent, and cuts with a smooth polished surface. The air cells are obstructed; the bronchial branches alone remain pervious, being only partially obstructed by a tumefaction of their lining membrane.

It very seldom happens that a lung is reduced universally to this tuberculous state, but is rather interspersed with such morbid degenerations. Under these circumstances, the blood vessels distributed to the affected lung are obliterated, in the substance of those morbid degenerations, as proved by injections; but they remain in the small portions of pulmonary tissue, that continues permeable in the midst of the surrounding changes of structure; and also in the bridles of cellular substance, which may pass through the latter.

Tuberculous Infiltration consists in the interstitial deposite of tuberculous matter in the substance of the lungs, which is followed by a closure of the air vesicles, and a condensation of the pulmonary texture. Like other forms of tuberculous degeneration, it also shows itself in other organs besides the lungs, so that it is not peculiar to them. It has been observed in the thickness of the digestive tube, in the serous membranes, and also in pseudo membranes. I have met with two cases of pulmonary consumption, where there was a species of hardness and elasticity along the whole alimentary canal, which I have never been able to give a solution of, unless it came from an interstitial deposite of tuberculous atoms. This notion is encouraged by the fact, that it is very common for the ulcers in the intestines of phthisical patients, to have small miliary tubercles at their bottom.

The colour of tubercles is affected by several circumstances: jaundice will tinge them, and especially when they are situated in the liver; adjoining mortification gives them a dark brown tinge: the black matter found in the lungs, by being blended with them, gives them a grayish colour, and causes the dispersion of black points in their substance.

Whatever may be the form under which tuberculous matter shows itself, whether disseminated, agglomerated, or infiltrated, it has one uniform termination—that of softening itself into a liquid state. This process begins in the centre of the mass, and always advances by degrees to the circumference. The preliminary change is into a soft, cheesy consistence; becoming more and more diffluent, until finally it obtains the thickness and liquidity of pus. In some instances, it has the consistence of well elaborated pus; in others, it resembles in a measure butter-milk, from one part being more fluid and serous like, while the other is opaque, and resembles curds or soft cheese. The latter is said to be especially the case in scrofulous subjects.

When the matter has become thoroughly softened, it finds its way into one or more of the bronchial tubes leading towards it. This is effected not by a separate process of ulceration, but by the tube itself and the adjacent vesicular structure of the lung having also undergone the tuberculous degeneration, by an infiltration into their structure. They consequently soften along with the primary tubercles. An excavation is thus formed by a discharge into the bronchia of the softened tubercle, and by its expectoration; which excavation becomes a permanent fistula.

It rarely happens that there is a single excavation; for as there are many tubercles scattered through the lung, they each, according to their state of maturity, execute the same process of softening either simultaneously or successively. The larger tubercles, or cavities, are for the most part surrounded by smaller ones, which are later in maturing, and as they progress, empty into the large ones. In this way the pulmonary structure, frequently, in the advanced stages of consumption, exhibits a collection of numerous excavations, communicating by means of tortuous canals or anfractuosities, which pass from one end of the lung to the other. The superior lobes of the lungs are most prone to this kind of destruction, and we often find them excavated into large tuberculous cavities, while the remainder of the lung presents its tubercles in the crude state. These pulmonary excavations are sometimes as large as the fist, and are occasionally so numerous that scarcely any part of a lobe is left except its periphery. They are often traversed by columns, resembling in shape the columnæ carneæ of the heart, and passing from side to side. These columns are smaller in the middle, and are formed of pulmonary tissue condensed, and infiltrated with tuberculous matter. Blood vessels, in some very rare cases, are found in the interior of these columns, but almost obliterated.

As a tuberculous excavation becomes emptied, its sides or periphery secrete and line themselves completely, with a false membrane, which is of an opaque white; thin, of a uniform surface, and of a soft, friable consistence. It resembles very much the false membrane which lines fistulæ in other parts of the body, and seems to be of an albuminous character. In some instances it is not a complete lining; but is rather interspersed in patches separated from one another, more transparent, less friable, and adhering closely to the parietes of the excavation; also the thickness is unequal, and it bears a closer resemblance to coagulating lymph. The lining membrane of this second form is occasionally found below the first; in which case the latter is loose and lacerated in several places. In some instances the pulmonary excavation is destitute of a lining membrane entirely; its parietes being formed by pulmonary tissue, red, hardened, and infiltrated with tuberculous matter at different degrees of development.

32

It is concluded, from these several circumstances,[*] that the lining membrane described first, is only the more perfect form of the second, which is finally changed into it; and that, when thus changed, its tendency is to become detached from the excavation, and to be replaced by one of a new production; and that, when loosened and lacerated, the lining membrane is discharged in the expectorations.

It is thought by Mr. Bayle, that the secretion from these lining membranes, forms the habitual expectoration of consumptive patients after the debris or wrecks of the softened tubercles, have been got up. This, though a very natural inference, is not fully established, for M. Laennec asserts that these excavations are frequently entirely empty; in which I agree with him: and that, when otherwise, the contained matter resembles much less the substance expectorated, than that in the bronchial tubes does. He therefore infers, that it is this bronchial mucus, augmented and vitiated by the irritation of the lining membrane of the lungs, which is really the expectorated matter. One thing I have frequently remarked, that the muciparous follicles of the trachea and bronchia are invariably much enlarged in consumption; and, like the follicles of other canals, indicate their irritation by this test.

There is a condition of the excavation which has obtained rather objectionably the name of encysted tubercle.[†] Its essence seems to be a mere conversion of the lining membrane into a semi-cartilaginous substance. In this state it adheres to the surrounding structure with great tenacity, and cannot be detached from it without dissection, or laceration. In some rare cases, an ossification of a partial kind in it has been observed.[‡] The cysts which surround tubercles, sometimes get into this semi-cartilaginous state before the softening of the tubercle. It occurs more frequently in the bronchial glands than elsewhere.

[*] Laen vol. i. p. 548   [†] Id 549   [‡] Bayle, p 22

As tubercles increase in volume, they push aside the large
blood vessels of the part, and flatten them in a measure, where
they assist in forming the parietes of an excavation.   Where
branches of these blood vessels penetrate into the tuberculous mass, they are obliterated* before the latter is matured,
and their orifices are so well secured that an injection of
them properly managed, will not penetrate into the excavation † The bronchia, on the contrary, become incorporated
with the tubercle, and finally dissolved along with it, and
their extremities retain a free communication with it, so that
it is rather uncommon to see even a small excavation which
has not several bronchial orifices looking into it.   These
tubes are scarcely ever opened on their sides, but have their
ends on a line with the walls of the excavation.

It is a very uncommon thing for death to occur from tubercles in the crude state, and before they have opened a passage into the adjoining bronchia. Hence, where we find subjects in this condition they generally have been victims to some
other malady of a more pressing kind; otherwise the tubercles are very numerous, and by the quantity of space they
occupy, interfere with the proper discharge of the pulmonary
functions.   When there are but very few tubercles, they are
sometimes all found in the state of softening; and emptying
into the bronchia.   But, according to my own experience
and that of pathologists generally, by far the most common
condition of the lungs at the time of death; is to have tubercles in the various stages of development and progress,
from the first evolution of a scarcely perceptible magnitude
and organization, to the state of pulmonary excavation.   We
hence find some of them as miliary grains, transparent, colourless, and looking like atoms of cartilage; others more
voluminous, opaque, and yellow in the centre; others softened into a curdy matter; others almost removed by expec-

* Baillie, Morb Anat , Albany. 1795, p 35
† Laen vol 1 p 547.

toration: and besides which, there are portions of lung infiltrated with tuberculous matter. Most commonly the greatest
devastation is in the summit of the right lung, which seems
to be particularly disposed to disorganization at this point.

It frequently happens that so long as the air is kept from
the tubercles, no very evident sign of their existence will be
present; but the admission of atmospheric air disposing them,
as it does all other animal productions or excretions, to putrefaction; they then become irritating, and cause hectic fever. Tuberculous collections with a sanious pus, are always
found in the substance of the lungs or in the pleura, when
the hectic fever has been violent, long, consumptive, and attended with fœtid excretions.*

Complications of Pulmonary Consumption with Maladies in other organs.

It is a matter of general observation, that phthisical patients seldom come to an end of their existence until they
reach the last stage of marasmus. It is from such extreme
emaciations that the name consumption has been taken.

This extreme emaciation is principally observable, in the
muscles and in the cellular substance and adipose matter: they
all disappear to such an extent as to be only the remains of
themselves. The skin is drawn tightly over the bones, and
observes their outline so nearly that the common expression
has been got from it, of an individual being merely skin and
bone. If it be pressed upon one place, by the position of the
patient for an undue length of time, it ulcerates and cannot be
healed readily again. On the sacrum large sloughs are thrown
off, which add much to the misery and horror of the patient's
situation. The nervous system remains of its ordinary volume, excepting the small particles of fat being absorbed
which exist in the sheaths of the nerves: but the peculiar

---

* Brossais, Phlegm. Chron vol. ii p 240.

texture of the nervous system, both brain and nerves, is never seen to greater advantage than in consumptive subjects, where the general exemption from fat, and the almost total disappearance of red blood, leave every fibre white, shining, and perfectly distinct.   The peculiarly healthy state of the nervous system will account for the unusually acute perceptions of both mind and body, which are seldom lost until the patient is almost in the last agony.

With the exception of the kidneys, my own impression is, that the glandular system of the abdomen is generally in a state of emaciation; when no particular disease manifests itself in them, causing their tumefaction.   The parietes of all the hollow viscera are evidently much reduced in thickness, as any one may readily ascertain who will examine them by inflation   M. Laennec is of a different opinion, both on this point and on the preceding, from me.   The bones remain of the same length, but diminish in circumference, and in the size of their articular extremities; the marrow is removed from them in great part, and serum takes its place: they become specifically lighter, and of a beautiful whiteness. They make, generally, very handsome and clear skeletons.

The shape of the thorax is evidently much affected: it becomes long and narrow, and the intercostal spaces are so much depressed, as to form long deep grooves between the ribs.   This is produced, in part, by the extreme emaciation of the patient, and in part by pleuritic adhesions, which are very common in the last stages of phthisis; and, as the volume of the lungs is then considerably diminished, the parietes of the thorax are pressed in by the weight of the atmosphere.

The volume of the heart seems also to diminish along with the quantity of blood: it loses all the adipose matter on its surface, and becomes remarkable for its smallness and for the firmness of its texture. The large blood vessels connected to it are generally of a healthy texture and highly elastic; and they contain, for the most part, clots of lymph, al-

most uncoloured by blood, and assuming their shape, penetrating even for some distance into their ramifications.

Such of the serous membranes as remain in their normal
state, have a polished brightness, and, like the skin, are almost ex-sanguine (ex sangué.)

The most remarkable, however, of the cadaverous appearances of patients, dying from pulmonary consumption, is the
very obvious tendency of the other viscera to a chronic disorganization, and most frequently from the development of
tuberculous disease, in some form or other.   It is therefore
very unusual to see a patient dying from pure solitary phthisis: almost invariably one or more of the other viscera have
responded to the suffering of the lungs.

The alimentary canal is very frequently the seat of these
pathological sympathies.   If the phthisis has been rapid, and
violently inflammatory; it is attended with a high grade of
gastric inflammation, marked by a deep redness of the mucous coat of the stomach, by contraction, and hardness of
this viscus, and by red patches in the mucous membrane of
the intestines.*   On the contrary, if its progress be chronic, and of the ordinary duration, great numbers of tubercles, about the size of mustard seed or smaller, will be
developed in the intestinal canal (especially the ileum,) beneath the peritoneum, and in the thickness of the mucous
and muscular coats.   These tubercles terminate in ulcerations, which proceed from within outwardly, spread into
one another, and become of various sizes, from a line or
two to that of one or more inches.   The ulcers have edges
elevated, ragged, and injected; and their bottom, when large,
is frequently formed only by the peritoneum: the perforation
of which sometimes take place, and would do so more frequently, if while the ulceration was going on within, a secretion of coagulating lymph was not thickening the out-
side of the intestine, so as to anticipate the progress of the

* Brouss vol. ii p. 240

ulcer, and raise a barrier against it. These ulcers are
described in the account of the mucous membranes. Notwithstanding this salutary provision to prevent a perforation
of the gut, it sometimes happens, that it is not sufficient; and
the stercoraceous matter being effused into the peritoneum,
causes an acute peritonitis with tympanites. Perforation,
however, does not necessarily expose the cavity of the abdomen; for where the ulceration can no longer be anticipated by the deposite of lymph on the surface, and in the
thickness of the peritoneum, that part of the intestine will
glue itself to an adjoining surface of intestine or of something else: and will thus gain a new barrier, which is either perfectly effectual, or else the perforation by progression will pass only from one fold of intestine into another,
so that the integrity of the peritoneal cavity is still maintained. These intestinal ulcerations generally give rise to the
colliquative diarrhœa of consumptive patients, though they
are not always followed by it, and especially if the colon is
not the seat of them, or only so to a moderate degree.

One of the most distressing sympathetic lesions of structure in phthisis, is an excoriation of the mouth and pharynx,
by aphthæ, which are also seen occasionally in the nose, in
the ears, and even on the vulva. They first begin by an alteration of the mucous membrane of the part, which becomes
red; and is covered with an innumerable quantity of small
white chalk-coloured plates: these plates at length fall off,
and the mucous membrane is seen to be excoriated, and with
a great number of fine ulcers, probably of its mucous follicles. These aphthæ differ from such as exist in acute fevers,
inasmuch as the latter first come as little transparent vesicles,
filled with serum, which burst and are then followed by
small white ulcers, with elevated edges and a conical base.
I have no doubt that these also are lesions of the mucous
follicles; but the difference is, that these follicles in the beginning of a complaint are in the healthy state, whereas
in consumption, they have been previously affected by the
tubercl

Scirrhosity, and tuberculous degenerescence of the mesenteric glands, are almost always the attendants of ulcerated intestines, in the same way as the bronchial glands are enlarged and diseased in phthisis. The opinion is generally received, and has been sanctioned by Bordeau, that phthisis frequently gives rise to fistula in ano; and that the latter exercises a salutary influence over it, and retards its fatal term. On this point M. Laennec, out of his immense experience and exact observations, states that he has seldom met with this coincidence, and that it has appeared most frequently without influence on its progress.* I may state, that my observations coincide with his.

The liver often sympathizes with the disorganization of the lungs. Sometimes it becomes yellow, voluminous, and fat. The presence of the latter is proved by its greasing the knife with which it is cut, and also by porous paper, when applied to it in a heated dried state, absorbing the fatty matter, and thus evincing its presence. The spleen is often hardened, surrounded by peritoneal adhesions, and has tuberculous matter in it. The kidneys are more exempt from sympathetic morbid derangement than other viscera.

The serous membranes often sympathize with tubercular consumption of the lungs. First of all, such patients are very subject to slight attacks of pleurisy, manifested during life, and on dissection after death. The contiguous surfaces of pleura are found adherent more or less generally: frequently the costal pleura, when free from the pulmonary, is covered with a layer of recent or of old coagulating lymph, penetrated with specks of blood, and roughened by filaments adhering to it. From eight to sixteen ounces of serum in the pleura are very common, showing clearly the inflammatory action which has been going on. Chronic inflammations of the peritoneum and arachnoidea are not uncommon. The pericardium also suffers sometimes.

* Op. Cit. vol. i. p. 560.

The heart, besides being reduced in size and increased in firmness of texture, is very apt to have small white plates upon its surface, of a fibrous nature, and readily passing to the state of cartilage.* They may be torn off easily, as they do not penetrate into its structure.

A lesion of the larynx is also very common in phthisis. On some occasions the lining membrane of it is only thickened and slightly injected; but on others it presents the appearance of aphthæ, like those of the mouth and pharynx, ending in ulcerations. Frequently the beginning of them is a small tubercle, in the thickness of the mucous membrane or beneath it. These ulcerations are of various sizes, from a small speck, to two or three lines in diameter; and they frequently penetrate the whole thickness of the mucous membrane, exposing thereby the cartilages of the larynx, and sometimes producing a caries of them, especially the arytenoids. The trachea and the bronchia, are also the seats of such ulcerations, but by no means so frequently as the larynx.

It is the occurrence of these ulcerations along the air passages which produces the hoarseness, and the gradual extinction of voice in consumptive patients.

The following tabular view from Mr. Bayle,† will present some of these coincident disorganizations in a more familiar way. In one hundred examinations of phthisical patients in the year 1804, (An. XII.) he found:

Larynx Healthy, in   -   -   -   83
   Do.   Ulcerated,   -   -   -   -   17
Ulcerations of Intestines, in   -   -   67
Alimentary Canal Healthy,   -   -   33

* Bayle, p. 62.   † Id p. 58,

Nature of Phthisis.

I do not propose to enter at large upon this subject, I therefore merely state in outline, that highly respectable authorities[*] assert, that the development of tubercles in the lungs is not an act of inflammation; but the result of a tuberculous disposition; and that, when inflammation is combined with it, the inflammation is of a date posterior to the tubercles. For my own part, I am not disposed to adopt this opinion. I rather view tubercles as a form of chronic inflammation, to which evidently all parts of the body are liable; but especially the lungs, from the peculiarity of their texture, and the quantity of lymphatic vessels entering into their composition. Like most other preternatural productions of the body, resulting from sub-inflammation of its tissues, tubercles, after having reached a certain state of maturity lose their feeble powers of life, and are removed by the process of softening described; which, if it took place on the surface of the body, would be called ulceration, from its analogy with it. It is at the same time admitted that some persons and families are more disposed to this chronic, or sub-inflammation of the lungs, than others; but the admission does not lead us farther, in regard to the primary nature of the malady, than a similar admission concerning sore eyes, or any other hereditary dispositions would do.

So long as the fact remains well established, that any one may by exposure become a victim to tubercular consumption; and, that it is always more prevalent where evident inflammations of the lungs are most common; the inference appears to me unavoidable, that it is not more ingenerate than any other of the thousand ills that flesh is heir to, and

[*] Laennec, vol. i. p 578, Bayle, Gendrin, &c.

that from the mode of its development and progress, it is a slow or sub-inflammation of the lungs, commencing generally, first of all, from an irritation of their mucous membrane. For a development of these arguments in a masterly and irresistible way, see Broussais Examen des Doctrines, from page 684 to 694; and Chronic Phlegmasia, passim.

CHAPTER XV.

IRRITATIONS OF THE HEART.

THE organic alterations in the texture and mechanism of the heart were formerly thought to be rather unfrequent; but improved and multiplied observations in later years, on this important class of diseases, have proved, satisfactorily, that they are by no means uncommon; that all periods of life are subject to them; that they are the almost inevitable inheritance of advanced age; and that they frequently lay the foundation of, or complicate other affections.

The essay of M. Corvisart* may be considered as introducing these subjects to the notice of modern pathologists, and demonstrating their importance. Its celebrity is well deserved, and though affected somewhat by an eccentric theory of the venereal disease being generally the cause of the organic alterations in the heart, it has stood well the test of time, and will continue to be esteemed for the facts and narratives which it contains. This book, like the more celebrated one of Morgagni, shows that facts stated with simplicity and honesty, are the property and the useful inheritance of all succeeding times, and that they may be applied as well at one period as another; a lesson for us when narrating symptoms and pathological appearances, to state them detached from all theories and notions, if we wish them to be useful to others.

All the tissues composing the heart are the subjects of disease and inflammation. The pericardium is liable to pericarditis and hydro-pericarditis; the lining membrane is

* Organic Diseases of the Heart, Philadelphia, 1812, translated from the French.

subject to inflammations acute and chronic, polypous concretions, and ossifications of the valves. The morbid alterations of the muscular structure are acute inflammations,
(Carditis;) and chronic ones, (Endurcissement, or hardening,) as in other muscles, Dilatation of one or all of its cavities, either partially or generally; Increase in their thickness, (Hypertrophy,) Diminution of their consistence,
(Ramollissement, or softening.) To these morbid states
may be added congenital malformations, as an imperfection
of its cavities, and an abnormal position of its large blood
vessels.

Pericarditis.

Pericarditis, called so from the membrane which enve-
lopes the heart, is an inflammation either acute or chronic,
of the serous membrane of the pericardium, and may be
either general, which is, perhaps, its most usual form, or
partial. It is, unquestionably, a disease of much more frequent occurrence than is commonly suspected, and is very
apt to be combined with irritations of the muscular tissue
of the heart, and with pleuritis. The leading anatomical
characters in this affection in the acute stage, are a concrete
fibrinous exhalation on both parts of the pericardium, a vascular injection of the latter, and a sero-purulent effusion into
its cavity.

The redness and vascular injection of the pericardium
which attends its inflammations is very rarely general: for
the most part, it is either partially in spots of various diameters; or punctated by numerous points of red blood,
grouped and scattered all over it. I have repeatedly seen
cases where, even this punctated redness was very faint
and limited. As in all other cases, almost, of acute inflammation in serous membranes, the pericardium itself is not
increased in thickness, tumid, or infiltrated, and the fibri-

nous layer which covers it may be pealed off readily, so as
to leave it smooth and apparently in a healthy state.

The fibrinous layer resulting from this inflammation, is
generally spread over the whole surface of the opposite
faces of the pericardium, both on the heart, and on its
large vessels as far as their line of junction, with the pericardium.   It is not of a uniform thickness as in pleuritis,
or regular on its surface, but is rough and flocculent; which,
no doubt, comes from the action of the heart drawing it out
into filaments, and making an attrition of the opposite
membranes.   This exudation of lymph is thicker than it is
in pleuritis, but has the same colour, a pale yellow; and a
consistence which preserves to it permanently, even when
removed, a membranous condition.

The serous fluid which is poured into the cavity of the pericardium while this fibrinous secretion is going on, is limped,
of a light citron colour, and frequently clear.   It is, however, in some cases found with fragments of the fibrinous
secretion floating in it, and also turbid from a mixture with
pus.   I have seen it in all these forms, limpid and clear,
limpid with flocculi of lymph or fibrine in it, and turbid
from a mixture with pus.   The distinction is, besides, of
no great consequence in a practical light, as the affection is
still essentially the same, and merely varies in the degree
of its violence in different persons.   There is good reason
to believe, that the quantity of serosity varies considerably
in the different stages of this complaint.   It is not unusual
at the beginning of the malady for it to amount to a pint;[*]
and in a case narrated by Corvisart, there were nearly two
pints.[†]   When the violence of the inflammation begins to
subside, the serosity is absorbed, so that frequently at the
termination of one of these attacks, the quantity left, has
been found very inconsiderable.   I have seen it amounting
to only three or four drachms, and even less.   It has been

* Laen. vol. ii. p. 653   † Op. Cit. p. 45.

very properly remarked, that here lies a distinction between
the anatomical characters of pericarditis, and of pleurisy
and peritonitis; for in the two latter, the quantity of serum
is generally fifteen or twenty times as great as that of the
fibrinous secretion.* The explanation may, I think, be afforded in the following way: from the limited extent of
the pericardium, and the subordinate influence which its
irritations exercise on other parts of the system; death from
it alone is rather unusual, at least in the early periods of
the inflammation, when the serosity is abundant; but the
reverse is true of the universal inflammations of the pleura
and of the peritoneum. The system perishes early under
their irritation, and consequently a proportionate quantity
of serum is found after death. If the irritation of these
membranes be only partial, and death follow at a remote
period, my impression from repeated observations is, that
the quantity of serum, as in pericarditis, is but small; allowance being made for the cadaverous percolation, which,
of course, will occur here as in all other cases.

The secretion from the pericardium is in some cases san-
guinolent, along with the sero-fibrinous· this, of course,
will affect the colour of the latter, and tinge it of a red colour, the intensity of which will depend on the quantity of
red particles of blood effused. It marks a higher degree of
inflammation still, which has been designated under the
term hæmorrhagic. When the latter is comparatively
mild, the redness of the fibrinous layer is not universal,
but merely in spots and punctated, or in points, as we often see it in pleurisy.

When a pericarditis is partial, that is to say, limits itself
to a single portion of the pericardium, the local phenomena
are the same as in general pericarditis; so that it is not worth
while to make a particular case of it.

When the inflammatory action of pericarditis has sub-

* Laen. vol. ii p. 654

sided fully, the fibrinous layer is converted by a process
of time, into cellular substance closely allied to the nature
of a serous membrane, and an adhesion is formed between
the opposite faces of the pericardium.   Frequently this
adhesion is so close, that the pericardium cannot be separated without dissection from the heart: on other occasions,
however, these adhesions are elongated, so as to allow of a
separation of one inch or more.   This is more frequently
the consequence of partial than of universal pericarditis.

In addition to these forms of pericarditis, it is not uncommon to meet with such as observe a more chronic and less
active character.   They are manifested by the internal or serous lamina of the pericardium, being highly and universally
reddened by small spots of blood interspersed over it and
very near one another, looking as if they had been laid on
with a pencil.   Most commonly with this appearance, there
is an absence of the coat of fibrine, and even when it does
exist, it is soft, thin, and resembles a layer of consistent pus.
There is, at the same time, a lactescent puriform serum filling up the cavity of the pericardium.   M. Laennec* is of
opinion that the close adhesions of the pericardium to the
heart, for the most part, come from this grade of inflammation when the secretion is absorbed, and that the long
adhesions are the result of more acute inflammation.

Sometimes tubercles show themselves in the false membrane, resulting from pericarditis; but they are of course the
consequence of a transition into the chronic stage.

On the surface of the heart we not unfrequently meet with
white opaque plates of from a few lines to two or three
inches in diameter, and of the thickness of a finger nail, they
have a soft semi-cartilaginous texture, and are placed superficially upon the serous membrane of the heart to which they
adhere very intimately, and sometimes seem to be identified
with it.   There is good reason to believe that they are the
result of chronic inflammation of a very low grade.

* Op Cit vol ii p 658.

In chronic pericarditis it is by no means unusual to find the muscular structure of the heart affected. As in other cases of chronic muscular inflammation, this state may be recognized by the hardness of the heart to the feel, by its whiteness as if it had been soaked in water for some hours, by its elasticity which will keep its cavities expanded, and by its easy lacerability. It is somewhat remarkable that M. Laennec, with all his excellence as a pathologist, should not have seen in these appearances an inflammatory action, but rejects the notion of the latter, merely because pus is not found between the fasciculi of its fibres, as if pus were an essential character of inflammation on all occasions.

A great difficulty in the treatment of pericarditis is the obscurity of its symptoms: several of the most skilful practitioners of Paris, as Laennec,* Recamier, and others, have declared that in their practice followed by a dissection of the patients after death, they have found themselves quite as often mistaken, as correct in a belief of the existence of this malady. Corvisart suggested that this obscurity might arise from its complication with other diseases which masked its symptoms; but the most simple cases have been found equally obscure with the combined ones. The probability therefore is, that pericarditis in many cases, exercises a very light and equivocal influence on the system at large, while in others a great disturbance is excited, which ends in death.

The latter cases may generally be known by a voluminous and loudly sounding pulsation of the heart, interrupted at intervals by reduced pulsations and diminished noise; this state is attended with an intermittent and contracted pulse, sometimes scarcely perceptible, and contrasting remarkably with the voluminous beat of the heart. The patient also suffers dyspnœa, pain, an unspeakable anguish, and is incapable of locomotion without its producing fainting; but these symptoms are not diagnostic, as congestions of

* Laen. vol. ii. p. 660.

blood in the heart and polypous concretions which result from them, give rise to the same.

The uncertainty of the symptoms of pericarditis exists both in the acute and chronic stage. M. Laennec, in commenting on this uncertainty, draws a happy and critical distinction between the words *divining* and *recognising* disease: the latter he thinks should not be employed when the signs are uncertain, and when it happens to the physician to find his opinions as often false as they are true.*

Contrary to the received opinions in medicine, it would seem, that old adhesions of the pericardium are of little consequence; for the authority just alluded to informs us, that he has opened a multitude of subjects, who had never made a complaint of disturbance in their respiration and circulation, and who had presented no sign of it in their last sickness, yet in whom there was an intimate and total adherence of the heart or of the lungs.

Hydro-Pericarditis.

This disease is an accumulation of serum in the pericardium, and varies in quantity in different subjects. When small it may be regarded as the effect of the dying state, or of that immediately consequent to death, and in this way it is sufficiently common; it is also not unfrequently connected with anasarca and other dropsies; but the pure uncombined hydro-pericarditis, without evidences of local inflammation, is very uncommon.

When it exists, the serum is of a citron colour, and is in quantity from one to two pounds; though Corvisart reports a case where he found eight pounds:† it is limpid, clear, and inodorous.

Dropsy of the pericardium, like its inflammation, is an obscure affection: sometimes no evident derangement of the

---

* Laen. vol. ii. p. 660.   † Op. cit. p. 63

system exists, and when symptoms do arise, they are common to it with other diseases. The stethoscope does not indicate it, except the accumulation amounts to at least one pint.* Some consolation may be derived for the obscurity of the diagnostics of this complaint, from the fact that pure dropsy of the pericardium is generally a consecutive disease; and consequently in its treatment we ought to look after the primary malady. In its nature it seems to be identical with hydrocele, and would, perhaps produce as little inconvenience, were it not from its mechanical interference with the offices of respiration and of circulation. Various operations have been proposed for its relief, consisting essentially in a puncture of the pericardium through the intercostal spaces, and the drawing off of the water. From the disease being rare, and the diagnostic unsettled, experience on this point is very limited and unsatisfactory. M. Laennec† has proposed perforation of the sternum with a trepan, just above the xiphoid cartilage, which would afford the opportunity of recognising positively the disease before the pericardium was opened. This operation being destitute of danger, seems plausible; and he has recognised also, that it might be useful when the disease was ascertained and the water let out, to throw some slightly stimulating injections in, to obtain a cure.

It is rather difficult to fix a standard of the precise quantity of serum which constitutes a hydro-pericarditis; for we seldom open subjects, in which there is not from one drachm to an ounce of transparent water in the pericardium. Corvisart has upon an average of a great number of individuals dead from every species of disease, suggested as a rule, "that when the serosity exceeds six or seven ounces, it should be considered a dropsy." If the quantity be less considerable, amounting to only a few spoonfuls, it is very probable, that the liquid has been effused during the last moments of life, and is an effect of the struggles with death.

---

* Laen. vol ii. p. 670   † Laen. vol. ii. p 671

Of Pneumo-Pericarditis.

This disease is a collection of *air* in the pericardium, and is stated by the French pathologists[*] to be not an unfrequent occurrence in the living body, and is often met with in the dead; care being taken in the latter instance not to confound it with the development of gas, one of the phenomena of putrefaction. I am not myself aware of having seen it, but the probability is, that like many other scientific observations, it has passed unnoticed when it did occur, from my attention not being especially directed to it, by previous information on the subject.

The quantity of air thus collected, is very variable; and its chemical nature has not been examined into. It co-exists with hydro-pericarditis most commonly, though it may be alone also. When the pericardium is opened, it escapes with a light whizzing noise.

Its signs in the living subject are doubtful and unsettled. It may sometimes be recognised by a resonance of unusual clearness upon the percussion of the lower part of the sternum, coming on suddenly; and by a noise of fluctuation determined by the pulsations of the heart, and by forced inspirations. M. Laennec states,[†] that in nearly all the cases where the pulsations of the heart can be heard at a certain distance from the thorax; the phenomenon is owing to a momentary development of gas, which is most frequently promptly removed; and whose presence in the pericardium does not give rise to any serious accident. In some very rare cases, the noise of the heart thus communicated has been heard at the distance of several feet, even in the adjoining chamber; but, it is very common to hear it at a distance, of from two to ten inches from the thorax of the individual.[‡]

---

[*] Bertin, Malad du Cœur Paris, 1824, p. 278.

[†] Laennec, vol ii p. 672.   [‡] Id p 454

It would appear that the palpitations of the heart called nervous, are generated in this way, and that a paroxysm is apt to be produced by walking quickly, or by ascending a flight of stairs. It is a state of comparatively little danger. In twenty subjects presented to M. Laennec, with palpitations which could be heard from two inches to two feet, only four had organic diseases of the heart: with the remainder it disappeared, and many of them returned to perfect health.

It is an axiom in pathology, that all the noises within the body heard by the naked ear, are due to the movements of some part which is in contact directly or indirectly with a gas. This notion corresponds perfectly well with a similar law in physics, for the experiment must be familiar to all, that a bell rung in vacuo does not produce sound by its vibrations, neither does it when surrounded by solid materia. Under this class of phenomena, we then rank palpitations heard at a distance, borborygmi in the intestinal canal, the crackling of the cellular substance in emphysema, the cracking of the joints in rheumatic affections by the development of air in them, the disease being called pneumo-arthrosis, the crepitation which follows contusions and fractures:* and the artificial cracking of the joints of the fingers by stretching them, a process which in eastern countries, where the art of bathing is carried to the highest perfection; can be extended by the adepts in it to every joint in the body, as I have been informed by a gentleman, who underwent the experiment, and who described it along with the warmth of the bath, as producing the most delightful sensations of indolence and exhaustion.

We proceed, in the next place, to treat of the diseases of the muscular substance of the heart itself, which may exist either alone or combined with the affections of the pericardium.

* Laennec, vol. ii. 457.

Carditis.

Carditis is an inflammation of the muscular substance of the heart, and is either general or partial. It very rarely presents itself in that acute form which generates pus, its inflammation in this respect closely resembling that of other muscular tissues. Meckel, however, saw it thus in a man of fifty years, whose heart had pus infiltrated between its muscular fibres.* M. Laennec met on one occasion with an abscess the size of a bean, in the parietes of the left ventricle; it was combined with pericarditis, and occurred in a child of twelve years; and in a man of rank who became a pauper from the disturbances of the French revolution, and died in the Hospital called La Charité, he found an albuminous exudation the colour of pus, and the consistence of the white of egg cooked, interposed between the fasciculi of the left ventricle.

I have myself never met with these forms of disease in the heart, and have reason to think from that circumstance, that they are very unusual, at least in this city. And if, with M. Laennec,† we consider the presence of pus as the only incontestable sign of inflammation, the heart will be found sufficiently exempt from such a malady I cannot, however, agree to any such limitation; it is carrying pathology centuries backward, and merging it in the period where heat, redness, pain, and tumefaction were considered the indispensable and inseparable phenomena of inflammation, and a common bile as its fixed and unchangeable type; a doctrine which has served more to mystify medicine, and to embarrass its principles than any other which ever existed. Let us for a moment glance at the inflammations of other tissues; do we not find their high irritations, frequently existing without pus in their interstices; the muscles

* Mem. Acad. Berlin, 1756, from Laennec, vol. ii. p. 555
† Laennec, vol ii p. 535

changing their colour, becoming brown, easy to tear, and sometimes converted into a soft mass without cohesion, and in a semi-fluid state? Do not the brain, the liver, the spleen, and other organs present the same condition in their irritations? On the contrary, if inflammations of less violence and more duration assail the same muscles, their natural brown is changed to a light olive or drab colour, they are harder to the touch, but at the same time tear much more easily than in health, and sometimes they undergo cartilaginous and bony degenerations, making them entirely useless as organs of locomotion.

If with the more improved school of pathology we admit these several conditions of organs as the evidences of inflammation, we can have no hesitation in applying the same principles to the heart; and we shall have as a consequence the acknowledged cases of carditis vastly augmented. For my own part, I am fully inclined to this course, convinced by these and other reasons of its propriety, and I therefore range in the same line, Mollescence, (Ramollissement;) Hardening, (Endurcissement;) Ossifications, Hypertrophy, Dilatation, and Aneurism, all of them being but modifications of the act of inflammation, depending upon its degree and stage.

Having settled this point, at least for the time, we may now proceed to discuss the other organic alterations in the texture of the heart.

Mollescence or Ramollissement of the Heart.

I have adopted the French term, in designating the diminished consistency of the heart, as rather more expressive than the corresponding English word *softening*. The softening of all the tissues of the body under the act of inflammation, is a French observation in pathology, made by Laennec,[*] and well deserves to be designated in the language of the country which first informed us of it. Having

* Laen vol ii p 535

adopted it elsewhere, I may, therefore, with sufficient propriety, apply it also to the heart.

This disease is recognised by the following anatomical
characters:　The heart is flaccid and collapsed, and so
weakened in its texture, that in squeezing it between the
ends of the fingers, they will penetrate into the ventricles.
It is seldom found gorged with blood, but is only half full
on the opening of the body.　Its colour, for the most part,
departs signally from what is natural, sometimes it is increased in intensity to a violet blue, which is especially the
case in severe continued fevers, but more commonly it takes
a yellow hue, analagous to that of dead leaves in the autumn.

This affection has been found both general and in patches:
sometimes it does not go beyond the circumference of a
single cavity, and it is very apt to exist along with dilatations.　Mr. Bertin* has stated his persuasion, that it never
exists without a pathological condition of the external or
internal membranes.

M. Laennec,† after rejecting the idea of M. Bertin and
Bouillaud, of this being an inflammatory affection, reasons
on it in the following exceptionable way: stating, That it
is an affection sui generis, resulting from a disturbed nutrition of the organ, whereby its solid materials diminish,
while the liquid or semi-fluid ones increase in proportion:
and that the means of curing it are directly opposed to such
as suit inflammatory affections.　That we often see muscles
softened to a moderate degree in a crowd of acute and chronic diseases, which state may be distinguished during life
by feeling them, and their firmness returning in a few days
afterwards, very suddenly.　M. Laennec admits at the
same time, that the softening of the heart is analogous to
the white softening of the brain, and to the gelatinous
transparent one of the mucous membrane of the stomach.‡

* Page 399.　　　† Vol ii p 540　　　‡ Vol ii p. 541

What is still more singular in him, as a profound and expe-rienced pathologist is, his admission that bones, cartilages, and fibrous tissues generally, become soft by inflammation from the quantity of lymph deposited in them at the time; but, on the contrary, the soft tissues, in which he includes the muscles, brain, and some others; that they harden. Thus, he makes the evidence of inflammatory characters to depend upon mere consistence. This is obviously opposed to what is now known on the subject; for consistence depends ra-ther upon the peculiar texture of the part affected, and the grade of its irritation, than upon what M. Laennec would call an affection sui generis: a mode of expression which, though seemingly candid and scientific, is merely a subter-fuge for all kinds of professional prejudice and blindness.

The symptoms of ramollissement of the heart are not of an exclusive kind, and are therefore common with those of other affections of the same organ. The leading ones are a pale and yellowish complexion, the skin dry and shri-velled, the lips without colour. If the affection be acute, the pulse is feeble, precipitate, and small, and there is a tendency to faintings; but if it be chronic, the pulse is feeble, soft, and languid. The impulsion of the heart is feeble, sometimes almost inappreciable, and the sound of its contractions is more dull, more obscure, and more ob-tuse than in the natural state; but they vary in their preci-pitancy, according to the disease being acute or chronic. As it is most frequently co-existent with dilatation of the ventricles, the sound becomes still less notable.

Induration of the Heart or Endurcissement.

The aggregate of examples of induration of the heart is so large, that this mode of its chronic irritation may be considered sufficiently common, and, like the softening of

35

the same organ, it is frequently attended with a dilatation of its cavities, and also with an increase in the thickness of their parietes. Lieutaud, in his Historia Anatomico Medica, and Morgagni in his Morbid Anatomy, have introduced many cases of it taken by the first from his contemporaries and predecessors, and by Morgagni, from his personal examinations of bodies; and in the present times, the cases reported are so abundant, that with my own private observations, this anatomical lesion is quite familiar.

The induration of the heart has been presented to anatomists, in various stages, from one slightly beyond the natural state, to a cartilaginous hardness, and even an ossific one partially. In the case of a female, aged fifty-five, recorded by Corvisart,* the parietes of the right auricle and ventricle were so much thicker than natural, and so compact, that they supported themselves without collapsing; were elastic, yielded with difficulty to pressure, and were spontaneously reinstated upon its removal. The cavity of the left ventricle was greatly distended, and its parietes had, at least, double the natural thickness. They were supported like an arch, and formed a very elastic fleshy box, which sounded when struck, like a dice box. The muscular texture of the ventricle retained its natural colour and appearance, and did not seem converted either into an osseous or cartilaginous substance; yet it was so indurated, that the scalpel, on cutting it, made a crepitating noise.

In another case related by M. Corvisart,† the patient being sixty-four years old, was taken with difficulty of breathing and violent suffocations, which lasting two months, induced him to enter the Clinical Hospital. The impulsion of the heart against the thorax was very strong, but there were no palpitations, and the pulse was small, concentrated, and irregularly intermittent.

Four months after the commencement of these symp-

* Op. Cit. p. 140.   † Op. Cit. p. 143.

toms the patient died; and was examined. The heart was much larger than natural, especially the right auricle and ventricle, and the opening between them was also dilated. The left auricle was very large, the ostium venosum dilated, and the mitral valves cartilaginous. The walls of the left ventricle were, at least, an inch in thickness, and very firm. The apex of the heart to a certain height, and in all the thickness of its substance, was cartilaginous; the columnæ carneæ were also cartilaginous.

It would appear from the report of M. Laennec,* that the resounding of the heart like a dice box when struck, and its hypertrophy generally go together: the induration, however, may exist, either with an increase or diminution of the cavity affected.

A universal induration of the heart has not as yet been observed in many cases; more commonly it is partial, and very seldom goes beyond one half of the organ: sometimes the external, and on other occasions the internal face of it is the seat of this change; and it may prevail, partially, in one of the cavities alone. In a case reported by M. Bertin, there was a softening of the right ventricle; and an induration of the left,† and in another, some of the columnæ carneæ were soft and others hard.

The colour sometimes is not changed at all from the natural standard.

* Vol. ii, p. 532.   * Page 404.

CHAPTER XVI.

IRRITATIONS OF THE HEART.

(Continued.)

HAVING in the preceding chapter considered the pathological conditions of the pericardium and some of the alterations in texture of the substance itself of the heart; we shall proceed in the next place to consider other modes of lesion which affect the capacity, thickness, and texture, of its cavities.

Dilatations of the Heart.

This malady is an enlargement of one or more of the cavities of this organ. In regard to mere capaciousness, it is met with to a slight degree in most old persons, especially such as have led irregular intemperate lives. In that stage it is not attended with much inconvenience, though the affection be permanent. It occurs also not unfrequently in young persons from the age of twelve to twenty-five; in them it is, I think, for the most part, temporary, and may be removed by reduced diet, by diminishing the quantity of blood, and refraining from violent exercise for some months. I have at least, in several cases, cured the symptoms indicative of it by such a course.

This affection is also called aneurism of the heart, and its precise state is somewhat modified in different cases. In one form it is attended with an increased thickening in the parietes of the cavity dilated; this is the most common: in another the parietes are much thinner, this is rather rare; frequently there is no sensible alteration in the thickness of the parietes; and lastly, a very rare form, and which, perhaps, above all the others, deserves the name of aneurism is, that where there is a pouch or cul de sac projecting from the cavity affected, and communicating with it.

As stated when speaking of the derangements in the texture of the heart, this condition of it is very frequently complicated with induration or ramollissement, and the colour is sometimes violet, and on other occasions more pale than usual, depending upon the acuteness or chronicity of the affection. It is, I think, more frequently found in the ventricles than in the auricles, and generally both of the former are dilated at a time. It is rather unusual to see a universal dilatation of all the cavities at once, though a specimen in the anatomical museum presented some years ago by Dr. Parrish to Dr. Wistar, is of that kind. A similar case is described by A. Burns,[*] where the heart cleaned from pericardium, lungs and fat, weighed two pounds, was larger than that of an ox, and all the cavities were equally dilated; but they, as well as the vessels, were of the usual thickness.

The causes which give rise to dilatation of the heart are often a resistance to the passing of blood through it, occasioned by some obstacle in the large vessels leading from it. This point M Bertin[†] says he has made out by observations extremely numerous. If the obstacle be permanent, as a contraction of the orifices of the large arteries, the dilatation itself will be permanent; but if on the contrary it be temporary, as that of a stasis of blood in the lungs, from inflammation or some particular exercise of them, then the dilatation is removed with the cause productive of it. I have, however, no doubt that even when there is no obstacle to the current of blood, if the heart get into a state of chronic inflammation

[*] Burns, Diseases of the Heart, Edin, 1809, p. 47.
[†] Bertin, Malad. du Cœur, p. 378.

in its parietes, its muscular fibres will lose their contractility somewhat, and will yield to the ordinary resistance of
the blood vessels, so that the cavities will become distended ·
and enlarged.

M. Laennec thinks that dilatation is more common among
women than men, owing to the parietes of their ventricles
being naturally thinner.

Hypertrophy of the Heart.

The term hypertrophy has been very generally applied
to express an excessive growth or disproportionate nutrition
of parts of the human body, without an obvious morbid
change of texture, and the heart like other organs is subject
to this condition of nutritive irritation.

This state is manifested by an increase in the thickness of
the parietes of the heart, and its cavities either remain stationary, or they may be enlarged or diminished, for there
is no rule on this point.   Generally the affection is bounded
to the ventricles and especially the left; the auricles but rarely participate in it, and are found commonly in their natural
condition.

M. Laennec[*] states, that he has in some cases seen the
left ventricle at its base twelve or eighteen lines in thickness.   This thickness, however, generally·diminishes towards the apex of the heart, and is seldom universal in the .
cavity. The columnæ carneæ and the chordæ tendineæ are
frequently disposed to participate in the affection. The muscular substance of the ventricle increases very much in the
firmness of its texture, and its colour becomes of a deeper
red.

The cavity of the ventricle often appears to have lost in
capaciousness what the parietes have gained in thickness; and
in some instances, where the heart was twice the size of the

[*] Loc. Cit. vol. ii. p. 499.

fist of the subject, the ventricle would scarcely lodge an almond.

In extreme cases of hypertrophy the heart has been found four times the size of the fist of the subject; as the fist is generally considered equal in magnitude to a heart perfectly healthy, the heart consequently had increased four times its natural bulk. In these instances its proportionate shape is much altered and its position is transverse; generally, in the cases which I have seen, it occupied principally the left side of the thorax, and shoved backwards the left lung. Allan Burns states, that he had seen a heart which weighed several pounds and yet the cavities were not more capacious than usual.*

The causes of hypertrophy are thought to be† habitual accumulation of blood in its cavities, either from moral or from physical influence, hence certain exercises of the organs of respiration, and their diseases give rise to it: it may, however, also come of itself. When it has existed for some time, it in turn influences the condition of other organs; giving rise to apoplexy, to encephalitis, and to cerebral congestions and irritations generally.‡ In this way have fallen three illustrious men, in medicine, Malpighi, Cabanis, and Ramazzini. It also disposes to bleeding from the nose. When the right ventricle is affected, pulmonary apoplexies and hæmorrhages result from the additional impulsion communicated to the blood, as it flows into the lungs.

Ossifications of the Heart.

Ossifications of the muscular structure of the heart are unusual. In my own sphere of observation, I have noticed but one instance of it, and that occurred in a double male fœtus where there were several other abnormal arrangements

---

* Diseases of the Heart. † Bertin, p. 349. ‡ Bertin. p. 351.

of the viscera, as most commonly happens, where two fœtuses adhere to one another.* M. Laennec, notwithstanding his very numerous pathological researches says, that he never met with an instance of ossified muscular structure of the heart. The celebrated Corvisart quotes no instance coming under his personal observation. M. Bertin's experience does not seem to exceed that of one or two cases, and those of a very limited extent in the ossification. As our collective experience together involves the result of many thousand cadaverous autopsies, it is clear that the instances are comparatively but few where this mode of disease occurs: not that the structure itself is incapable of it, but that the ossification incommodes so much the functions of the heart in conducting the circulation, that life is extinguished generally in the very early stages of the disease, before it has become well marked.

Cases, however, do occur from time to time. Several of them are narrated succinctly by Lieutaud,† taken from different writers. These ossifications were, for the most part, partial, and found stuck away in the thickness of the muscular substance, especially of the ventricles and in their septum. In some instances, from the small quantity of animal matter in them, they resembled calcareous concretions more than organized ossifications.

Albertini met with a case of ossified auricle; the late Allan Burns saw a perfect ossification of the ventricles; Haller was called upon to see a young man immediately before death, in whom there was no pulsation of the radial arteries, though that of the carotids was very perceptible. On dissection the heart was found of its natural size; the inferior part of the right ventricle was ossified, and the most fleshy parts of the left ventricle; also the valves of the aorta and pulmonary artery. In the journal of medicine for 1806, in

---

* North Am. Med. and Surg. Journal, vol. ii. p. 395.
* Anat. Museum for Preparation.
† Lieutaud, Hist. Anat. vol. ii. p. 59.

Paris, the following highly interesting case is communicated by M. Renauldin. A student of law, of severe attention to his studies, joined to an abstemious course of living, and aged twenty-three years, experienced at last continued headache, frequent dyspepsia, with a respiration habitually somewhat difficult. Being attacked with peripneumony, he recovered; but afterwards, on the slightest exercise, he experienced lively and frequent palpitations of the heart, and was in other respects so infirm that he was compelled to keep his bed. He at length died. On dissection, the lungs were found sound; but on attempting to cut the left ventricle, a great resistance was experienced, occasioned by the entire change of this part into a real petrifaction, which had a gravelly appearance in certain places, and resembled in others a saline crystallization. The granuli of this species of gravel were very near one another, and became larger as they receded from the surface of the ventricle; so that internally they were continuous with the fleshy columns. The latter were also petrified, were much augmented in size, and looked like stalactites placed in different directions. The thickness of the left ventricle was also augmented. The right ventricle was sound. The large arterial trunks of the heart were also sound, but the temporal, the maxillary, and a part of the radial on each side were ossified.

The ossification of the heart in this case was of very unusual extent, and is probably narrated in too unqualified a manner; as we cannot conceive how the ventricle could pulsate, if it were entirely changed into a petrifaction. The account, however, is admitted by the French pathologists, Corvisart, Laennec, and Bertin, as correct and authentic, being quoted by them as such. Also, as the state of the left auricle is not alluded to, the probability is, that it at least retained the natural structure, and supplied in part the deficiency of the circulating powers arising from the vitiated state of the left ventricle. A very remarkable instance of this kind will presently be quoted from Allan Burns.

An inferior degree of induration, amounting to a cartilaginous change of texture, is more common than ossification.
Several instances of this kind will be found recorded by the
gentlemen whose names have been so serviceable to me in
the composition of this paper.* It occurs indeed not unfrequently on the internal face or periphery of the ventricles,†
especially the left; in the form of cartilaginous plates, which
seem to be identical with the lining membrane, and interposed between it and the muscular substance of the heart.
M. Kreysiz has reported a case in which he found such an
incrustation ossified.‡

Upon a review of the several circumstances connected with
ossifications of the substance of the heart, it would seem that
they are to be ranged in the same line with the indurated state
formerly alluded to; the commencement of the affection being
hypertrophy or a nutritive irritation, the middle stage induration, and the terminating one ossification, which of course
must be rare as the patient inevitably perishes in a vast majority of cases before this stage is reached, from the heart
not being able to carry on the circulation. As every journey, however long, is composed of intermediate steps, so
are the disorganizations of the heart: the differences between
the steps are almost imperceptible, but the two extremes
are at the widest points of separation; so that it scarcely appears possible for the same line of march to connect them,
and yet such is the case.

Bordenave reports, that he met with a person whose heart
was almost completely ossified. I am not, however, in possession of the details of this case, having got it from Portal.§
Mr. Allan Burns, from circumstances of an unaccountable
kind, considering the limited opportunities of dissection in
Scotland, speaks in very familiar terms of derangements in

---

* Corvisart, p 138, et seq   Bertin, p 401.   Laennec, vol. ii. p. 566.
† Laen. vol. ii. p. 568.
‡ Laen. loc cit.
§ Anat. Medicale.

the structure of the heart, which have come under his notice.   Yet he is generally considered, by his countrymen
and others, very good, and sufficiently accurate authority to
be freely quoted.   In one case, he says that he found the
ventricles mere calcareous moulds, and in another, both of
them were cartilaginous; but in only one case, has he found
an auricle in any degree deranged· meaning, I presume, in a
similar manner, he has never met with a single instance, in
which both the auricles and the ventricles were at the same
time affected. *

A case reported by him is equally, if not more astonishing than those of Bordenave and Renauldin; and, having every evidence of accurate and cautious statement about it,
goes far to prove, that the auricles have great power in sus-
taining the circulation, when the ventricles are incapacitated
from it by a gradual change of structure.   It occurred in a
poor woman aged sixty, and named Margaret Henderson,
who was treated in the Glasgow Hospital for dyspnœa, anxiety in the chest, and attacks of breathlessness, during which
she became of a livid hue.   She was under the continued necessity of a semi-erect position, with feeble and intermittent
pulse for a few days before her death, though previously it
had been regular.

On dissection, the pericardium was found loaded with an
enormous quantity of fat, and of an opaque dusky hue, with
ragged spiculæ of bone projecting from its surface, and
making it very irregular.   It adhered closely to the parts
around, and seemed incorporated with the substance of the
ventricles.   Over the whole extent of the latter it was ossified; and the ventricles themselves, except about a cubic
inch at the apex of the heart were ossified, and as firm as the
skull, the ossified part forming a broad belt.   Some of the
columnæ carneæ were also changed into solid bone.   Both
auricles were healthy, but thicker than usual; and, so far as

* Op Cit p. 127.

the examination of the remainder of the vascular system extended, it also was healthy.   The preparation was given to Dr. Munro.[*]

Mr. Burns remarks, that the ventricle may be ossified, and may be as rigid as stone: and yet the blood may find its way into the arteries, and be fairly circulated through all the parts of the body, provided the auricle remains healthy. But as there are no valves between the auricles and the veins, a considerable quantity of blood becomes refluent on the contraction of the auricle; and thereby produces a pulsation in the neck, and an undulation in the epigastrium.   In these cases, an evident provision is made for the inaction of the ventricles, by the muscular structure of the auricle, being invariably augmented, firmer and stronger.

In plate 5th, of Baillie's Morbid Anatomy, is represented a heart considerably enlarged, and with an ossification, which covered from fifteen to twenty lines in breadth of the right auricle and ventricle; and extended from the inferior end of the descending cava, to the apex of the heart, being in all five inches or more in length. The original communication of the case, was by Dr. Simmons.[†] It radiated at each end in broad digitations, which there increased its extent very considerably.

The facts now quoted, will be sufficient to illustrate the ossific tendency of the muscular structure of the heart, in its chronic irritations; and that, however, improbable it may be at first sight, yet, the circulation of the blood is consistent with an inaction of the ventricles, in consequence of the auricles assuming a vicarious function.

Polypi of the Heart.

There are two kinds of productions found in the heart, and designated by the term polypus.   One is very com-

[*] Loc Cit. p. 128
[†] Medical Communications, vol. 1. p. 228.

mon, especially in chronic complaints, where there is a great deficiency of red particles in the blood; and is an inorganized accretion of the fibrine or albuminous part of the blood, precisely such as takes place in similar cases, where blood is drawn from the arm into a cup, and is allowed to settle. This appearance, from phlebotomy in old dropsies, is often mistaken for active inflammation; and seems, indeed, to justify the use of the lancet to any extent: whereas it is in fact, only an indication of the paucity of the red globules, which are not in sufficient number to colour the fibrine, and to prevent its uniting in a homogeneous mass.

Such accretions of fibrine, are found most generally in the right side of the heart, and are colourless very frequently. They extend themselves into the large veins, and into the pulmonary artery, following its branches; but they have no other connexion with the heart, than that of being entangled in the columnæ carneæ, and in the irregularities of its interior surface. Generally, their formation is subsequent to death, but there are strong reasons for believing, that they sometimes form a long time before this event. Besides many others of a subordinate but satisfactory character, there are some very prominent and conclusive. They are the extreme tenacity of these accretions, which have a firmness, but little less than that of muscle; a colour of various shades from a light flesh one to a violet; whereas the recent accretion is easily torn, and is of a uniform colour: then there is an evident tendency to a vascular organization of the accretion,* as in many other abnormal productions. Lastly, the fleshy columns of the heart have been found flattened considerably by them, which could not occur after death.

The second kind of polypus is absolutely attached to some part of the substance of the heart, by a continuation of structure. As observations of this kind, many of which are on

* Laennec, vol. ii. 595.

record, are questioned by some writers, a direct evidence
on the subject will be more satisfactory than a chain of reasoning; I therefore refer to a preparation which was for some
time in my charge, and which I have repeatedly examined
carefully.* This patient was twenty-six years of age, and
suffered the extirpation of a scirrhous testicle the size of an
ostrich egg, in the Pennsylvania Hospital, September, 1819.
He died in eight months afterwards, from the scirrhous affection being repeated to an enormous extent, in the lymphatic glands of the loins; at least, this is the inference I obtain
from the Drs. description, and from having seen two cases
in many respects similar.

Dr. Coates goes on to state, that the vena cava was distended to an enormous size, and nearly filled by the polypus,
which measured five inches and a half in length, and nine-
tenths of an inch in thickness, tapering gradually to both
ends.   It adhered apparently to the anterior side of the
vena cava; but when torn away, left the surface smooth.   It
was afterwards apparent, that the connexion was by means
of processes of the same nature, extending into a number
of small veins entering into the cava on that side, from the
scirrhous tumour in the abdomen.   The two ends of the polypus were firmly attached, the lower one to the bottom of
a cavity with smooth edges, and which was probably the remains of an obliterated vein.   The upper end of the polypus was by accident cut off before its attachment was seen,
in consequence of the heart being removed; but it was afterwards ascertained, that it adhered to the edge of the Eus-
tachian valve, by a strong dense pedicle resembling the
lining membrane of the auricle and vein, and three lines in
diameter.   The texture of the polypus was fibrinous, dense,
and firm.

In 1822, a girl of sixteen was admitted into the Hôtel Dieu

* See the Phila. Journal of Med. and Phys. vol. iv. p. 336, for the year
1822. paper by Dr. B H. Coates.

of Paris, for two enormous tumours upon the right shoulder, and in the arm pit of the same side. Having died
there, she was opened. The right auricle of the heart was
found filled in great part, with a soft gelatinous clot, having
in its centre vesicles filled with a semi-concrete fluid; and it
was traversed by an infinitude of vessels injected of a bright
red or black. This polypus extended into the right ventricle, into the ascending and the descending vena cava, and into
the right subclavian and jugular veins, and confounded itself
in a measure with their parietes, which were much dilated.

A man aged thirty-six years: entered into La Charité, in
1817, for symptoms of aortic aneurism, under which he
died. On examination, the right cavities of the heart,
besides having fresh coagula, contained shreds of a fibro-
albuminous matter organized, and adhering so strongly to
the parietes, that they could only be separated by lacerating
them. These shreds prolonged themselves into the ascending and descending cava, and almost obstructed the orifice
of the pulmonary artery.*

These cases ought to put the question at rest about the
formation of organized, and adherent polypi in the heart.
They have been found more commonly on the right side,
in the right auricle; and the venæ cavæ; probably from
the partial stasis of blood, which sometimes, perhaps frequently occurs there, especially in diseased lungs   The
fact besides is sufficiently familiar, that in large aneurisms,
the stasis of blood which occurs in them, occasions a deposite of the coagulating lymph in concentric layers. There
are indeed, but few of the large blood vessels of the body,
which have not been found obstructed by such coagula.
Haller* saw, in a woman of forty years, the ascending cava
between the emulgent, and the iliac veins shut up by an adherent coagulum, and the current of blood was passed up-

* Bert. p. 448.
† Opus. Pathol. Observ. p 23.

wards by the right spermatic vein; which was in a state of
extreme dilatation.   M. Laennec, has met with three cases
of the ascending cava, obliterated by a coagulum adhering
to it for three or four inches, in such way as to allow a very
partial circulation upwards: the carotid artery has been found
occupied by similar coagula;* also the aorta.†

The case seems in fine to be sufficiently made out, that
besides the polypi, or accretions of the fibrinous part of the
blood, which follow death, similar accretions occur during
life.   And that many of them have been found organized in
the heart, and in the large blood vessels, both arteries and
veins; and adhering by a continuity of substance to the parietes of these cavities; sometimes obstructing them completely, and turning the current of blood into other channels.

* Bertin, p. 446.   Laennec, vol. ii. 591 to 592.
† Am. Med. Jour. No. 5.

CHAPTER XVII.

IRRITATIONS OF THE HEART.

(*Continued.*)

OSSIFICATIONS OF THE VALVES

THE partial ossification of the valves of the heart is a very common affection in old age, and frequently presents itself also in the middle term of life. It is known to every anatomist, that the orifice of communication between the auricles and the ventricles is defined by a fibrous ring, from which the tricuspid and the mitral valves spring; and that in the case of each orifice, the muscular fibres of the corresponding side of the heart form loops, the extremities of which, as a general rule, are attached to the fibrous ring forming the orifice. The fibrous structure of the ring is continued into that of the valve, and the loose margins of the valve are attached by a continuation of the fibrous structure, called chordæ tendineæ, to the projections of the muscular structure of the heart called columnæ carneæ.

A fibrous structure also forms the orifice of the pulmonary and of the aortic artery, and this fibrous structure is continued measurably into the semi-lunar valves. The basis of all the valves of the heart being thus laid in fibrous structure, their mechanism is completed by their surfaces being formed by a continuation of the thin, smooth, and shining serous membrane, which lines the cavities of the heart, and of the blood vessels. This combination of fibrous and of serous structure has been denominated by

Corvisart fibro-serous,* and is supposed, from its particular character, to be the cause of the indurations and ossifications, so often found in the valvular structure of the heart: the fibrous matter exhibiting the same tendency there, that it does in other parts of the system.

The ossifications, however, in the heart, as in other parts of the body, which attend a pathological state, present this difference from the ossifications arising from the physiological tendencies of the body. In the latter, the precursor of bone is mucilage, and then cartilage; but in a diseased condition, the deposite of bone is not preceded in this way. It is indeed primary: the calcareous matter brought to the part by the circulation, seems to be absolved abruptly and instantly from the laws of vital affinities, and to be governed by those of mere physical chemistry; which occasions its deposite in masses, either in plates of a small size, or in grains resembling, strongly, an imperfect crystallization. The quantity of animal matter in these bony deposites, is most commonly at its minimum, and scarcely appreciable. The grit, so often found in the pineal gland, is a striking example of this; and we frequently have the ossifications of the valves of the heart quite as unalloyed. It is, therefore, from general and well marked similitude, that such concretions are familiarly called grit, and stone. An irritated state of secretory surfaces gives rise to the same phenomenon. The calcareous matter in the secretion seems to be absolved suddenly from the laws of vitalism, and to be immediately subjected to those of crystallization; as far as this process can go on, with other matters intervening between the atoms to be crystallized. The difference, however, in this case is, that the concretion does not adhere to the surface which secretes it, but is washed off, perhaps, as soon as it is formed.

In many cases of calcareous deposite in the heart, the

* Org. Dis. of the Heart. Phil. 1812. p. 158.

atoms are not aggregated, but seem rather to be deposited in the interstices of the part; very much in the same physical state, however, as when they are aggregated, and leaving the inference that these atoms are also deficient in that proportion of gelatine which usually enters into the composition of bone. In several experiments which I have tried on the subject, I have been struck with the efficiency of a mucilage in preventing the precipitation, and the consequent return to a crystallized state of a strong saline solution. This will explain why the calcareous matter of bone, does not present itself in a sort of crystallized state; while the enamel of the teeth, which have scarcely an appreciable quantity of animal matter in them, evidently have their atoms arranged on the plan of crystals. Under these considerations, the question very naturally arises, whether fibrous membranes in a state of irritation have not a disposition to secrete calcareous matter to the exclusion of gelatinous? and whether it is not owing to this trait, that calcareous concretions almost pure, are more common on them than in other parts of the body.

The most frequent situations of these ossifications of the fibrous structure of the heart are, the mitral valve between the left auricle and left ventricle; and the semi-lunar valves at the orifice of the aorta. Ossifications, though sometimes witnessed on the tricuspid valve, and on the semi-lunars of the pulmonary artery, are yet rather uncommon, and co-exist generally with an unnatural communication between the right and the left sides of the heart,* from which M. Bertin has drawn the inference, that the arterial blood has much to do in the production of them by its irritating influence. Unusual, indeed, as pathological changes are there, the cartilaginous induration is more common than the osseous. Ossifications of the semi-lunar valves of the pulmonary artery, and of the tricuspid valves, have been seen by

* Bert. p 217.

Morgagni, by Corvisart, Bertin, Laennec, Burns, and several others; so that there ought to be no doubt of their occasional occurrence, though they are almost incomparably
more rare than those of the left side. This infrequency
of ossified valves on the right side of the heart, induced
Bichat to deny its occurrence there on any occasion.
For a summary of some such observations, of a very interesting kind, M. Laennec may be consulted with advantage.*

 The anatomical characters of valvular ossifications are as
follow: When the valves are entirely affected, they frequently are enlarged so much as to form a sort of irregular
pad around the orifice to which they belong, and at the same
time the orifice is diminished in its diameter; sometimes,
indeed, reduced to a few lines. The ossification is originally formed in the thickness of the valve, and it, for some
time, will be smoothly covered by it; but in the progress of
its growth, the asperities of the ossification pierce the valve,
and are then exposed naked to the current of blood. The
valve in this state is sometimes so ragged, that it looks at
a little distance like an irregular jagged ulceration, and
when felt, is rough and hard to the hand, strongly resembling
small fragments of stone in the multitude of its asperities.

 The most usual form in which we see ossifications of the
aortic valves is in small graniform masses in greater or less
number, and placed at their base; or in their edges, especially where the corpuscles of Arantius are. I have in several
instances seen an ossification about the size of a grain of
wheat in the angle between two adjoining valves, and adhering to their margins, in such way as to prevent their
accurate closure, on the re-action of the artery. It is not
uncommon to see the osseous induration extending all
along the base of the semi-lunar valves, and thus forming
an almost continued circle: the removal of which, would

* Vol. ii p 573.

be attended by that of the valves from the identity and close connexion of the two.

Where these several mechanical conditions of ossification have increased much in size, the valves become permanently and rigidly fixed in their positions, and are not changed from them except very inconsiderably; certainly not enough to check the reflux of the blood from the aorta, while the latter is re-acting on its contents.   Even small ossifications will present the rigid closure of the valves, and produce some derangement in the circulation, as was found to be the case with the late Dr. Wistar, where there was an ossification at the junction of two valves.   The progress of ossifications of the semi-lunar valves, is sometimes such, that it leaves only a small orifice for the passage of the blood. Morgagni saw in a gul of sixteen, who had been sick from birth, the valves of the pulmonary artery so ossified, swollen, and united, that there was scarcely space enough to admit a small bean.   Corvisart has often seen constrictions from this cause of the large arterial orifices, and I have myself, not unfrequently met with them.   He relates* a case, an abridgment of which deserves being introduced at this place.   A washerwoman, aged 73, was put under his charge in 1803. Six years before that, she had while walking, experienced such difficulty in breathing, and palpitations of the heart, that she was obliged to stop short.   The frequent renewal of these symptoms, with œdema of the legs, and irregular pulse, compelled her to seek refuge in the Hospital, at the time stated.   She had been there but thirteen days, when she died, apparently suffocated.

On examination after death, her heart was found not much larger than usual, and there was half a pound of serum in the pericardium.   The left ventricle was so hard and elastic, that it retained permanently, a nearly cylindrical shape. The mitral valve, along with the corresponding ostium ve-

* Page 172.

nosum, were ossified at several points.   The semi-lunar
valves of the aorta were indurated, ossified, and thickened
in such a manner, by the calcareous deposite between their
laminæ, that they were fixed in their state of depression;
and their loose edges approached so as to come in contact,
and block up the aperture of the vessel.   The current of
blood would thus have been completely obstructed, had not
one of the valves still retained merely enough flexibility at its
base, to permit an opening of only one or two lines, for the
blood to pass through.

In regard to the valves placed between the auricles and
the ventricles, their induration is found also in all the stages
and states, from a cartilaginous to an osseous condition.   The
cartilaginous state is sometimes confined to the chordæ tendineæ, and to the fibrous ring at the base of the valve; and
presents the appearance of a smooth, but unequal circular
pad, which constricts the ostium venosum.   On other occasions this cartilaginous, or fibro-cartilaginous change is found
along the margins of the mitral, and tricuspid valve, and
diffused through their thickness.   In its texture it resembles
strongly the semi-lunar cartilages of the knee joint.

The osseous induration of the mitral, and tricuspid valves
is varied in its position and mechanical shape, in the same
way with the cartilaginous; and like it is formed primitively,
between the two laminæ of the valves.   It is, however, disposed to much greater inequalities of thickness: and not unfrequently its rough points are denuded, and so ragged, that
they look like a caries.   In ossifications of the edges of the mitral valve, their jagged edges are sometimes found adherent:
and indeed blended together to such an extent, that the orifice between the auricle and ventricle, is converted into a
sort of narrow canal or slit, into which a large quill cannot
be easily introduced.

Vegetations of the Heart.

These are wart-like productions, from the lining membrane of the heart, which are observed to grow from all its valves, and from the auricles, particularly the left. They are met with much more frequently on the semi-lunar valves of the aorta, than elsewhere. These productions, by their number and the size to which they grow, sometimes form a serious obstruction to the circulation of the blood.

They strongly resemble common warts, especially such as arise from a venereal cause on the organs of generation, and in their vicinity. It was from this resemblance, that M. Corvisart, took up the notion of their venereal origin, and suggested the advantage, when their diagnostics could be established, of instituting an antisyphilitic course of treatment. I may merely state, that this idea has not been adopted; and, that they are not supposed by the pathologists of the present day, to be caused by syphilis. Their colour is commonly of a yellowish white with a tinge of red; and their size varies from that of a millet seed to a pea. Their surface is not unfrequently rough, so that it resembles a strawberry, from the multitude of little tuberosities upon it; and sometimes they are elongated into cylinders. They exist in greater or less numbers in different subjects, and are sometimes so abundant as to give a granular appearance to the valve, or surface which they cover.

Their texture resembles very closely, that of the polypi of the heart; consequently some of them have about the consistence of coagulated lymph, while others are much more firm. They frequently contain in their centre a dark spot, as if produced from blood, and sometimes a clot of blood is actually found there. They adhere with considerable tenacity to the lining membrane of the heart, wherever they arise, and seem to be continuous and identified with it: when soft, they may be scraped off with the handle of the scalpel; but when hard they require cutting to be removed.

These vegetations, or warty excrescences from the lining membrane of the heart, have been variously accounted for. M. Laennec* says, that they arise from an irregularity in the motion of the blood; and being formed out of precipitated coagulating lymph, they become organized by a process of absorption, and of nutrition, analagous to that which occurs in false membranes. On this point, M. Bertint remarks, that he has no doubt of such being the case sometimes; but he also thinks, that they may come originally from inflammation, followed by an albuminous secretion from the lining membrane. This is indeed rendered the more probable, from serous membranes when inflamed presenting the same kind of albuminous granulations. Moreover, as the inflammation of the left cavities of the heart, and of the aorta is more common than that of the right cavities, and of the pulmonary artery, we are led to the inference, that as these vegetations are found more frequently in the former, so they are the result of inflammation in a majority of cases. My own experience on the subject, is too limited to permit me to decide, which of these authorities ought to prevail. I have no doubt, that they are both right in regard to particular cases.

There are other species of vegetations found within the heart, and called by M. Laennec globular, from their shape. I imagine that they are very rare, as I have never met with them; yet as they constitute one of the interesting pathological conditions of the heart, it will be proper to say a word or two concerning them. They are of a spheroidal or oval shape, and vary in size from a pea to a pigeon's egg. Their exterior surface is even, smooth, and of a yellowish white; they contain sometimes matter resembling half fluid blood, on other occasions pure blood, or that kind of fibrinous sub-

* Laennec. vol II p. 620   † Bertin. p. 919.

stance which occupies old aneurismal sacs, they have also been found with a sort of puriform matter in them.

These globular productions are found most usually at the inferior part of the ventricles near their apex, and in the sinus of the auricles; and they invariably adhere to the parietes of these cavities. Their adherence is accomplished by means of a pedicle of a very irregular form, which is interlaced with the columnæ carneæ, and may sometimes be detached from them without rupture.

It is very difficult to account for the mode of their formation: it would seem almost as if the matter in them was of an irritating quality to the lining membrane of the heart, and that the latter took on a secretion of lymph for the purpose of enclosing it in a cyst, so as to render it harmless. M. Laennec states, that the first time he ever met with it, he was reminded of a singular case reported by a fellow student of his as follows: A girl in a moment of violent grief swallowed an ounce of arsenic, but escaped very unexpectedly from its effects. The following year, being in a similar state of mind, she took arsenic again, but was not so fortunate in escaping. On examining her body, after death, the effects of the recent dose were obvious on the stomach; and besides them a cyst was found, which seemed just detached from the vicinity of the pylorus, where the traces of its adhesion were still perceptible. This cyst contained an ounce of arsenic crystallized, and had the consistence of an ancient false membrane. It was supposed to have been formed around the arsenic by the sudden inflammation which followed the first dose, and that the patient owed the preservation of her life to its enveloping the poison.

Rupture of the Heart.

This is rather an unusual affection, but it every now and then happens in consequence of a violent effort; of a fit of anger, and other strong emotions. Dr. Physick informed me that he knew a man of seventy, who, having married a young girl; the night of the wedding he died suddenly in bed, and on examination it was ascertained to have proceeded from a rupture of the heart. Many cases of ruptured heart have been found connected with its previous ulceration at the spot; hence some anatomists are disposed to think that ulceration is its most common cause. Rupture has also been found to arise from aneurisms, from softening of the heart, and from blows on the chest. It also occurs where the parietes of the heart have been thinned by an excessive dilatation.

In the winter of 1821-22, a gentleman aged about forty, by profession a lawyer, in passing through his kitchen stopped to say a word to the cook. He drew a sigh and fell down dead. On examination, a small triangular laceration was found in the front of the right ventricle, through which the blood had escaped. The part was shown to me afterwards by the late Dr. Lawrence: but, on the death of the latter, the preparation was by some means lost.

The large blood vessels of the heart are also subject to rupture within the cavity of the pericardium. M. Portal has seen a rupture of the descending cava at its junction with the right auricle, in a young woman who died suddenly in a cold bath.

I have narrated in chapter 10th, in consequence of its connexion with the history of the natural colour of the gastric mucous membrane, an interesting case of rupture of the aorta occurring under my own observation. To this the reader is referred again for an account of the change of structure in the part, and of the appearances generally on dissection.

If we consider the natural thinness of the auricles between the musculi pectinati, and that of the right ventricle in certain spots where there is a large quantity of fat covering the heart, it seems rather remarkable that rupture of the heart is so uncommon an accident. This, however, is not only the case, but the right ventricle is not so often ruptured as the left; neither are the auricles so often ruptured as the ventricles

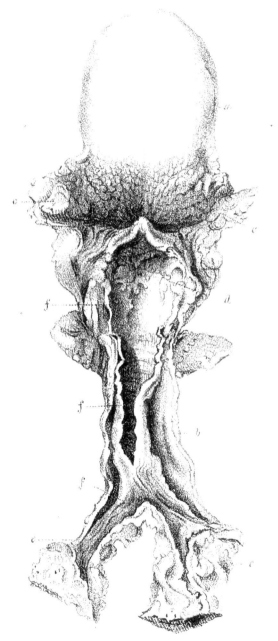

CHAPTER XVIII.

DISSECTIONS, ILLUSTRATING THE PATHOLOGY OF THE THORAX.

Croup.

THE following dissection exhibited, with remarkable distinctness, the state of the respiratory organs in this affection. The history of it, as communicated by Dr. Jackson, the attending physician,* is as follows: E. M. a healthy, robust infant, aged one year, was seized, Feb. 1st. 1829, with catarrh and inflammation of the tonsils. Emetics and purgatives were administered; they operated favourably, and an apparent amendment ensued. On the 5th, the respiration became stridulous and laboured—venesection with the warm bath ad deliquium was practised, which again produced an abatement of the symptoms. On the morning of the 7th, Dr. Jackson was called into consultation on the case: the respiration was then exceedingly laboured; accompanied with the peculiar sound of croup; stridulous, dry, and unattended with any mucous rattle; cough dry. The tonsils were enlarged, a small ulcer on each; the fauces were red, but had no appearance of membranous exudation, as is often seen in cases of croup commencing in cynanche tonsillaris.

Sixty leeches were applied to the throat, and a warm bath administered, with three grains of calomel every half hour—after the leeches, a blister to the throat. No im-

* Amer. Jour. No. 8. August, 1829.

provement was manifested.   In the evening, twenty drops
of hive syrup every hour were added to the former treatment, and calomel, one grain every hour.   At the same time
muriatic acid was applied to the fauces by means of a brush,
as recommended by Bretonneau; in the belief, that, although
no exudation was discernible in the fauces, it existed in the
larynx, and blocked up the glottis, into which the air was
introduced with great difficulty.

8th.—Some improvement—mucous secretion established
in fauces and trachea, the respiration easier and less stridulous.   Mucous ronchus, or rattle, throughout both lungs;
thorax resonant; pulse frequent; cheeks flushed.   Blister
directed to each side of the thorax—calomel, with hive syrup continued.   A secretion of viscid mucus in fauces,
copious during the day—and was removed by swabbing—
bowels opened several times during the day; discharges
dark green—pediluvium at night, with poultices to legs.
During the day, infant more animated and lively.

9th.—Became much worse in the night: in exploring the
chest, the mucous ronchus or rattle, that existed the previous day, had disappeared, and no respiratory murmur was
distinguishable, yet the chest was resonant on percussion—
respiration exceedingly laboured, and requiring strong muscular exertion—continued to grow worse, and expired suffocated towards noon.''

*Autopsy, February 9th, twenty-four hours after
death.*—Present Dr. Jackson; weather cold, and no visible
putrefaction.   On opening the thorax, the lungs did not
collapse, though there was no unnatural adhesion.   Interlobular emphysema existed throughout the lungs, which was
manifested by bubbles of air collected on their surface in
clusters, and in strings or chaplets following the division of
their lobuli.   One of these strings traversed completely the
circumference next to the ribs, of the left inferior lobe.
There was also a considerable emphysema around the root
of both lungs.   Throughout the inferior lobe of each lung

there was a high sanguineous congestion, such as exists in the acute stage of peripneumony, and which gave a solidity approaching to the sanguineous hepatization. This congestion was of a greater intensity at and about the root of the lungs. The remaining lobes were of a light spongy texture, and, except for their emphysematous state, seemed sufficiently fit to carry on respiration.

The emphysema had passed into the anterior and superior mediastinum behind the sternum, and thence below the fascia profunda cervicis, into the root of the neck, up the trachea to the larynx.

Having taken out together all the respiratory organs, and laid open the trachea and bronchia, there was found a perfect and entire lining of coagulating lymph, extending from the superior margin of the glottis, through the larynx, trachea, and bronchia, into the lungs. This membrane became thicker and thicker in its progress downwards; and could be traced satisfactorily into the secondary branches of the bronchia. It adhered with tenacity to the larynx, and upper half of the trachea; but not so much so as to prevent its being pulled off in a state perfectly distinct. In the lower part of the trachea, and in the bronchia, the membrane was so loose, that it separated with the greatest facility, but retained perfectly its tubular shape.

The mucous membrane of the larynx, trachea, and bronchia, beneath this lining, was highly injected with blood, and inflamed, presenting an appearance rather rougher than common. In the bronchia it was of a scarlet colour, which increased in intensity the farther the bronchia penetrated into the lungs, until their ramifications became so small, as to prevent their being satisfactorily traced. The augmentation of colour was very abrupt, beyond the terminations of the lining membrane of lymph. The ramifications of the bronchia contained a sero-purulent fluid mixed with air. For an illustration of this case, see Plate IV.

*Ulceration of Epiglottis Cartilage, and of the margins
of Glottis; Disseminated Tubercle, and Emphysema
of Lungs; Scirrhous Liver.*

A gentleman, aged about fifty, rather free in the use of
alcoholic drinks, supposed to take about a pint daily in common, has had for some time symptoms of dyspepsia, attended with borborygmus, &c., a short time before death, his
bowels became very irritable. The circumstances, however, which seemed to lead immediately to death, were inanition, and extreme marasmus, arising from an inability to
swallow any thing without great difficulty, and extreme
pain, and a disposition of the pharynx to return the food
to the mouth. He was also troubled with excessive and incessant coughing, and expectorated a reddish mucus, having
a fleshy appearance. He had no night sweats, no hectic fever, no pain about the thorax, excepting a continued one
which seemed to be at the root of the neck just above the
clavicles. There was nothing unusual in his respiration, or
in the sonoriety of his thorax when struck.

The autopsy was made, November 30th, 1828, about thirty-six hours after death, along with his physician, Dr. S.
Jackson.

Exterior aspect.—General pallidness, and extreme marasmus, with some putrefaction about the abdominal muscles.

Neck.—Pharynx and œsophagus healthy, the epiglottis
cartilage was removed by ulceration down to a level almost
with the root of the tongue; its ulcerated edge was bare, and
the mucous membrane in a ragged state, having separated a
little from the ulcerated edge of the cartilage. From the
epiglottis, an ulceration, of the doubling forming the upper
margin of the glottis, extended on each side to the arytenoid
cartilages. The rima glottidis was larger than usual, and
the blood vessels about the glottis and root of the tongue
seemed to be in a state of chronic congestion.

Thorax.—The heart of common size; the tricuspid, the mitral, and the aortic valves had undergone a partial cartilaginous degeneration; the two last more than the first. Aqua pericardii about one ounce; white concretions of lymph in the right cavities of the heart.

Lungs presented disseminated tubercles throughout: the intervening pulmonary structure being still respirable. In the summit of the right lung were some small pulmonary excavations, from eight to twelve lines in diameter, and there was a pleuritic adhesion at the same place. Lungs were also congested and heavy. At their lower edges there was a well-marked interlobular emphysema; there were no tubercles there.

Abdomen.—Liver diminished one-half in size, of a light yellow colour, and looking as if each of its acini had undergone a tuberculous change. The gall bladder filled with a thick ropy mucus coloured deeply by bile. The mucous coat of the stomach had the light slaty tinge indicative of its chronic phlegmasia, but no unusual vascular appearances. The small intestines, especially the ileum, presented several chronic ulcers of various sizes; some of which had almost perforated it. The large intestine sound. Other viscera of abdomen not obviously altered.

Head not examined.

Peripneumony, with Tubercles and Emphysema of the Lungs.

A black man, aged about thirty, had suffered during the winter with violent cough, of five months' duration. He died suddenly with symptoms of difficult breathing, which lasted only a day or two. I examined him on the 13th of May, 1829, along with Dr. Togno, his physician.

The thorax, before it was opened, gave out a heavy, fleshy sound on the right side and beneath the sternum. There was not much emaciation, the muscular system being well developed

The abdominal viscera were universally sound; the stomach on its mucous coat was of a light pink colour.

Thorax.—The right lung presented universal but old pleuritic adhesions. Its substance was red, carnified, or nearly solid, and irrespirable. It presented, when cut into, some small cysts of puriform matter and many small tubercles in the first or semi-transparent state about the size of a pin's head. The volume of this lung was diminished one-third in its size. The left lung did not collapse on opening the chest; much of its vesicular structure was solidified and red, with the same sort of transparent tubercles diffused through it. The emphysema of the lung was very conspicuous on this side of the thorax, and was manifested by very small globules of air covering its surface under the pleura, and which could not be made to disappear upon pressure. It is probable that this emphysema produced the sudden death.

The heart was more than a half larger than common, in all its cavities; and the left ventricle was in a state of hypertrophy. The substance of the heart was whitish and hard; its cavities not being disposed to collapse. It had that sort of induration of structure, which is the frequent attendant of its chronic irritations. There was a white patch of ten or twelve lines in diameter, on its front surface.

The right auricle and the two ventricles were filled to distention with a white, firm coagulum of fibrine; which was interwoven with their irregularities, and extended for a foot or more into the contiguous large vessels, to wit, the venæ cavæ, the pulmonary artery, and the aorta.

Chronic Catarrh, and healed Tubercles.

November 4th, 1827. Magdalen Asylum. Examined for Dr. Meigs.—A man about fifty years old, who had served as waiter and guardian there. His case had not been regularly attended to, so that the symptoms were not much known; except the principal one, that of his having suffered from catarrh for many years.   I found the lung on the left side healthy in its structure, but with very extensive adhesions to the thorax; which gave it, on percussion, a sort of semi-obtuse sound.   On the right, the periphery of the pleura was sound; but the lung was tumefied in its centre, with a few small tubercles in it, not evolved: and at the apex of the same lung there was a cicatrization, such as is represented by Laennec.   At the bottom of the cicatrization was a knot six or eight lines in diameter, which seemed to be the remains of an old tuberculous mass, or of a pulmonary cavity.   The preparation is in the Anatomical Museum.

Phthisis Pulmonalis.

Mr. S. has been under the treatment of Dr. Isaac Hays for the last two months, for pulmonary consumption.   He had no cough, no expectoration, no pain in the breast, the leading symptoms have been progressive emaciation, reaching at last to an extreme point, and most profuse perspirations at night.   So far from diarrhea, his bowels have been constipated.

Examined February 1st, 1828, twenty hours after death: present, Drs. Hays and Samuel Jackson.

Thorax.—Lungs adhering universally on both sides, so that we had to tear them off from thorax; pleura pulmonalis, and costalis identified by the adhesion, so that the pleura costalis was stripped from the ribs, on raising the lungs to examine them.   Lungs hard, inelastic, and literally filled with crude tubercles, from one to three or four lines diameter: some few of them had begun to soften, and they were, for the most part, distinct from one another.   A very small quantity of permeable, respirable lung was found at the under part of the inferior lobe of each lung; but so little, that it was a matter of surprise, that he could have lived to such a stage of disease.

39

Heart of healthy size and structure.   Surface had on it at the apex, a white patch of nine lines in diameter, somewhat fungous; and there was another white patch, oblong, but not fungous, on the right auricle.   A white, or drab coloured coagulum in right auricle, extending into venæ cavæ, a similar one in right ventricle, passing into pulmonary artery, and following its ramifications.

Abdomen.—Peritoneum healthy, stomach contained one quart of gas.   Mucous coat smeared with mucus, and of a light pink tint; some large veins in the cellular coat in patches.   Thickness of mucous coat normal, and its consistence was also normal at the small curvature, but somewhat softened at large.   At cul de sac it was so soft, that it could be scraped away with the finger.

Small intestines healthy.   Large intestines; coats attenuated: mucous coat so soft, that it could be removed by scraping with the back of the scissors.   Small ulcerations, with elevated, ragged, injected margins, and white unequal bottoms, reaching to the cellular coat, surrounded the loose edges of the ileo colic valve.   No ulceration elsewhere. Vascular injection in the region of the ileo colic valve. Elsewhere the large intestine was semi-transparent, and of a light pearl colour.

Liver healthy.

Phthisis Pulmonalis.

Mr. G., aged about fifty years.

External Appearance.—Marasmus to the last degree, thorax long, narrow, intercostal spaces sunk in, pectoral muscles drawn into axilla, muscles shining through skin. Abdomen drawn in towards spine.

Thorax.—Heart of common size, right auricle filled with blood, more than half of which was a transparent yellow fibrine, extending into the right ventricle, and looking as if it had been formed some time before death.   Ossifications of small size about the root of the aorta, and semi-lunar valves. A polypus, seven or eight inches long, half an inch in dia-

meter, transparent and yellow like the preceding, was drawn
from the aorta, and was found with branches corresponding
with those from the arch of the aorta.   About half an ounce
of yellow transparent serum in pericardium; no inflammation of latter.

Lungs.—Old strong adhesion, universally connecting the
periphery of lungs on each side of thorax to the pleura costalis.   Many dry tubercles in each lung, from a line or two
to eight or ten in diameter, several empty pulmonary excavations from dissolved tubercles on each side.   The lower
portions of the lungs did not contain so many tubercles and
excavations as upper; but still they were numerous.

Abdomen.—Peritoneum healthy generally.

Stomach.—Mucous coat somewhat thicker than usual,
and looking as if it had suffered very generally from old
phlogosis, a patch near pylorus, about three inches diameter,
where the vascularity was very considerable.

Small intestine.   Duodenum healthy.   Jejunum and
ileum abounding in large ulcers of mucous coat, which went
around the circuit of the gut, and were from twelve to eighteen lines wide.   On the peritoneal surface, corresponding
with these ulcers, there had been a secretion of recent coagulating lymph; as if to wall up, and to repair the cavity of the
intestine.   Where these ulcers on the different folds of the
intestine were contiguous, the intestines adhered to one another by the coagulating lymph.

Large intestine.   The beginning of colon on internal face
covered for some five or six inches by ulcerations, also the
adjoining part of ileum, the remainder of large intestine
healthy.

Mesenteric glands much enlarged.   Other viscera of abdomen healthy.

Mr. G. had a pleurisy twenty years previously.   His health
had been declining for the last two years.   His symptoms
were principally pain in the abdomen, but no diarrhea.   He
had a slight cough, and not much expectoration.

The head was not examined

Phthisis Pulmonalis in an Infant aged three months.

An infant son of S. G., aged three months, about three weeks ago was seized with catarrhal symptoms, manifested by frequent cough, distressed respiration, quick frequent pulse, fever. There was no disposition to perspiration at any time during its malady It was treated by low diet, repeated bleeding, leeching to the thorax, a blister, purging, and dia-phoretics.

Autopsy, Dec. 16, 1827, assisted by the attending physician Dr. Shoemaker.

External Appearance—By no means emaciated.

Thorax.—The sub-cutaneous cellular adipose substance over the left pectoralis major, had a common phlegmonous cavity of about one drachm in capaciousness; supposed to have arisen from the blister. The greater part of the pus had been discharged by an ulceration of the skin. No well marked secretion of lymph bounded the abscess; the fat contiguous to it was like adipocere, and the little granules of it were separated from one another. The pleuræ were per-fectly sound and contained no serum. The lungs were packed throughout their whole substance with crude tuber-cles, which had pushed the air cells aside: some of the tuber-cles were insulated, and other in clusters; the single tuber-cles were from a quarter of a line to three lines broad, and the clusters were of various sizes none of them exceeding in extent three or four lines. These tubercles were interspersed through the lung so as to resemble a plum-pudding, and to leave but small interstices between them for the air vesicles. The lungs were rendered so hard by the abundance of the tubercles, that they collapsed but very little when the thorax was opened. None of the tubercles were in a state of sup-puration; but, by pressing the lung, a purulent matter or mu-cus could be squeezed to the surface in small quantities. No inflammation of lining membrane of trachea, glands about the bifurcation of the latter hard, tuberculous, and considerably enlarged.

Heart.—Pericardium contained ℥ij, of light coloured transparent serum, but had no sign of inflammation. Heart healthy; right auricle filled with a coagulum of red blood. Foramen ovale admitted at upper margin a common probe.

Abdomen.—Peritoneum healthy. The liver of a light yellow, gall bladder contained a thick tar coloured mucus with bile. Stomach and intestines entirely healthy: there seemed to be scarcely any red blood about them; for inside and out they were almost white, or at least of the lightest sienna ground. There was not the slightest tendency to ulceration in the mucous coat of the small intestines, or mark of irritation; neither were the mesenteric glands in any way enlarged. Head and spine not examined.

Phthisis Pulmonalis.

Mrs. R., aged forty, has for several years been subject, during the winter, to inflammation of the thorax, which kept her in a delicate, emaciated state. This winter she has had repeated hæmorrhages from the lungs, marked by the usual symptoms; and a short time before she died, she lost much blood from piles, which inflamed and ulcerated.

February 9th, 1829, I examined her in the presence of her attending physicians, Drs. James and J. Randolph.

Thorax.—The left pleura contained a pint and a half of turbid serum; of a dark colour, as if tinged with blood, and slightly inspissated with pus: the pleura itself was healthy, excepting several specks of ecchymosed blood under it, both on the thorax and lung; it was also rather opaque: left lung healthy. Right lung had an old peripheral adhesion all around it. It was generally sound and healthy, but a space of the under lobe four inches square, had a puruloid infiltration into its substance, mixed with small tubercular excavations, and with the natural air vesicles.

Heart.—Healthy in texture and size; but the parietes of the ventricles were reduced to one third of the usual thickness.

Abdomen.—Viscera sound, no ulceration in intestines. The internal coat of the stomach had not the villous appearance which is usual, but rather a smooth, white, porcelain-like condition, interspersed with veins containing black blood. She had not, it appears, been incommoded by gastric symptoms.

In the omentum majus, and along the great curvature of the stomach, under the peritoneum, were several spots a few lines in diameter, of ecchymosed blood, which with the ecchymosis under the pleura, showed the disposition of the hæmorrhagic irritation of the mucous membrane of the lungs, to be repeated elsewhere.

She was four months gone in pregnancy.

Pleuritis, and Meningitis from Measles.

An infant daughter, aged fourteen months, of Mr. F. was seized, six weeks ago, with measles, in a mild form, from which she seemed to have almost recovered. A fortnight ago, severe catarrhal symptoms came on, followed, after a few days, with strabismus; but no delirium or local heat of unusual degree about the head. The heat of the skin, generally, was very great. During the progress of the disease, the child was bled, and was also leeched on the temples.

Head.—Dura mater adhered with great tenacity to the bones, as is common at this period of life. The arachnoid membrane over the whole circumference of the encephalon, was of a yellowish purulent colour, from the deposite beneath it of a matter which seemed to be pus, serum, and coagulable lymph mixed; and which had, therefore, a gelatinous consistence. Upon separating the convolutions of the brain, the same kind of matter was found extending to the very bottom of them all, and in some places forming

purulent foci, between the contiguous surfaces of the pia mater.   This observation would seem to prove, that the affection
was of the pia mater, and that the secretion occurred from
its surface which is most free, to wit, the one next the arachnoidea.   If it had been an affection of the arachnoidea, we
should scarcely have seen the secretion of pus penetrating
to the bottom of the convolutions of the cerebrum; but it
would be on the free surface of the tunica arachnoidea, from
a principle common to inflamed membranes, to wit, that of
secreting their morbid productions from the free surface.

The brain was in a soft mushy state, and had many vascular points about it, giving the appearance of congestion.
There was a drachm of turbid serum in each ventricle; under the posterior part of the velum interpositum there was
the same sort of sero-purulent effusion just alluded to.

Thorax.—Lungs white like those of a veal, and did not
collapse much on opening the thorax.   Some slight accumulation of blood about their roots; but the structure was
soft, spongy throughout, and by no means hepatized.   No
serum in either pleura.

The right pleura presented a recent and easily lacerable
adhesion of its posterior part, between the lung and chest.

The pleura costalis universally on that side had been
highly inflamed, and was completely imbued with red blood
which had been extravasated into its texture.   Some of the
patches of blood were a complete ecchymosis of ten or
twelve lines in diameter running into one another.   In the
posterior inferior part of the pleura, a layer of recent coagulable lymph, four or five lines thick, and from two to three
inches broad existed, adhering by one surface to the lung,
and by the other to the pleura, and having a vascular communication with both, at least, so the specks and points of
blood on its surface led me to infer.

The heart was healthy.

The viscera of the abdomen were very pallid, and the
hollow ones semi-transparent.   The mucous coat of the sto-

mach and large intestines could be scraped off very easily with the thumb nail, or the handle of a scalpel. The muciparous glands were not visible. The liver was of a dull yellow colour.

Abdominal viscera in other respects healthy.

Pleuritis, Peripneumonia, and Pericarditis.

H. E., aged twenty-two months, was taken with cough and hoarseness on the 26th of January, 1826. His mother supposed it to be croup, and administered antimonial wine so as to vomit him six or seven times. I was called in a day or two afterwards. His symptoms were then hoarseness, occasional cough, laborious and hurried respiration attended with an unusual elevation of the thorax during inspiration; pulse frequent, small, and not strong; not much heat of skin. Between this period and his death, which occurred Feb. 2nd, he was treated with frequent cathartics, with expectorants, and with diaphoretics. He was blistered largely on the breast, and had spirits of turpentine rubbed upon the parietes of the thorax. A close examination of him three times a day did not, on any occasion, indicate the necessity of bleeding.

Autopsy.—Left lung hepatized throughout by inflammation; pleura of the same side had on its costal circumference a coat of coagulating lymph, one and a half lines thick. Right lung healthy in its structure, a coat of coagulable lymph on the pleura costalis opposite to this lung.

The pericardium contained half an ounce of serum, and had suffered universally with recent pericarditis, which showed itself in a general lining of coagulating lymph.

Brain somewhat congested; slight watery effusion under tunica arachnoidea of upper surface of hemispheres. No water in ventricles beyond what might be accounted for from infiltration after death.

Pleuritis and Carditis.

In the dissection of a mulatto boy aged fifteen, I found the pleura costalis on the left side adhering universally to the pleura pulmonalis by a recent layer of lymph, which, by the infiltration of serum into it, was reduced to a yellow, thin, gelatinous mass four lines in thickness, and resembling dropsical cellular substance.

The pleura on the right had also been inflamed, but the adhesions were trifling, and it contained about twenty ounces or more of a yellowish transparent serum.

The texture of the lungs was sound. The heart was enlarged at least one half beyond its common size, in the case of each cavity, and had a hard elastic condition, such as occurs to it, when there has been an inflammation in its substance. The pericardium was sound.

Hydrothorax.

In the dissection of a male subject aged fifty, Dec. 1824, the following condition of the viscera existed: Three quarts of water in left pleura; left lung collapsed. Pleura costalis and diaphragmalis studded over and coated with coagulable lymph. The right pleura contained eight ounces of water; the pericardium three ounces, but there were no signs of coagulable lymph in it.

The abdomen contained one quart of water with a small quantity of pus. Intestines and stomach anasarcous, a few shreds of lymph on intestines. Lower and upper extremities very much distended with anasarca, left lower extremity much more so than the other.

Ventricles of brain contained three drachms of serum.

Albumen in considerable quantity, detected by heat in the serum of the pleura, pericardium, and abdomen. Little or none in extremities, or in that of brain. Much in urine.

*Hypertrophy and Enlargement of Heart, followed by
Sudden Death from Agitation of Mind.*

A shoemaker aged about fifty, complained for two or three
years of pain in the left breast from time to time, when over
fatigued or exposed. Retaining his flesh, he was considered
by his friends as hypochondriac. In the afternoon of March
22nd, 1823, he took a walk, and, on his return was informed
of his having lost by theft, a pair of boots and a pair of shoes.
He was much agitated at the news; in a little time complained of feeling unwell; requested to be conducted to his
bed, and in ten or twelve minutes afterwards died.

Dr. Huston having been called in at the moment of his
illness, administered some sp. corn. cerv. to him with no effect.

Autopsy forty hours after death.—By squeezing on
the chest, a considerable quantity of frothy mucus, amounting to several ounces, was discharged from his mouth by
Dr. H. some time previous to the examination.

Exterior Aspect.—Perfect rigidity of limbs, settling of
much blood on the back of the neck, and about upper parts
of chest. Lips blue and congested.

Respiratory Apparatus.—Sound of thorax somewhat ob-
tuse to percussion, on left side near middle. Lungs of a deep
bluish or modena from the great congestion of blood in them;
collapsed only inconsiderably on opening of thorax; trachea,
bronchia, and lungs filled with frothy mucus. The capillary veins of the serous or sub-serous tissue distended almost
to hæmorrhage. The same in regard to mucous membrane
of whole respiratory apparatus; also to lungs, trachea, larynx,
and root of tongue. About three ounces of straw coloured
serum in each pleura. Nothing like tubercles or derangement of lungs, except from the recent accident.

Circulatory Apparatus.—Heart enlarged to nearly twice
the natural size, with hypertrophy and dilatation together.

Aorta from orifice to innominata enlarged to two or three times its usual capacity.   Internal membrane thickened, softened, and cartilaginiform, interspersed with specks of beginning ossification.   Middle coat also increased in thickness, but diminished so much in density that it yielded as if it were half rotten; external coat sound.   Semi-lunar valves thickened as if from chronic inflammation, but no ossification in them.   Blood collected in abundance in great vessels, but still fluid; a pint of it was discharged, before the thorax was opened, from the veins of the base of the cranium, the brain having been previously examined.

Abdomen.—Viscera in a healthy state.   The gastric mucous membrane throughout, of a uniform light claret colour, or perhaps speaking more exactly, like a recent stain of claret upon white linen; with the exception of the summits of the rugæ, where a deep claret colour was prevalent along each one of them.   The stomach contained his dinner, which seemed to have been of soup and bread, and an inspissated thick coat of mucus was spread over it.   When this was removed, small punctated patches of red blood were seen in the capillaries of the mucous coat.   This is sometimes mistaken for inflammation.   The mucous membrane of natural consistence and thickness: I could not, however, tear it up in shreds after the way spoken of by Louis; though with the end of the scalpel slid along, I could raise it.

The brain was highly congested with blood, as in an apoplectic state, but there was no extravasation.   A chronic thickening and inflammation of the arachnoidea was perceptible on the summits of the hemispheres: at the posterior part of the velum interpositum and in lateral ventricles. Two or three drachms of serum were found in each lateral ventricle.   The commissura mollis was absent, as is commonly the case, where there are effusions of water in ventricles.

Hypertrophy of Heart, and Mollescence of Stomach.

Jan. 13th, 1829.—The Rev. Mr. ——, aged forty-three, of a large stature, six feet, and robust in proportion, from an early period of life has been subject to palpitations of the heart, which are said to be hereditary in the family. For the last two years dyspepsia was added to his other complaint; and he was reduced very much. A few weeks ago he had some dropsical effusion into the lower extremities, which after a while disappeared. A few days before his death he was seized with an inflammation of the scrotum and testicles.

Autopsy thirty-two hours after death, in the presence of the attending physician, Dr S. Tucker, and Mr. R. Dorsey, student of medicine. Weather cold.

Abdomen —Enormously distended with flatus: muscles of, somewhat putrefied. Colon in its whole length distended almost to bursting with flatus; and, on an average, from three and a half to four inches in diameter. On the ascending part, a patch of recently extravasated blood, two inches in diameter, existed on the peritoneal coat. It probably came from a vessel ruptured by the over distention. The colon contained liquid fæces of a yellow colour, which adhered to its parietes.

Small intestines also distended with flatus, and contained a yellow, bilious fæces.

Stomach distended with flatus. There were several dark spots on it, such as occur in old gastric affections; and its veins were moderately injected with blood. The whole mucous coat of its left half was in such a state of mollescence that it could be scraped off readily with the thumb-nail, being only in a slight degree more tenacious than common mucus, and it was there of a kind of chocolate colour. The other half of the mucous coat had a slight greenish tinge;

and the boundaries between it and the mollescence were well defined by a change of colour and of consistence.

Spleen healthy.

Liver healthy, but rather light-coloured.

Thorax.—Lungs, texture of perfectly sound: an old pleuritic adhesion over several inches of the right one. No congestion of blood in them.

Heart but little inferior in size to a small bullock's heart; all its cavities were dilated, and had their parietes thickened; the ventricles to twice the natural thickness, and the auricles to three times. Vessels of the heart healthy.

There was a slight pericarditis manifested by some films of coagulated lymph; and by a turbid serous effusion, amounting to about two ounces.

The other cavities not examined.

Inflammation of the Internal Membrane of the Heart and Aortitis, with Chronic Pleuritis and Pericarditis.

Anne Ebner, aged fourteen, a domestic in the family of Mr. Otis, portrait painter, has for some time had unpleasant symptoms about the thorax; the leading one of which was difficulty of breathing on ascending a flight of stairs, or upon severe exercise, and irregularity in the action of the heart and in the pulse. Having died, I examined her about twenty-four hours after death; being assisted by Drs. Samuel Tucker and Charles D. Meigs.

Universal adhesion of the pleura costalis to the pleura pulmonalis, apparently for the most part of ancient standing. The heart in mass, larger than that of the largest male adult. Universal adhesion of pericardium to the heart; the substance of the heart of a whitish colour, hard and elastic. Each of the cavities of the heart dilated to twice or three times the natural standard. The left ventricle rather more enlarged than the other cavities; hypertrophy of all the cavities. The lining membrane of each, of a white, shining appearance, and thicker than usual. In the left auricle, for the extent of two square inches, on its inferior surface, the lining membrane was studded with small granulations of coagulating lymph. Hypertrophy of the mitral valves. On the auricular side they were covered with small granulations of coagulating lymph.

The aorta, near its root, had a distinct layer of coagulating lymph, which could be raised up in shreds, being peculiarly distinct from the lining membrane of the artery.

The same appearance was visible in the pulmonary artery, but the layer of lymph, not quite so separable from the lining membrane, as in the aorta.

The right lung congested in its upper lobe.

The peritoneal coat of the liver thickened, and covered with coagulating lymph. The ascending cava was free from any investment of coagulating lymph. The mucous coat of the stomach, of the small, and of the large intestines, red and congested, the jejunum, of a red rose colour.

The liver considerably enlarged.

There were no evidences of inflammation in the lower part of the aorta, and in the small vessels.

This is one of the few instances, of genuine and indisputable inflammation of the lining membrane of the heart and aorta, that I have met with. It was here not so much indicated by redness, as by the effusion of coagulating lymph. In Dec. 1828, I met with a subject of advanced age, where the aorta internally was so highly inflamed, as to be of a deep lake or crimson colour.

Pericarditis.

Alms House, July 10*th,* 1827.—William Johnson, a coloured man, middle stature, had, on my taking charge of the surgical department, scrofulous indurations of the lymphatic glands on each side of the neck, larger than a hen's egg. He had, also, a suppurating lymphatic gland in the right axilla. I treated him for about two months with iodine, and derived no very obvious results.

About the first of this month, he complained of more debility than usual, and of a loss of appetite; his bowels became loose. Three or four days before his death, the latter symptoms increased into a dysentery, and he died very suddenly on the night of the 9th inst.

I examined him about ten hours after death. The lymphatic indurations of the neck were suppurating.

Thorax.—A pint of red serum in the pleura on one side, the other side healthy. Universal pericarditis, consisting in a red spongy coat of coagulating lymph; nearly one quart of water tinged red by blood in pericardium. There had been no symptoms apparent to the medical attendants of local affection of the heart, not even pain; and no well marked difficulty of breathing, except the day before his death: though, from the appearance, I should suppose, that the disease had been on him for, at least, two or three weeks.

Abdomen.—Nothing remarkable about it, except the mucous coat of the colon, which was tinged of a sooty or lead colour, as in cases of old inflammation.

A Case of Rheumatism with Metastasis, producing Carditis, Pericarditis, Peripneumonia, and Pleuritis.

A young lady in Market Street, " A. B., aged eight years, of a delicate habit, began on the 16th November, 1827, to complain of a cold; that is, she had a slight sore throat, cough, and a general soreness over the body. She was dieted, and took a dose of castor oil by the direction of her mother.— 17th.—She remained pretty much the same. 18th.—Her feet and hands were observed to swell, and were very slightly inflamed, though not painful· they were sore to the

touch. 19th.—The first day of my visiting her. She
complains of a severe pain in her right groin; a small tumour is observed here, the soreness of this part excessive.
Purged with calomel and magnesia, and the part bathed
with warm sweet oil. 20th —The pain and soreness of the
groin much mitigated; but the chest is suffering from severe
pain accompanied by great oppression Was blooded; the
blood very sizy. 21st.—All her symptoms much relieved.
22d.—Pain in the groin nearly gone; could bear the part
touched, and move her limb without much suffering.   In
the evening I was sent for, but being engaged, I requested
my friend, Dr. Hays, to visit her for me.   He found her
sitting on her mother's lap, being unable to lie down.   She
complained of pain in the region of the heart, with difficulty of breathing.   Her pulse was frequent, but not corded;
the respiration was short, pain being experienced, when an
attempt was made to draw down the diaphragm.   A metastasis of the disease having evidently taken place to the
heart and diaphragm, revulsives were ordered with the hope
of relieving these parts.   A large sinapism was applied over
the chest, which afforded prompt relief, and on my visit the
next morning I found her free from pain.   During that and
the two succeeding days, she improved so much as to be able
to be about; and nothing but a little debility seemed to remain.   But on the twenty-fifth, she exposed herself several
times, by walking, without additional covering, through a
long, cold entry, by the ill-directed advice of the servant,
in whose charge she was left for a few hours: the consequence was, that on Monday the 26th, she was attacked
with a severe pain at the extremity of the xiphoid cartilage, accompanied by great distress in respiration, and total
inability to lie down   I ordered a sinapism applied over
the pained part, which very promptly relieved her. 27th.
Her stomach much harassed by sickness and vomiting; the
groin free from pain, as was the part upon which the sinapism was applied yesterday.   After the stomach had conti-

nued for an hour or two in the situation just stated, it would suddenly be reconciled, and the top of the left shoulder would now be the seat of excruciating pain, which in turn would become easy by a return of the disease to the stomach, which would now be sick as before; or the pain would fix itself in the left side near the margin of the false ribs; and thus the affection would alternate a number of times in the twenty-four hours. 28th.—Stomach very sick, with some difficulty of breathing. In the after part of the day, these symptoms became very much more severe; so much so indeed, that there was now violent and frequent vomiting. A white tenacious mucus in considerable quantity was eventually thrown up, which, at the moment, afforded great relief. I was present at this time; and from the great abatement of her distress, I indulged a hope it would be permanent; but in about an hour after I had left her apparently much improved, I was suddenly called to her; and before I could reach the house, she was a corpse.

" During the whole progress of this disease, the arterial system was but little affected: the pulse, with the exception of the last day, was neither frequent nor tense; yet it bore evacuations remarkably well, as far as they were pursued. Bleeding, leeching, and purging, were in turn ordered: as were, with some vigour, blistering and the repeated application of rubefacients.

" The cough, which attended through the whole course of the complaint, was always found to be augmented, whenever the chest became the seat of attack. Expectoration was difficult, requiring numerous efforts to bring up a small quantity of white tenacious mucus; but this little always appeared to afford some relief.

" It was truly astonishing to see with what suddenness the disease would shift its seat, and with what severity it would affect the part to which it would translate itself. When the stomach became the seat, it would instantly produce violent sickness, and sometimes pretty severe vomiting, which would continue for several hours. After this, it might, in an instant, be transported to the diaphragm, lungs, or pleura. When here, she would experience severe pain, great difficulty of breathing, and almost incessant coughing, and an inability to lie down.

"From these parts it would return to the stomach, attended by the usual consequences of extreme sickness, or distressing vomiting; or, more fortunately, it might take its flight to the point of the shoulder, where it would tarry the longest, and of course with the lesser inconvenience. On the twenty-eighth, it attacked the stomach with unusual violence; and after the severe vomiting mentioned above, it seized upon the heart, and death almost instantly followed. For after it had left the stomach, she desired to be seated upon her mother's lap, where she had not been more than five minutes, before she shrieked violently from pain seated in the region of the heart; she stiffened all her limbs by a sudden effort, and in a moment died.

"It is worthy of remark, that the child's parents are both sufferers from rheumatism, and that she had several times before been attacked with the disease; and also that eighteen months before her death, she had had chorea Sancti Viti, which continued for three or four months, and was cured by the repeated administration of purgatives, principally cremor tartar and jalap in combination."[*]

Autopsy, thirty-eight hours after death, in the presence of her physicians, Drs. Dewees and Hays.

Exterior Aspect.—Colour as usual after death; no great marasmus; pupils dilated; expression of countenance tranquil.

Head.—Membranes of brain natural; cerebrum natural; cerebellum somewhat softer than usual; not a drop of water in ventricles of brain.

---

[*] Amer. Jour. Med. Sciences, vol. ii. p. 473, communicated by Dr. Dewees.

Medulla Spinalis.—Membranes natural; it seemed harder than usual, and its elasticity was so considerable that it would suffer an extension of two inches, followed immediately by an equivalent contraction. The rugæ on its surface very perceptible. Its elasticity was independent of the dura mater, for it continued in the same when the latter was slit up both before and behind. The dura mater contained about two drachms of fluid, one half of which was blood, and the other the serum peculiar to this cavity. The upper and the lower enlargements of the medulla spinalis, (renflements,) where the nerves of the upper and of the lower extremities come off, were unusually developed.

Thorax.—Heart twice as large as usual, and adhering by a thick coat of lymph to the pericardium, excepting a small extent of the right ventricle, and the whole of the right auricle. Two ounces of straw-coloured serum in pericardium. The texture of the heart was sensibly altered; its parietes being almost universally thickened; of a light colour, about that of veal flesh; so rigid as not to collapse after the manner of a healthy heart upon the evacuation of its contents; and cutting in the crisp semi-cartilaginous manner peculiar to inflamed muscles. I did not detect any inflammation of its lining membrane: the right cavities contained coagula of red blood.

The left pectoralis major muscle had been the seat of pain; it was found not altered in colour, but the texture had undergone the same pathological change with that of the heart. The pleura of the region behind it, had some filaments of coagulating lymph passing between it and the corresponding surface of the lung. The whole circumference of the pleura on both sides of the body had lost the smooth shining condition of the normal state, presented here and there specks and pellicles of lymph, and was slightly turbid. Each cavity contained about two ounces of a straw-coloured, transparent serum.

The thymus gland was natural, being about the size of it in early infancy.

The right lung was heavy, fleshy, and had lost one half of its spongy character; the blood being infiltrated into its cellular substance, and identified with the organ.   The left lung was also partially solidified with blood, but by no means to so high a degree as the right, for its spongy character still predominated: it was pushed to the back of the thorax by the augmented heart.

Abdomen.—Peritoneal surface universally healthy.

Stomach.—Of a pink colour on its mucous membrane, especially along the ridges and sides of the rugæ; being two or three degrees lighter than that of Mr. W. J., reported at page 122.   It seemed entirely healthy, and had abundant rugæ.

Small Intestines.—Duodenum healthy; the jejunum and ileum, in the greater part of their extent, were reddened by a turgid state of the capillary veins, but there was neither ulceration, ecchymosis, or thickening.   They were smeared with mucus, and had some appearance of irritation, but possibly the latter might have arisen solely from retrograde congestion, by the arrest of the circulation at the heart. The congested state of the lungs would favour the opinion; but in that case one would infer that the stomach also should have been congested with venous blood, which was not the fact.

Large Intestines.—Spasmodically contracted, and contained only mucus.

Liver.—Peritoneal coat somewhat turbid, a little thicker than natural, and abounding in large, distinct absorbents; granular substance, (acini,) not so distinct as usual, hard, cohering strongly, and somewhat intermixed with that resisting yellowish matter, constituting what has been called the fat liver.*   Had this state of the liver a connexion with the

---

* Having once tried it by experimenting, I am of opinion that this matter is not adipose, but a modification of coagulating lymph.

chorea, or with the long course of purging instituted for the cure of the latter?

Gall Bladder.—Contained a thin, yellowish mucus; cellular coat increased to three lines in thickness by the infiltration of a gelatiniform fluid.

Spleen healthy. *Kidneys* not examined.

CHAPTER XIX.

GENERAL PATHOLOGY OF NERVOUS SYSTEM.

THE very extensive distribution of the nervous system, its intimate intertexture with all the solids, and the continued requisition by the latter upon its influence, for the due performance of their functions, render it among the most interesting tissues of the body.

One of its most striking features, is the variety which it exhibits in the different classes of animals. In man and the mammalia it consists of a cerebrum, a cerebellum, a pons varolii, medulla oblongata, and medulla spinalis, and from these, numerous cords pass to all parts of the body. The brain in man is much greater in proportion to the spinal marrow than in any other animal, and the spinal marrow predominates much in its thickness over the nerves which proceed from it. In some fishes the brain scarcely exceeds in size the medulla oblongata. In the molluscæ there is only a brain, which sends off nerves as radii from a centre, to ganglions scattered over the body, almost as large as the brain itself. In insects the brain is scarcely larger than one of the numerous swellings of the spinal marrow, and sends off its nerves in the same way. In polypi there is no regular and distinct nervous system, and hence it appears that the lower we descend in the scale of animals, the less this system is to be found concentrated in a particular region, and the more it is diffused over the whole body.

This general view of the invariable presence of the nervous system in different animals, proves the necessity of its existing in order that animal life may be possessed: and it

also exhibits another important feature, that it is susceptible of a great variety of exterior modifications, without
having its essential characters impaired. It is also observed,
in regard to this system, that the less it is accumulated in
centres, the less important its integrity is to the life of the
animal; for example, a toad or a tortoise has comparatively a
small brain, which exercises so slight an influence on the
general condition of the animal, that its removal will not
prevent life from being sustained in its usual relations and
vigour, for many months afterwards.   There are many species of worms and insects, which on being cut into two or
more parts, each of those parts becomes an independent animal, possessing its own sensations and distinct powers of
life. And many of the zoophytes, on being divided into very
small pieces, from the general diffusion of the nervous principle in them, have a distinct existence communicated to each
section.   It is only when we approach the higher orders of
animals, that the integrity of the nervous system and the
presence of its central parts, become indispensable to life;
and that this necessity is more strongly perceived, the larger
that the brain is, in proportion to its ramifications.

The foregoing facts render it probable that the nervous
system is analogous in all animals: and we may conclude it
to be nearly the same in all parts of the same animal, from
the metastasis of function which occasionally has occurred
where a sense has been lost either naturally or by accident.
It would seem, therefore, that the varieties of its functions
depend upon the peculiar character and arrangement of the
organ supplied with nervous matter.   We are also furnished
with another idea from examining the state of the nervous
system in different animals; namely, that, as in polypi, &c.,
a new animal can be generated from a section of an old one;
so it is evident that each part possesses integral properties,
and consequently must have the principles or modifications
of its nervous system blended together: but in man and all
other mammalia, these modifications have each their parti-

cular throne or habitation, as the eye that by which we see, the tongue that by which we taste, and so on of the other senses.

We find, moreover, by experiment, that other locations of functions take place in the latter animals, that the brain is the seat of intelligence, the medulla oblongata of the principle of respiration, and that the medulla spinalis is the immediate seat of life to all other parts. Be it allowed that such localities of vital functions do exist, of which there seems to me to be so little doubt, why may not the different parts of the brain afford settled positions to the moral faculties, as asserted by the phrenologists?

It has been considered probable, that nearly all of the nerves have an increase of matter, as they get farther from their origin in the brain or spinal marrow: this accounts for the sensibility met with every where on the surface of the body, so diffused and minute in its division, that the finest needle cannot be introduced without causing pain. Though it be true, that this opinion of the extreme terminations of nerves being larger or containing more matter in the aggregate, than the trunks from which they emanate, is opposed by the common appearances on dissection; for there we find that as ramifications pass off the nerve is diminished: yet it is difficult to explain the universal sensibility of different organs, without supposing some such arrangement. The fibres of muscles, the surface of the skin, and other sensitive parts, may possibly, receive something like a coating of nervous matter. If this be the case, the medulla derived from the brain and spine is sufficient to furnish the whole body, as it may possess a plasticity and ductility somewhat like that of gold: which the natural philosophers tell us is such that a grain of the metal may be beaten out to cover a surface of several feet square; and one cubic inch is sufficient, to gild completely a wire; long enough to surround the globe.

The celebrated Hunter, in his view of the vitality of the

blood, admits unequivocally the general diffusion of a nervous matter through the whole system, though he does not
undertake to describe the mode of arrangement.   His words
are, " I consider that something similar to the materials of
the brain is diffused through the body, and even contained
in the blood: between this and the brain a communication is
kept up through the nerves. I have therefore adopted terms
explanatory of this theory; calling the brain the *materia
vitæ coascervata,* the nerves the *chordæ internunciæ,* and
that diffused through the body the *materia vitæ diffusa.*
Of this latter every part of an animal has its portion. It is,
as it were, diffused through the whole solids and fluids,
making a necessary constituent part of them, and forming
with them a perfect whole; giving to both the power of preservation, the susceptibility of impression, and from their
construction, giving them consequent reciprocal action.
This is the matter which principally composes the brain;
and where there is a brain, there must necessarily be parts
to connect it with the rest of the body, which are the nerves;
and the use of the nerves is to continue, and therefore convey, the impression or the action from one to the other.
These parts of communication must necessarily be of the
same matter; for any other matter could not continue the
same action.

" From this it may be understood, that nothing material
is conveyed from the brain by the nerves, nor, *vice versa,*
from the body to the brain: for if that was exactly the case,
it would not be necessary for the nerves to be of the same
materials with the brain; but as we find the nerves of the
same materials, it is a presumptive proof that they only
continue the same action which they receive at either end."

Conceding this *materia vitæ diffusa* to be a coating of
nervous matter over the whole structure of the body, we can,
from its degree of profusion, estimate, and even anticipate,
the sensibility of different organs; the latter quality being small when the matter is sparingly diffused, and highly

exquisite, when it is abundant.   In this view of the subject, we see the reason for the accumulation of the pulpy nervous matter of the retina; the materia vitæ diffusa has to appear there in the form of a continuous membrane, in order that a delicacy of sensibility might be given to the organ, suited to receive an impression so inconceivably feeble, as that occasioned by the matter of light.   This latter substance, travelling at the immense velocity of two hundred thousand miles in one second, though it has been concentrated in focus upon focus, with a view of determining whether in such a condensed condition it possesses any appreciable momentum, has always escaped the test of the most delicate instruments.   An organ of this exquisitely refined sensibility, is alone capable of responding to a stimulus so exceedingly subtile, that it is even questioned whether it is matter, or merely a quality of it.

The structure and expansion of the auditory nerve, a pulpy distribution on the internal surface of the labyrinth, resembling the retina, affords a parallel, in some measure, to the optic, by depending for the performance of its peculiar functions on a degree of sensibility, capable of feeling the most delicate vibrations of the air.

It is not important at present to enter further into the investigation whether the nervous principle is supplied to each molecule of the body or not, the fact that each part has sensibility being sufficient.   But the question is, whether this sensibility be inherent in every part of the human frame; or distant, and its origin to be looked for elsewhere? The following experiments will, I think, prove the latter hypothesis.

SECTION I.—*Experiment on the Nervous System.*

The admirable work of Le Gallois on the principle of life, has formed the basis of many interesting inquiries on this subject in different quarters of the world, and from the general result of his observations and experiments, the following conclusions seem to be established.

First, That the principle of all inspiratory motions, resides in that part of the medulla oblongata which gives rise to the nerves of the eighth pair.

Secondly, That the principle which animates every part of the body, resides in that part of the medulla spinalis, from which the nerves of that part originate.

Thirdly, That it is likewise from the medulla spinalis, that the heart receives the principle of its life and of its power; but in the whole medulla, and not in a circumscribed portion of it.

With the view of testing the accuracy of these conclusions, the following experiments were executed some years ago. They were undertaken with no desire to establish particular theories or to controvert them, but merely to arrive at sound and useful inductions, and to compare them with the statements of the celebrated French physiologist just named.*

Experiment 1st —Took a kitten four days old, and divided the spinal marrow between the occipital foramen and first cervical vertebra; this instantly stopped respiration. The animal was much agitated, and gaped frequently. At the end of ten minutes, when sensibility had almost ceased, the larynx was divided from the os hyoides, and the lungs artificially inflated   By continuing the inflation for five minutes, the animal was evidently much revived.   At the end of twenty-five minutes (sensation and the power of motion continuing,) the spine was divided between the tenth and eleventh dorsal vertebræ.   At thirty minutes each of the parts thus separated retained sensibility and motion: but all sympathy between them was destroyed, as an impression

---

* These experiments and some others, were performed with the assistance and in behalf of two candidates of the University, Elias Buckner of Virginia, and the late J. P. Freeman of Philadelphia, who subsequently made them the subjects of their inaugural essays

made upon the fore parts produced no effect upon the hinder, and *vice versa.* At forty minutes, the posterior extremities were insensible: at forty-five minutes the anterior parts manifested sensibility when violently pinched: at fifty-two minutes no signs of life remained. Artificial respiration was kept up by intervals till this time. From the quantity of blood lost, and the appearance of the heart, it was pretty certain that death resulted from the hæmorrhage. At sixty minutes, the action of the heart continued, although its cavities were completely emptied of blood, and filled with air.

Experiment 2*d.*—Took a rabbit four days old, and divided its spinal marrow between the occipital bone and atlas, with a needle. Respiration was immediately suspended, and the animal became convulsed, struggled, and gaped; its strength rapidly diminished, and in three minutes life was almost extinguished. Artificial inflation of the lungs being now commenced, in two minutes the animal was much revived, and became still more lively as the process went on. At seven minutes from the commencement of the experiment, a wire was passed through the whole of the spinal column, which immediately extinguished the sensibility and motion of the whole body. With a view of ascertaining the condition of the circulation, a hind leg was amputated, which furnished no blood, and the femoral artery, on being exposed, was found flaccid and empty. Blood was slowly discharged from the veins. The head showed signs of sensibility and life by gaping, as if in a respiratory effort.

Experiment 3*d.*—Took a rabbit of the same age as in the preceding experiment, and under similar circumstances we divided the spinal marrow in the same place: respiration was immediately suspended. In two and a half minutes the animal had almost expired. Artificial respiration was now commenced, and in half a minute afterwards, sensibility returned and the animal revived: we continued the inflation for six minutes, with the effect of full restoration to the ge-

neral functions of life. During this period, whenever a cessation of the inflation occurred, the animal lost its sensibility
and struggled as if for breath.—We now made an incision
between the last dorsal and first lumbar vertebræ, and through
this opening was passed a large wire, down to the end of the
spinal column. The lower extremities were immediately
deprived of sensibility and life: the circulation was also suspended in the parts, as amputation of the hind leg produced
no hæmorrhage. The inflation of the lungs being continued;
two minutes afterwards we passed the wire through the upper portion of the spinal marrow, and sensibility and life,
with the circulation, were immediately destroyed in the upper extremities.

Experiment 4th.—The spinal marrow of a kitten was
divided as in the preceding experiment, and the same phenomena occurred; namely, instantaneous suspension of respiration, tremors over the whole body, gaping of the mouth,
&c. At the end of ten minutes, sensibility became almost
exhausted, and the inflation was commenced, which being
continued four minutes, revived the animal. The carotids
were now laid bare, and the circulation was seen to go on
rapidly. But on suspending the inflation for a few moments,
the action of the heart became much enfeebled, and the blood
assumed a dark colour, which soon changed to a florid, on
resuming the inflation. This was repeated several times,
and always with the same result.

At the end of thirty-eight minutes the carotid and vertebral arteries were tied up, and decapitation performed between the third and fourth cervical vertebræ. A few drops
of dark blood issued from the vertebral arteries, which increased in quantity, and changed in colour, upon inflating
the lungs. The mouth continuing to gap, at forty-five minutes the thorax was opened; in doing which, such was the
acuteness of sensibility and the power of motion in the animal, that its legs were confined to prevent its struggles.

The action of the heart went on violently, and during the

suspension of the inflation, its left cavities were filled with dark blood, which soon changed to florid on resuming the inflation. At fifty minutes a leg was amputated which yielded a few drops of blood. The inflation was persevered in for a few minutes, and the animal revived astonishingly, sensibility being manifested on the slightest touch.

At sixty-five minutes we destroyed the cervical parts of the spinal marrow, by passing a wire through the vertebral canal to the first dorsal vertebra. Upon inserting the wire great pain was evinced; but as soon as it passed down, all sensibility became extinct in the anterior, while it still continued in the posterior extremities, though it was much diminished. At seventy minutes the wire was pushed through the whole spinal canal, and instant extinction of all the symptoms of life took place. The inflation was resumed for several minutes without any effect. At seventy-seven minutes the heart contained dark blood, and feebly pulsated when we left it.

Experiment 5th.—Laid bare the larynx of a kitten, and separated it from the os hyoides—the cranium was next removed and the cerebrum extracted, which produced no important effect. The cerebellum was then taken out, and the animal still continued to respire perfectly and freely for ten minutes It stood strong and firmly on its feet, exhibiting symptoms of violent pain, and making several efforts to cry, with partial success. At the expiration of seventeen minutes the medulla oblongata was extracted, which put an immediate stop to respiration. At twenty minutes we commenced the inflation of the lungs, which being continued for eight minutes, the animal was observed to be dead, evidently from the loss of blood.

Experiment 6th.—Took a rabbit four days old, and removed the upper portion of the cranium. The brain was then cut off in slices, and though a considerable quantity of blood was lost, the animal still retained strength to stand and to crawl about. The cerebrum and the cerebellum being re-

moved in the same manner, respiration still continued.   In
eight minutes, we removed the medulla oblongata, when respiration immediately ceasing, the animal became weak and fell
down, showing little sensibility.   Three minutes afterwards,
we inflated the lungs, and in one minute the animal was much
revived.   In two minutes we examined the contents of the thorax, and finding the action of the heart to continue, a wire was
passed through the spinal marrow, which was followed by an
immediate cessation of sensibility and of the circulation.   But
it is to be observed that the heart continued to dilate and
contract feebly.   ·

Experiment 7th.—After dividing the spinal marrow of a
kitten, between the last dorsal and first lumbar vertebræ, a
probe was introduced, and all the spinal marrow destroyed
as far as the first dorsal   The action of the intercostal muscles immediately ceased—a laborious and imperfect respiration was carried on for a few minutes, which was succeeded
by gapings.   Sensibility appeared completely lost in the
body, and in four minutes afterwards much impaired in the
anterior, though it was still considerable in the posterior extremities.   At five minutes we commenced inflation, and at
seven minutes the posterior parts were sensible to the least
touch, the gapings still continuing.   At ten minutes we destroyed the lumbar portion by running a wire down the canal to the tail.   This produced an instant loss of sensibility
in the hinder parts, while the anterior continued still sensible.   At fifteen minutes the spinal marrow was divided at
the first cervical vertebra, which produced no obvious effect.   At seventeen minutes, sensibility was still perceptible
in the anterior parts, and gaping continued.   At eighteen
minutes, we destroyed the cervical portion, when life immediately ceased.

Experiment 8th.—Dissected down and put ligatures upon
the sympathetic and par vagum nerves of a kitten.   The animal appeared to be in the most excruciating agony; and soon
ceased to cry and to breathe, though it made strong efforts

to do both. At the end of five minutes the ligatures were removed, and the larynx exposed: the rima glottidis was rigidly closed, which accounts for the stoppage of the breath. At the end of eleven minutes, when the animal appeared entirely exhausted, a tube was passed into the trachea, and inflation commenced. After a few strokes of the piston, the animal began a voluntary respiration through the blow-pipe. At twenty-five minutes the spinal marrow was separated at the first cervical vertebra, which put an immediate stop to respiration. At thirty minutes sensibility continued strong, when a probe was passed in at the cervical vertebra, and run through the whole length of the spine, which produced an immediate extinction of life in every part.

Experiment 9th.—Laid open the abdomen of a kitten, and tied up the aorta just below the cœliac artery. In ten minutes sensibility was much impaired in the posterior extremities, though by no means extinguished. The posterior extremities were now separated from the body between the first and second lumbar vertebræ, and when thus separated they exhibited sensibility for two minutes. At twenty minutes the animal stood on its fore feet, respiration and circulation being pretty free. The spinal marrow was now divided at the first cervical vertebra, which, as usual, produced a suspension of respiration. At twenty-three minutes we commenced inflation, and at twenty-five minutes amputated a leg, which afforded a little blood. At twenty-seven minutes decapitation was performed. Three minutes afterwards we recommenced inflation, and the anterior parts exhibited signs of sensibility when pinched; the head gaped. At thirty-three minutes destroyed all the spinal marrow, which extinguished life entirely. At forty minutes we opened the thorax, and observed the heart pulsating; and on wounding the aorta, dark blood issued.

Experiment 10th—Opened the abdomen, and put ligatures under the aorta and vena cava, leaving them loose. We next dissected down, and tied up the carotid arteries and jugular veins, separated the larynx, and introduced a tube for the purpose of inflating the lungs, through which the animal breathed. In ten minutes we divided the spinal marrow at the first cervical vertebra, which put an immediate stop to respiration. At the end of fourteen minutes we commenced inflation, and at seventeen minutes decapitated, and continued the inflation. At twenty-two minutes the ligatures were tied, which had been previously fixed on the aorta and vena cava, and then we cut off the posterior parts at the last dorsal vertebra. At thirty-nine minutes sensibility was very manifest, the inflation being continued. At forty-two minutes we opened the thorax, and found the heart to beat regularly and strongly. One of the internal mammary arteries having been divided accidentally, bled freely per saltum. At fifty minutes, the circulation going on vigorously, the venæ cavæ were seen carrying dark blood to the heart, and the pulmonary veins returning vermilion-coloured. The auricles contracted synchronously, and emptied themselves completely. The ventricles did the same.

At fifty-five minutes, sensibility was very much impaired. One leg, being amputated, did not bleed, although the action of the heart appeared regular and vigorous. At fifty-seven minutes, the aorta being cut, bled freely of vermilion-coloured blood, which caused a gradual diminution in the action of the heart. At sixty-two minutes, however, it had so completely ceased, as not to be excited by the point of a needle; though on blowing air into it from the vena cava, its contractions were feebly renewed.

It appears to me, that the foregoing experiments pretty clearly establish the validity of the three positions assumed. That the medulla oblongata is essential to voluntary respiration—that the spinal marrow is immediately connected in its functions with the vitality of all the parts to which it sends nerves, and that the heart is indebted to the spinal marrow for its ability to carry on the circulation. To cor-

43

roborate these points however more fully, let us review the bearing of the several experiments.

First, In the first, second, third, and fourth, as the object of inquiry was to ascertain the influence of the medulla oblongata on respiration, a section was made with a needle just below the occipital bone, and a suspension of breathing immediately took place. This proves that the organs of respiration are put in motion by an influence derived somewhere from within the cranium, and that however indispensable the integrity of the phrenic and the intercostal nerves may be to their action, still the primum mobile is not in them or the parts of the spinal marrow to which they belong.

Next it was desirable to ascertain what part of the encephalon maintained the process.

Experiments fifth and sixth prove it to be the upper part of the medulla oblongata, near the origin of the par vagum and glosso-pharyngeal nerves; for in each of them the successive removal by slices of the cerebrum and cerebellum did not arrest respiration. The moment, however, that the medulla oblongata was injured, a stop to this process was the consequence.

We are thus led to a beautiful and important conclusion in physiology: one which, from the unequivocal character of the proofs brought to its support, is justly entitled to the greatest attention; and which ought to enter into all our reasonings upon the symptoms connected with apoplexy and other affections of the brain attended with compression of its substance. It is highly probable, from the cavity of the cranium being completely filled, that any deposites of blood within it by increasing the aggregate mass of contents, or any diminution of its capacity by a part being depressed, which is equivalent thereto, will cause itself to be felt throughout the substance of the brain: the compression being communicated not only to parts immediately contiguous, but also, by a juxta-position of particles, to the

whole mass.   If this reasoning be correct, we may understand in what manner respiration is affected by compression on the medulla oblongata, notwithstanding the effusion
or depression may take place at a very remote situation
from it.   Conceding this, is it not proper to make perforations in the cranium, to relieve compression, by allowing
the brain more space, though we may not be assured that
the effused fluid will be exposed?

In relation to this part of our subject is an observation
made in experiment eighth.—A ligature placed on the par
vagum stopped respiration, by producing a spasm of the
rima glottidis; and a blow-pipe introduced into the trachea,
simply by keeping the passage for the air open, restored the
function.

Secondly, As regards the influence of the spinal marrow
upon the life of other parts.   In experiment second, a wire
passed through the whole of the spinal column, immediately extinguished sensation, motion, and circulation throughout the body.   In experiment third, a wire, passed through
the lumbar portion of the spinal marrow, destroyed life in
the lower extremities.   The same injury inflicted on the
dorsal portion produced the same effect on the upper extremities.   Experiments fourth, sixth, seventh, eighth, and
ninth, all demonstrate the same principle, by similar results.

Thirdly, In regard to the manner in which the action of
the heart is kept up. *   The greater part of the experiments
show the circulation to have ceased along with the destruction of the spinal marrow: But the seventh, taken with the
other, brings forward an interesting fact, namely, that the
action of the heart is not sustained by any particular portion of the medulla spinalis, but by the whole of it, each
section contributing its nervous influence.

---

* By action of the heart is meant that degree of vigour in it necessary
to maintain the circulation, and not simply its diastole and systole.

In one set of experiments we have seen the circulation sustained by the upper part of the medulla spinalis, the lower being destroyed, while in another by the lower part of the medulla spinalis, the upper being destroyed; and in the seventh, the circulation was kept up by the extreme portions, that is, the cervical and lumbar, the dorsal being demolished.

Connected with the influence exercised in this manner over the heart is a singular circumstance. To keep up a vigorous circulation where one part of the medulla spinalis is destroyed, it appears only necessary to curtail its extent. This may be done either by putting ligatures on the great arteries, or what is still more surprising, by cutting off the head of the animal. To conclude, it will be seen by the result of these experiments, that whether the nervous matter is diffused through the whole system, as believed by Mr. Hunter, or not, the fact is equally well established that the spinal marrow and the medulla oblongata give to it life and activity.

Shortly after the publication of Le Gallois's Memoir on the seat of the principle of life, an English physiologist of distinction, Wilson Philip, undertook to prove that Le Gallois's experiments were invalidated by his own, and that when an animal was previously stunned by a blow on the occiput, and his medulla spinalis destroyed by hot iron, or dissected out, that the results were different from a destruction of the same by pushing a wire down the spinal canal. To test the validity of these objections, the following experiments were executed, which, in their result, tended to establish still more fully M. Le Gallois's opinions.

Experiment 11*th.*—A rabbit was rendered insensible by a blow on the occiput, but not motionless, so that the breathing still continued. The medulla spinalis opened, and destroyed by a wire, as hot as one of a size for the experiment could be kept. On introducing it afterwards through the foramen magnum into the brain, the breathing immediately ceased. The femoral artery was laid bare, about two or three minutes after respiration had ceased. The beating of the artery was evident. On opening it, a dark-coloured blood flowed from it freely. We now had recourse to artificial inflation of the lungs. When it had been employed for half a minute, the blood which continued to flow copiously from the artery, became of a highly florid colour. The other femoral artery was then opened, from which florid blood also flowed freely. When about an ounce of blood had flowed from the vessels, the inflation of the lungs was discontinued, and the blood again flowed of a dark colour. It continued to flow from the femoral arteries altogether for seven minutes. Three minutes after the blood had ceased to flow from them, the artificial respiration being continued, one of the carotid arteries was opened, from which a florid blood flowed in a copious stream, to the amount of a drachm and a half. The flow from the carotid artery ceased in eleven minutes after the femoral artery had been opened. Most of the blood was now of course evacuated. A good deal had been lost in opening the spine, which always happens. The left auricle and ventricle were found nearly empty· the blood which remained in them was florid. The right auricle and ventricle were full of dark blood.

Experiment 12*th.*—Took a rabbit twelve days old, and rendered it insensible by a blow upon the occiput. We then opened the spine, and passed a hot wire into the brain and through the whole extent of the spinal marrow. Sensibility and voluntary motion were immediately destroyed. We now exposed the carotids: their appearance pale and rather flat: we divided them: blood discharged slowly, and of a dark colour. We now commenced artificial inflation of the lungs: no change in the colour of the blood produced: the quantity discharged was about half a drachm Examined thorax: motion of the heart continued. Two minutes after resorting to artificial respiration, no effect was produced by it on the action of the heart. We now opened the abdomen,

and exposed the aorta: on cutting it, the blood which flowed
was dark. Recommenced artificial respiration: no change produced in its colour The action of the heart had now almost
ceased, and was not invigorated by continuing respiration.

Experiment 13*th.*—A rabbit, same age as above, was
rendered insensible by a blow upon the occiput. We opened
the spine, and passed a hot wire into the brain, and then down
the spinal marrow. Respiration ceased, and sensibility and
motion were lost. One minute afterwards we exposed the femoral artery and divided it—blood followed of a dark colour
and small in quantity. Two minutes after we commenced
artificial respiration, and continued one minute and a half.
Blood not changed in colour. We next exposed the carotids,
and divided them: about ten drops of blood were discharged;
colour dark. Examined the thorax; action of the heart continues; continued respiration; no flow of blood from the carotids; action of the heart not increased by continuing respiration. Two minutes after we divided the curve of the
aorta: the heart incapable of throwing the blood out of it,
though its action continues. We then opened the pulmonary
artery just where it comes off from the ventricle: blood was
discharged and the ventricle emptied itself.

The result being the same in all our experiments, I have
no doubt but that they will be confirmed should they ever
be repeated. Dr. Freeman and myself were convinced of
the truth of what Le Gallois published, and of the incorrect-
ness of the opinion of Philip. That he has been deceived
in his experiments, we are inclined to believe; and that they
are erroneous is sufficiently apparent. It requires an exact
knowledge of the parts, together with a familiarity in piercing
the spinal marrow, to perform the experiment with rigid
accuracy, of which we were apprized by an accident which
befel us. In executing one of our experiments, we were
surprised to find that its result coincided with those of
Philip, and was in opposition to those which we had previously performed. We were desirous of knowing the cause

of this unexpected occurrence, and, upon examining the spinal marrow, we found that we had pierced only through a small portion of its extent, the remainder being untouched. The wire may pass on the posterior part between the spine and membranes, and the sensation communicated to the hand of the operator will very much resemble that arising from passing it through the spinal marrow itself. Is it not probable then, that Dr. Philip has been thus deceived in regard to his having penetrated through the spinal marrow? for it is probable that if he had, he would have been led to advocate the opinion of Le Gallois, and to add his testimony to that of others.

Section II.—*Sympathies.*

As it is very generally conceded by physiologists, that the nervous system not only makes us acquainted with external objects, but is also a means of reciprocal intelligence between the several organs, parts, and tissues of the body;* so we find its morbid derangements very quickly manifested by disturbance in the functions of other systems, especially the muscular. Some of the most striking sympathies, however, of the nervous system, are of its different parts with one another: thus, for example, when one side of the encephalon is affected with phlegmasia, scirrhus, tubercle, or apoplectic effusion; the symptoms frequently extend themselves to both sides of the body, producing epileptic convulsions, coma; want of, or diminution of intelligence; and several other symptoms, in which the two symmetrical sides of the body equally participate.

The two nerves of the same pair are very prompt in their sympathies. When one of the optic nerves is disordered, the other is apt to get into the same state. A neuralgia, beginning in a nerve of one side, frequently extends to the congeneric one of the other, as in sciatica. Nerves on the

* Broussais' Prop ix 10, &c.

same side, and filaments from the same fasciculus, sympathize with one another very readily: thus, as Bichat states,*
an injury done to the frontal nerve, has sometimes been followed by blindness from its affecting also the optic, and
numbness in the whole arm sometimes follows the puncture
of one of the cutaneous nerves in bleeding.

As the texture of the brain and of the nerves differs, it
will suit best to study, separately, the consequences of their
inflammations and morbid changes

The irritations of the central portion of the nervous system are attended, almost universally, by some fault in the
faculties of intelligence, sensation, and locomotion, or rather myotility; and it is principally from the indications derived from these sources, that the information of the practitioner can be made up   Perspiration, circulation, and digestion are only affected in a subordinate degree.

The state of the intellect may be ascertained by the mode
of answering interrogatories, and the general deportment.
The mind will, in different cases, be exhibited in all its conditions, from a universal delirious excitement, to a stupor,
rendering it perfectly torpid, and incapable of action.   Some
individuals, of a phlegmatic turn, are, by disease, rendered
gay and animated, and exhibit more intelligence than in
health.   Some have the intellectual operations a little clogged.
Others have a hallucination bearing upon a particular object
or train of ideas.   In short, whatever may be the attributes
and faculties of mind, and the ideas and deportment naturally connected with them, they are more or less, generally
perverted, exalted, or depressed.   It is not my business to
give the detail of this branch of symptoms, and I therefore
pass to the consideration of others, with the simple observation, that intellectual excitement is, in a majority of cases,
the precursor of intellectual depression, but sometimes the
latter precedes the first, and then follows it again.

* Anat. Gen vol. 1 p 198

The sensitive apparatus, consisting in the senses and in the skin, also present a strongly marked order of symptoms. The sight, the hearing, the smell, taste, and touch may one or all be perverted, exalted, or diminished. The state of each sense is to be tried by its appropriate excitants: the eye by a strong light, the ear by loud sounds, the nose by odorous bodies, the mouth by sapid ones, ink for example, and the skin by pinching. And as all of these functions are double, so each side of the body is to be tried by excitants of suitable strength. Most frequently, there is a sentiment in the brain of local pain or uneasiness, and sometimes a similar phenomenon will be evolved in some of its dependencies, either the senses or the skin.

It is stated* that the inflammation of the central parts of the brain, as the fornix, the corpus callosum, and septum lucidum evolves, sometimes a sensibility of the skin, of the trunk, making the slightest touch painful and intolerable.

In regard to the state of motility of the muscular apparatus, it is much affected in many places. The iris has the pupil either dilated or contracted unusually, remains fixed in its position, or undergoes unusual vibrations. The globe of the eye is changed from its axis, sometimes there is a paralysis or spasmodic contraction of the eyelids. The mouth may be drawn to one side, or its motions and those of the tongue and lower jaw perverted or paralyzed; sometimes the head is drawn forcibly backwards, or inclined to right or left, or one or more of the muscles of the neck is contracted; occasionally, the larynx is drawn upwards and downwards continually.

The muscles of the trunk, suffer momentary spasms, affecting respiration; sometimes the trunk is bent backwards, or to one side, very nearly forwards. The muscles of the limbs, also, experience the influence of the irritations of the central portion of the nervous system They may be either

* Martinet, p 63.

in a state of rigid contraction; or feebleness and relaxation, as in paralysis; or they may retain that kind of fixidity, as in catalepsy, which causes them to remain precisely in· the position in which they are placed, either by the agency of some one else, or by the original spasm.

It is asserted that paralysis of the muscles of the upper extremities with or without rigidity, is owing to a lesion of the thalami nervorum opticorum, and the posterior lobes of the brain; while a similar paralysis of the lower extremities is occasioned by a lesion of the corpora striata, and of the middle lobes.

It was remarked but a short time ago, that the functions of digestion, circulation and respiration, were only subordinately affected in diseases of the brain. The principal perversions of the stomach will be found in want of appetite, and in vomiting; sometimes there is constipation, and on other occasions, especially as the disease advances into its last stages, an involuntary discharge of fæces. The pulse is swerved from its natural condition either by increased or diminished frequency, and by its rythme; the frequency is increased in the early stages of phlegmasia, and decreased in the later periods; and when there is extensive extravasation or disorganization of the cerebral pulp. The respiration may be slow, quick, deep and full, or feeble, regular or interrupted: it is difficult, when the medulla spinalis is affected, and this difficulty augments as the affection advances into the cervical region; until it may amount to absolute suffocation, when it gets into the region of the origin of the phrenic nerves.

One of the most remarkable consequences, and most invariable too of irritations of the medulla spinalis, especially; but also of the brain; is the influence manifested upon the urinary apparatus. The bladder loses its power of contraction, and becoming paralytic, the urine discharged is merely what overflows. Frequently, however, before the accumulation reaches this point, the pain from distention is so excessive, as to require catherism.   The secretion from the kidneys is reduced in quantity, of a dark colour, and of a disagreeable ammoniacal fœtidness; sometimes so intense, that it requires the utmost resolution in the operator to stand his ground.   This urine is frequently found mixed with mucus and filaments of lymph, and discoloured with blood, all arising from the irritated state of the lining membrane of the bladder.

Very great efforts have of late years been made by the continental pathologists, and especially the French, (Flourens, Serres, Delaye, Rostan, Bayle, Foville, and Pinel de Grandchamp, Rolando, &c. &c.;) to determine exactly, by the lesions or perversions of the intellect, of motion and of sensation, the location of the lesion in the central nervous system; and it must be conceded that the comparison and approximation of a considerable number of cases goes far to substantiate their general conclusions.   M. M. Rolando and Flourens, have founded their opinions upon vivisections or ablations of different portions of the encephalon of animals. Owing, however, to the very unnatural state in which animals, thus used, are situated, there are always strong objections to such inferences; accordingly, the conclusion of the first, that the cerebellum was a voltaic pile, presiding over locomotion, and of the second, that it was merely the regulating organ of motion, as well, also, as their joint opinion, that the cerebrum is the organ of consciousness or sensation, have been received very coolly by most physiologists, and utterly rejected by others.   For my own part, I have but little hesitation in asserting, that a disease, whose symptoms are well observed during life, and whose pathological changes are closely inspected at a suitable time after death: is by far the most unequivocal way of ascertaining the functions of the part affected; and in the rigidness of its inductions, is immeasurably superior to a vivisection, where fear, pain, and irritation modify phenomena.

It appears from the observations of M. M. Delaye, Foville, and Pinel Grandchamp, that in the lesions of intelligence, the surface of the cerebrum formed by its cineritious matter, always has suffered some pathological change; whereas, in the lesions of locomotion, the injury is either in the medullary matter, or in the masses of the cineritious, which are deeply situated.   Their testimony, added to that of M. Serres, has gone to establish the fact already briefly alluded to, that in the exclusive palsies of the arm, or rather of the thoracic extremity, the throne of the affection is the thalamus nervi optici, and the medullary matter diverging from it   And that the palsies of the abdominal extremity come from a morbid condition of the corpus striatum and the adjoining medullary matter.   M. Serres has also advanced the opinion that an apoplexy of the cerebellum extends its influence to the penis so as to produce a priapism, which continues even after death.   He, however, has not witnessed this fact himself, but gives it out on the authority of others. It is also stated on the same authority, that injuries of the crus of the cerebellum are manifested by deranging the locomotive power of the opposite leg.

The vitiated structure which has been witnessed on the surface of the brain as attendant on intellectual disorders, is most commonly an increased or diminished consistence, an unusual adherence of the cineritious matter to the pia mater, so that in drawing off the latter, the cineritious matter follows it in flakes; and another change of it, is a marbling of various hues of red.   In acute mania the red colour is intense, but in fatuity or chronic mania, the colour is much lighter; and in protracted cases so indistinct, that there is some difficulty in distinguishing between the cortical and the medullary substance.

From the dissections of Rostan,* it appears that the mode of lesion is not of so much consequence in giving rise to certain symptoms, as the part of the brain which is the seat

---

* Ramoll. du cerv. p. 252

of it.   Hence bloody effusions, hardening, softening, scirrhus, &c., in identical places, are followed by identical symptoms, maiking the influence of the more interior parts of the
cerebrum upon certain muscles.   In simultaneous vitiations
of intelligence and myotility, both the surface and the interior of the cerebrum have, after death, been found affected.
And in one case where an individual had suffered from a
blow on the head which gave rise to exostosis, from the interior of a parietal bone: the symptoms in the development of
the exostosis, and the consequent compression of the brain,
were observed first in the intellect by a diminution of memory.   In the mean time the locomotion was unimpaired,
but subsequently hemiplegia took place, and the individual
died from the progress of the tumour, which was found after
death.   It is very easy under such circumstances, to explain
the succession of symptoms: the intelligence was weakened
in the first instance from the surface of the cerebrum being
the part first pressed upon, and the motility was subsequently impaired, as the pressure was propagated through
the surface to the more interior parts.

   In a considerable number of cases, where the motility of
the arm was more or less impaired than that of the leg, a
corresponding grade of alteration existed in the structure
of the thalamus and of the corpus striatum; the thalamus representing the arm, and the corpus striatum the leg almost
invariably.*

   These observations of the French school, make the train
of intellectual and physical symptoms following affections of
the brain extremely intelligible and interesting.   M. M. Foville and Pinel Grandchamp have gone farther still.   Availing themselves of the discovery of Mr. Charles Bell, of the
anterior nerves of the spinal cord being those of motion, and
the posterior being those of sensation, and associating with
this happy idea, the fact that the anterior cords of the me-

Rostan, loc. cit

dulla spinalis expand into the cerebrum, while the posterior ones expand into the cerebellum, they have found by experiments that there is the same difference between the sensibility of the cerebrum and cerebellum, that there is between the anterior and posterior fasciculi of spinal nerves; consequently, the cerebellum may be considered to preside over sensation, as the cerebrum does over intelligence and motion. These experiments are supported by some pathological ones of Lapeyronié and Petit de Namur. *

* Rostan, loc. cit. 255.

CHAPTER XX.

IRRITATIONS OF ENCEPHALON.

PHLEGMASIA, OR ACUTE INFLAMMATION

THE most frequent form of encephalic irritation is sanguineous congestion, without the rupture of a blood vessel, and it is presented in a vast number of grades, of more
or less intensity. The type of this irritation most often
witnessed on dissection, is as follows: the integuments of
the head, as you cut through them, are found to contain in
their veins a great quantity of fluid blood, which runs off in
a streamlet from below; the pericranium is highly injected,
and the bones of the vault of the cranium retain a very sensible redness, when they are torn off, and held between a
light and the eye. The dura mater is also filled with blood,
which, owing to the opaque, fibrous character of the membrane, is not so evident in the shade of its colour, as in the
multiplicity of the drops of blood on its surface where the
bone has been torn off; and in the tendency of these drops,
from their size and abundance, to coalesce, and even to form
streamlets. The veins of the pia mater are also turgid with
blood, and many of its arteries have some blood left in them.
Along the course of the principal veins, we frequently meet
with small patches of ecchymosed blood between the brain
and the pia mater, or under the arachnoidea.

When a section is made through the substance of the
brain, there exude from the cut orifices of the vessels, small
drops of blood, of a size proportionate to that of the vessels
themselves. These drops in many cases of congestion, are

so numerous as to variegate strikingly the exposed surface, and so near one another, that many of them coalesce by their mutual attraction.   In a congested brain, it is more-over rather difficult to make a clean cut of it; meaning thereby, such a one as will not be smeared with blood, by the sweep of the knife blade, as it passes along the incised sur-face.   In cases where the congestion is rather more advanced, there is an infiltration or ecchymosis of blood in very small red points, and as M. Gendrin* says, commonly united in groups, which may be distinguished by their resembling stains; by their irregular fringed or denticulated edges, and by their having a deeper tinge in the centre, than at the cir-cumference.   According to the same authority, these spots are frequently grouped or clustered along the course of the principal arterial trunks, which traverse the substance of the brain; and are occasionally so confluent as to form a species of marbling, varying in its hues from a light to a deep red, and penetrating irregularly in different directions.   In this latter grade of congestion, the consistence of the brain is not much affected in the places alluded to: it is rather more dense and less viscous than usual.   It is upon the limits of these inflammations, however, that some slight softening of the central pulp is manifested; which may be ascertained by comparing it with other parts, and especially with that dis-eased.   M. Gendrin remarks, that he is disposed where an increased humidity and viscosity is well marked, to ascribe this softening to an infiltration of serum upon the limits of the inflammation; and, that this conclusion is sustained by the contiguous pia mater, also presenting a considerable in-filtration.

In phlegmasiæ of the brain, of a comparatively moderate degree, which have run their course in a week or ten days, and where the superfices is only or principally affected; the corresponding cortical substance is much increased in its

* Histoire des Inflammations, vol II p. 114.

consistence, highly injected, and strewed with numerous small dots of extravasated blood, which when the inflamed part is smoothly incised with a knife, communicate a red, granular or gravelly appearance. The pia mater, and the arachnoidea also manifest strong pathological changes; the former being red, injected, and easier to tear than usual, while the latter has a serous infiltration beneath it, and is thickened, and opaque, having sometimes a layer of coagulating lymph upon it. In these cases it is difficult, perhaps impossible, to ascertain whether the primary inflammation has been that of the brain itself, or of its meninges. The discrimination is not very important to practice, as the same indication is presented in both instances, to subdue the inflammation by active depletion, and by rigid abstinence.

The phlegmasiæ of the brain, are generally attended in the first stage with acute local pain, but this sensation as they progress disappears, and is succeeded by more or less stupor. The inflammatory alterations of structure never exist to an equal amount throughout the whole substance of brain; but are manifested in patches, or distinct portions, the centre of each of which exhibits the principal force of the inflammation. From this centre, to the circumference, the indications become more and more moderate, until they are insensibly lost in the surrounding healthy structure. These patches of inflammation are red, but their hues are, in different individuals, from a vermilion to a scarlet; and are interspersed with small masses of blood.

From the consistence of the part being augmented, it becomes more elastic, and more capable of resisting an effort to lacerate it; and when lacerated, it does not tear more readily in one direction than in another. In this respect it differs materially from a healthy brain, especially when the latter has been prepared by hardening it, in alcohol or in acids. The degree of consistence, however, which is exhibited in an inflamed brain, as far as the observations of pathologists show; seems to be subject to remarkable variations

45

and changes, as I shall presently have occasion to mention.
It exists in all the grades, from a hardened, elastic and resisting body, to a state of semi-fluidity; in which the latter is
generally surrounded by the former.   When the inflamed
portions of brain are near its surface, they adhere more
strongly to the arachnoid membrane than sound parts do;
hence in attempting to tear off the arachnoidea, and consequently the pia mater, flakes of cerebral substance will follow, which are traversed by capillary vessels, engorged
with red blood.   The red discoloration attending this grade
of cerebral inflammation, cannot be removed by ablutions of
water.

The following case, will illustrate what sometimes occurs
in the active inflammations of the brain.   A man of sixty
was brought to the Hôtel Dieu of Paris, with the following
symptoms: remarkable diminution of the functions of the
senses; dull delirium; general sensibility retained, a slight
hemiplegia on the left side, with a manifest rigidity of the
muscles; respiration and pulse natural.   For six days the
symptoms remained stationary; they then became aggravated, and the patient died, with a stertorous respiration.
On inspection, in the middle of the right hemisphere a portion of the medullary substance, was found reduced into a
putrilage; and the circumference of this focus was hard, inflamed, and injected of a purplish red   There were about
two spoonfuls of serum, in each of the lateral ventricles.*

The hardness which takes place in inflammations of the
brain may be alone, or it may surround such a collection of
softened, disorganized, cerebral matter as has. been just
spoken of.   It frequently alters so completely the texture,
and appearance of the brain, not only in consistence, but apparent constitution, and colour, that its vestiges are scarcely discernible.   The hardened part is of almost a uniform vermilion tint, and of a density enabling it to resist

---

* Gendrin, vol. ii. p. 119, from Delavauterie Diss. Paris, 1807.

no inconsiderable force when applied to its laceration. While dwelling on these pathological changes, I must beg, that what I have already stated, may be constantly kept in mind, to wit, that such changes are always partial, and never general in the acute cerebral phlegmasiæ; and, that the diseased part, whether it be hardened or softened, highly vascular, or less so, will be found blending its confines gradually and insensibly into the surrounding healthy structure. In other words, these phlegmasiæ are not exactly circumscribed, but their indications disappear from the centre or principal point, by a progressive degradation to the circumference, until at the latter it becomes difficult to distinguish what is morbid, and what is healthy.

When *Softenings* follow these inflammatory indurations of the brain; they are distinguished from softenings, depending upon a mere infiltration; either by having floating in them some masses of the indurated matter; or, what is more common, by having a part or all of the pulp surrounding them, in a state of induration. The distinction between the hardened and the softened matter, at their surface of contact, is well marked by the mollescence commencing abruptly, and by its being more complete there, than elsewhere. The colour of the softened putrilage, is from a light red to a deep claret ground. It is fluid, and has most of the traces of its original organization extinguished, with the exception of some engorged shreds of vessels, which frequently have adhering to them small masses of indurated and reddened cerebral substance.

M. Gendrin* remarks, that according to his observations the softening (Ramollissement) is modified by the degree of inflammation, and the peculiar texture of the part assailed. For, " when the inflammatory congestion is strong, and the disease is seated in a vascular part of the brain, as for example in the corpus callosum; filaments and clots of

blood are arrested in, and as it were incorporated with the
softened red pulp, by which the latter receives a red striated
appearance.   When the inflammation has remained for some
time at a moderate degree, the softened matter is always insulated, by a layer of highly inflamed tissue, presenting a
strong vascular injection, and a certain density.   The softened pulp is then more or less discoloured, is more deli-
quescent or mixed with a colourless serosity, which seems
to occupy small spaces in its thickness.   It is chiefly upon
the limits of the focus, that one observes these modifications, which are the marks of a beginning separation, and
absorption of the disorganized pulp.   When by the progress of the inflammation, the suppuration is fully accomplished, the softened pulp becomes of a grayish red; and
approaches more and more to the appearance of the pus,
which sometimes separates itself in drops in its thickness."

It occasionally happens, that the pus resulting from an
inflammation of the brain being collected into a focus, along
with the softened and disorganized portion of the tissue; a
false membrane is formed which circumscribes them and constitutes a sac, including them completely.   I have a preparation of this kind where the sac is nearly a quarter of an inch
thick, and was formed in the very centre of the pons varolii of an infant.   It is from this source that cysts and indurations, resembling cicatrices, are derived.   We every
now and then read cases, where these purulent circumscribed
foci have supplanted very extensive portions of cerebral
substance.   Several are reported by Dr. Abercrombie.[*]
In the Journal General de Medicine, tome vi, a case is narrated, where all the right hemisphere was converted into a
purulent focus without odour, and destitute of all traces of
the primitive organization of the brain; excepting the cortical substance, which was firmer than common, and of a
punctated redness.[†] Morgagni, Portal, Lieutaud, and a host

[*] Dis. of Brain, p. 93, et seq   [†] Gend. vol. ii. p. 140.

of minor writers contain similar accounts. As, however, my object is rather to draw inferences from a multitude of satisfactory and authentic observations, than to narrate these observations one by one, I have to refer such as desire it, to the original works themselves.

The summary then of what has been stated is, that acute inflammations of the brain are marked by vascular congestion of the whole organ; and especially by a punctated, or striated redness of the place 'affected, and also by increased hardness. That these conditions vary more or less, according to the intensity of the inflammation. That the latter terminates in a softening finally, in which pus and cerebral substance are blended together, and constitute a mass of a semi-fluid consistence; and that this mass varies according to the proportion of red blood in it, from a light red or pink colour, to a dark, deep one, of the colour and appearance of claret lees.

CHAPTER XXI.

IRRITATIONS OF BRAIN

(Continued.)

CHRONIC OR SUB-INFLAMMATION

This inflammation, like the corresponding condition of other tissues, is frequently indicated by the indurated state of the part affected. The induration becomes exceedingly well marked, when it constitutes the periphery of an old laceration or wound of the cerebral tissue, as in some cases of apoplexy, or of mechanical violence. Chronic inflammation is also often attended with a well marked augmentation, in consistence of the whole mass of the brain.

In the autumn of 1824, a young gentleman amused himself in discharging his pistols at a collection of cats, who, to the great annoyance of his father's family, were continually making irruptions into the back yard, and disturbing the household. Unluckily for him, while he held in his hand a charged pistol, having some occasion to bend forward, the pistol went off, and lodged a ball in his forehead. Dr. Physick was sent for, who found the bone shattered, and the ball lying loosely upon the surface of the brain. The patient was, of course, stunned by this injury, and it was thought by every one, that his death was at hand. The fragments of bone and the ball were removed, the dura mater was found lacerated, and a portion of the substance

of one hemisphere, near the falx major, was wounded down
almost to the corpus callosum, so that the surgeon could readily insinuate his finger that far.

A course of the most rigid treatment was immediately
instituted. It consisted in large and repeated evacuations
of blood from the arm, cathartics; and the lowest and most
abstemious regimen. By the virtues of this management,
he not only did not die at that period of the injury, but
to the surprise of every one, he was finally reinstated upon
his feet; the wound in his forehead closed, and he, being a
lawyer, resumed his professional labours. Being of an active and robust frame, and attached to athletic exercises.
he found his health so far restored, that he returned to all
his customary recreations, but observed, during this period,
a regulated diet, and avoided alcoholic drinks.

On the expiration of nine or ten months, he found himself
so well that he began to assume greater latitude in his diet,
and, on an occasion, ate heartily of pot pie. The consequence of this excess was vomiting, a convulsion, and indications of an inflammation of the brain. The medical treatment of the first instance was resumed by Dr. Physick, and
his aliment reduced to the smallest quantity consistent with
life. He lingered in this way for several weeks, became
extremely emaciated, had several repetitions of his convulsions, and finally died. I examined him after death.

The membranes of the brain were natural in point of texture, and almost destitute of red blood. They looked clean,
white, and healthy universally, excepting the injured part
where the ball entered. The medullary substance of the
brain was perfectly white, but of a consistence almost equal
to that of a common healthy brain hardened in spirits of wine,
and cut beautifully smooth, leaving a polished surface. Its
fibrous arrangement was as distinct and well settled as the
fibrous arrangement of wood, not leaving the possibility of
doubt on this as the natural structure of the brain. It also
had scarcely a vestige of red blood in it. The cortical sub-

stance was of a very light yellow or ash colour, many shades
lighter than what is common to it, and approximated to that
of the medullary. This strongly marked consistence of the
encephalon, its very white colour and destitution of red
blood, it occurred to me, were the result of the great loss of
blood and the very low diet; for the patient from the period
of his relapse to his death, had used scarcely any thing but
barley water. If so, this may be considered the normal condition of the brain under great privation of food. About
the year 1817, I had remarked similar appearances in a
German woman, who, it is supposed, along with several
other passengers, was through the inhuman avarice of the
ship owners, almost starved to death on her voyage to this
country, and actually died a short time after arriving, from
the effects of privation and ill usage.

The old cicatrix of the forehead was still very visible, and
was situated on the termination of the hairy scalp. A few
days before death, it had ulcerated and discharged some pus.
The lost bone had not been regenerated but in part; consequently an adhesion existed between the skin and the dura
mater, and the latter again adhered to the brain. Below
this adhesion the primary injury of the brain existed as an
abscess of fifteen lines or more in diameter, but the purulent
matter had been very generally discharged through the ulcerated cicatrix. The parietes of the abscess, were highly
indurated cerebral substance, with a very large proportion
of coagulating lymph, forming thereby a cyst. The injury
had been inflicted near the summit of the left hemisphere
just at the side of the falciform process of the dura mater,
and the latter served to form the internal face of the abscess.

Another case illustrative of this indurated state of the brain
in its chronic irritations occurred to me in 1824. A
gentleman brought his wife to this city to be treated by Dr.
Physick for mental derangement. The disease had manifested itself five or six years previously in a way and under
circumstances the narration of which may be passed over as

not essential to our present purpose. She had been lethargic in intellect, as well as in body, for two months previous to death; her infirmity having subsided into that state, from one of considerable acuteness and activity. A few hours before death she recovered sufficiently to recognise the friends around her, and to express her opinion of the fatality of the complaint.

Autopsy Dec. 25th, day after death. —The tunica arachnoidea on the upper surface of the cerebrum, was thickened and separated by water, from the top of the hemispheres. The brain had the firmness of the fresh brain of a sheep, which every one who has attended to the circumstance, must know to be many degrees harder than the human brain. There was a drachm of serum in each lateral ventricle; the fornix was unusually hard and membranous, and a hydatid the size of a pea existed on each side of the plexus choroides. In separating the opposed sides of the thalami nervorum opticorum, their adhesion was so strong and tenacious, that a part of the right thalamus was torn off. An ounce of serum was found effused between the base of the brain and of the cranium.

The following are the notes taken at the time of the dissection in the winter of 1820–21, of a female adult maniac who was brought into the dissecting-rooms of the university. On the anterior face of the os frontis, inclined to the left side of the middle line, was an osseous protuberance, and on the posterior face, somewhat above the orbitar processes, the surface was very rough. The dura mater adhered universally to the interior of the cranium with such tenacity, that it could not be separated without laceration. The pia mater had but very few of its vessels distended, or rather occupied with blood; and such as were so, were much contracted.

The lateral ventricles of the brain contained a small quantity of serum. The pineal gland was enlarged to four times its normal size, and was converted into a cyst containing a watery fluid. The medullary substance throughout the brain

46

was preternaturally firm. The tuberculum superius and pos-
terius of the thalami were very much enlarged. The fornix
was much diminished.

To these instances of induration of the brain, I will add
a fourth. George Woods, (seaman,) a man of from forty to
fifty, apparently; was admitted into the Philadelphia Alms
House in October, 1820, with general palsy of five months'
standing, said to be the consequence of a wound on the head
from a cutlass, received many years previously. It was
stated, but I know not whether upon sufficient authority,
that the accident occurred in the Mediterranean before Tri-
poli In February, 1822, he died and I examined him.
There was a universal and extensive emaciation: extreme as it
was, the left pectoral extremity exceeded all other parts of
the body in this, for the marasmus seemed to have left nothing but skin and bones.

An oblique depression, half an inch deep, existed across the
fore part of the sagittal suture: it was two and a half inches
long, and an inch and a quarter wide. This depression was
covered by a cicatrix in the skin, below which there was a
deficiency or hole in the cranium, filled with a thin layer
of old ligamentous matter. The dura mater adhered closely
to this ligamentous membrane, and so did the cicatrized integuments. The bone at the edge was three-eighths of an
inch thick, and smoothly bevelled down to the dura mater
by the action of the absorbents. There was no depression of
the bone on the inside of the cranium, consequently the
brain was not compressed.

A very slight adhesion existed between the dura mater
and the pia mater, from inflammation at the summit of the
right hemisphere. The brain was extremely hard to the
feel, as well as on cutting it. The lateral ventricles contained
a little more serum than usual, and the anterior tubercles of
the thalami were very projecting. The pineal gland contained the customary quantity of grit, and had on its anterior

part, between the roots of the pedunculi, a congeries of grit-
ty matter a line and a half wide, consisting of small particles
slightly agglomerated.   There were several hydatids on the
margins of the plexus choroides.   Nothing unusual at the
basis of the brain.

From the facts now adduced, as well as from such as might
be selected in numbers from the most approved writers on
pathology, it is sufficiently clear, that chronic inflammations
and irritations of the brain are attended with either partial or
general induration of its substance in some cases, and frequently the nearer we are to the focus of the inflammation, the
greater is the induration.   In the first case it was seen that
this induration is sometimes at least, so permanent and so
blended with coagulating lymph, as to continue, notwithstanding the adjoining suppuration; and thereby to form a
cyst or bag for the latter, as in common phlegmon of the
cellular substance.

This indurated condition seems to be the consequence of
a low degree of chronic inflammation; for when it passes this
grade, the inflammation, instead of determining an augmentation of density, is followed by ramollissement and disorganization.   Where some degree of acuteness either attends
upon or supervenes upon a chronic inflammation, the cerebral tissue assumes a characteristic reddish yellow colour, in
the softened portion.   In recent cases, the red is pale, and
in the more advanced there is a grayish pale yellow.   The
quantity of red, however, will vary according to the normal
vascularity of the part, and according to the degree of congestion of the vessels.

When chronic inflammation is followed by suppuration,
the pus is not always assembled into a focus, but becomes
infiltrated through the adjoining cerebral tissue, disorganizes
it, and communicates to it a grayish green colour, derived
from the yellow colour of the chronic inflammation and from
the green one of the pus.   The disorganization is so com-

plete, that all trace of a fibrous disposition in the medullary part of the brain is lost; as fully so, indeed, as it is lost in the softenings from acute inflammation.

When suppuration is not brought on by the supervention of acute upon chronic inflammation, the induration is sometimes almost cartilaginous. M. Rostan[*] has quoted a case to that effect from M. Droullin. A widowed woman, aged seventy, of considerable obesity, was brought into the hospital for considerable pain all over the head. Her intelligence and myotility were both impaired, and she finally died, at the expiration of a year, in a state of profound coma. On examination, a patch of blood as large as the palm of the hand, and of the thickness of a penny, was found on the dura mater on the summit of the hemispheres: the arachnoidea was raised up by an effusion of serum. The brain was congested with blood, and the medullary substance, especially that of the right hemisphere, was of a hardness approaching that of cartilage. The strongest pressure with the fingers on the optic nerves could not injure them, and the same was the case with the pons varolii.

Cancer of the Brain.

The symptoms of this affection during life, do not present any well marked difference from those of other cerebral diseases; and the pathological appearances are strongly analogous to those left by chronic inflammation, upon which an acute one has supervened. In a dissection made by M. Rostan,[†] an ovoidal tumour was found on the confines of, and protruding within the right lateral ventricle. It was of a deep red colour in some places, and grayish in others, and its consistence was partially hard, and in other parts soft. The substance generally of the right hemisphere was softened, and interspersed with rose-coloured patches. The an-

* Rostan, loc. cit. p. 401.   † Id p. 408.

terior internal part of the left hemisphere was of very great
firmness, and crackled under the section of the scalpel; it
was of a light rose colour, and presented a shining surface.
There were some appearances about the corpora striata of an
apoplexy; that on the right side having its tissue infiltrated
with a bloody effusion, and that on the left being diminished
in volume, and having a cicatrix in its centre.

Hydatids of the Brain.

Hydatids are cysts containing a transparent yellow fluid,
like serum. They are most commonly formed in the plexus
choroides; and, when there, seem to be, as Dr. Abercrombie*
has stated, a mere collection of water in the loose cellular
substance connecting the vessels. It is a very common thing
in the adult brain to see a vesicle of four or five lines in diameter adhering to the outer margin of the plexus choroides
of each side; and not unfrequently, in old persons, a chronic
inflammation or irritation is found in the cyst, thickening
its parietes, and productive of a calcareous deposite in it.
Sometimes these cysts are very numerous, of various sizes,
and are strung in clusters along the plexus choroides. From
the frequency of their occurrence, I am not disposed to think
that in the main, they are productive of inconvenience to
the functions of the brain, except where they compress it
by their size. These hydatids, or cysts, as they may be
more properly termed, are among the most common pathological appearances: any one who wishes to read cases of
them, has only to turn to Morgagni on the Causes and Seats
of Diseases, to Portal on Medical Anatomy, to Lieutaud's
Historia Anatomico-Medica, and to Baillie's Morbid Anatomy.

There is, however, another kind called acephalocysts, of a
much more rare occurrence, and which appears to be an ant-

* Diseases of the Brain. p 317

mal of a very simple structure, consisting in a membranous sac containing a fluid, and having a life of its own. It has been found both in the ventricles, on the surface of the brain, and in its substance. I am not aware, however, of having ever met with a case of this description in my own private dissections. M. Rostan[*] has seen it but once; in which case the hydatid was as large as a pullet egg, and was situated in the left lateral ventricle, but distinct from the plexus choroides. He also quotes a case furnished by M. Droullin, and presented in a woman of seventy, where the cyst beginning at the basis of the brain near the thalamus nervi optici, penetrated the fissure of Sylvius, and after a tortuous course, amounting in all to about five inches, terminated in a small pouch, being its pedicle, in the inferior part of the middle lobe. The part of the brain adjoining the transit of this cyst was softened.

The acephalocysts can scarcely be confounded, except by a very superficial inexperienced observer, with those indurated cysts, principally formed of coagulating lymph, which constitute the parietes of old bloody effusions, or of suppurations in the substance of the brain. They may be well distinguished by the transparency of their coats and by the pellucid fluid which they contain.

Tubercles of the Brain.

This disease, though there are many cases of it reported, and especially by Mr. Abercrombie,[†] I am not disposed to view as one of very frequent occurrence. Their physical appearance is nearly the same with that of tubercles of the lungs, or spleen, or liver, or indeed of any other organ. When in the crude or growing state, they are observed in the several gradations of size, from a line or less in diameter, to an inch or more: they are whitish, semi-transparent,

[*] Rostan. p. 412.   [†] Abercrombie, loc. cit p. 166 to 182

when fresh, and of a hard cartilaginous feel. They have been found attached to the membranes of the brain, arising from the surface or bottom of its convolutions, and in its thickness. Like the tubercles of the lungs, when matured they become of an opaque white, and are softened or converted into a purulent cheesy matter. Their progress is slow; hence arises a very remarkable feature in their character, that the symptoms do not, for a long time, evince a severity proportionate to the mischief done in the structure of the brain. On a sudden, frequently when least expected, inflammation of an acute kind supervenes upon the contiguous part of the brain, and the patient is hurried off by a rapid dissolution, sometimes of an apoplectic type, and on other occasions resembling hydrocephalus The leading trait of tubercles in the brain would seem to be an intense head-ach, resembling what is called sick head-ach, attended with more or less periodicity, and an obstinate vomiting. Paralysis, convulsions, torpidity of the limbs, and lesions of intelligence, are rather occasional symptoms than constant ones.

Tubercles of the brain are said* to occur in persons and in families having a tendency to tubercles in other organs, and they are occasionally complicated with other affections of the brain. On dissection, there is often found either extensive effusion or extensive ramollissement of that part of the brain in which the tubercles are situated.

The following cases will illustrate the character of tubercles in the brain. C. Henry, aged two years, (a coloured child,) was admitted into the Alms House, Nov. 5th, 1827, for paralysis of the left side, and a declining state of health besides. This state continued with but slight improvement, till the early part of the subsequent March, when he was seized with what seemed to be a mild remittent fever. This fever lasted from the 13th to the 19th of March, when he died. It was treated with occasional doses of calomel and

* Aber p 167

other cathartic medicines, and with the warm bath. The following details presented to me by a highly intelligent and zealous resident student, Mr. Henry S. Levert, under whose charge the patient came, will show the progress of the symptoms.

The day of his attack the application of the warm bath was directed; and he was restricted to the use of barley water, which was also continued the succeeding day with advantage. His fever being considerable on the third day, the warm bath was repeated, and he was purged with Calomel iij. gr. P. Rhei. v. gr. On the fourth day there was no mitigation of symptoms, and there was a continual motion of the right hand, by throwing it across his breast. He was purged that day with Calomel, gr. vi., followed in the evening with a dose of castor oil.

On the 17th day of the month, the fifth of the attack, he was stupid and motionless, excepting an occasional closing of the fingers of the right hand. The pupil of the right eye was dilated, that of the left natural. The pulse was full, intermittent, and slow. The symptoms being hydrocephalic, he was blistered over the whole head; rubbed in the groin with mercurial ointment, and had one grain of calomel administered every two hours during the day. On the eighteenth his state was nearly the same, but the globe of the right eye was turned to the outer canthus. He died that night about three o'clock.

On examination, this subject was found with the ventricles of the brain much distended with water; and the substance of the brain was soft. There was a spherical tubercle, of from eight to ten lines long in the thickness of the pons varolii, which had grown between its laminæ, and separated them from one another, and another of the same size in the right thalamus nervi optici. Moreover, there was a tendency to such tumours in other parts of the brain.

A second case of tubercle of the brain, was presented to

me November 23d, 1827, in a patient of Dr. S. Tucker, whom I was called upon to examine. The autopsy took place twenty-one hours after death. The history is as follows: Mr D. aged nineteen, having been unduly exposed to a hot sun about three years ago, it was followed by a severe bilious fever attended with delirium.

Two years ago he was seized with epilepsy, the paroxysms of which continued to recur at intervals of three or four weeks, till the time of his death. Occasionally he exhibited marks of insanity.

Five or six months ago he was also assailed with tubercular consumption, attended with copious expectoration. The emaciation became extreme before death. The following appearances were presented on his examination:

Head.—Membranes of the brain natural, except the pia mater, which was somewhat congested. The entire substance of the encephalon unusually hard. A drachm of water in each lateral ventricle. In the middle of the right hemisphere, just above the level of the corpus callosum, there existed a spherical scirrhus or tubercle, about one inch in diameter, extremely hard, and arising from the bottom of a convolution. The medullary matter around it was soft and brittle, and did not adhere to it except very slightly: it had raised up the pia mater in developing itself.

Thorax.—The heart was natural, but contained some whitish coagula of blood. The superior half of each lung was disorganized by indurations, tubercles, and by pulmonary excavations communicating with the trachea The inferior half of each lung contained a few tubercles, but it was not disorganized. The apices of the lungs adhered to the pleura.

Abdomen.—Its peritoneal surface, and that of its viscera was healthy. The stomach and colon were crisp, as if they had been tanned for a short time, in a diluted acid or alum water. The glands of the mesentery were enlarged; and in addition to such as are usually seen, great numbers

17

about the size of mustard seed were developed near the intestines.   Numerous patches of red inflammation, looking like the precursors of ulcers, existed on the mucous coat of the intestines.   There were several ulcers from two to five lines in diameter in the small intestines, and a few in the large.   There was no perceptible ulceration in the ileo-colic region.

The stomach was not ulcerated, was moderately distended with gas; had its mucous coat in numerous rugæ, and of a sienna or bright brown.   The liver, spleen, and kidneys were healthy, and contained but very little blood.

CHAPTER XXII.

IRRITATIONS OF THE BRAIN

(*Continued.*)

MOLLESCENCE OR RAMOLLISSEMENT

PATHOLOGISTS are as yet not agreed whether this is an inflammation, or rather a result of it; or whether it is a specific and distinct affection of the cerebral tissue. Unquestionably, inflammations of the brain, like those of other tissues, terminate frequently by a softening of the part affected; but such pulpy collections have their origin indicated, as stated in the preceding chapter, by being surrounded and enclosed by an indurated mass of cerebral substance, or else by a cyst of coagulated lymph. But the ramollissement to which I here refer, is not shut up, and marked by an enclosure of lymph, or of indurated cerebral substance; for it comes directly in contact with the surrounding sound part, or else is insensibly lost in it. The colour, itself, is in some cases nearly, or perfectly white; and is seen in all gradations, from that to a deep brown or red, resembling the lees of claret wine. In respect, therefore to colour, as it is identical in both modes of softening, and subject to great varieties, no distinction can be obtained from it. The probability is in both cases, that the colour is derived from the quantity of cineritious matter, and of red particles of blood in the softened pulp.

To the accurate and excellent Morgagni* we are indebted for, perhaps, the earliest well written account of this pathological change in the structure of the brain.   His statement is as follows: A woman, named Jacoba, of common condition in life, (and who, by the way, enjoyed the honour of having her name set down by Morgagni, by reason of her having thirteen ribs,) being in the fifty-ninth year of her age, was seized with apoplexy, followed by fever of a violent kind.   Being brought to the Hospital, it was observed that though unable to speak, she yet understood; for she spontaneously extended her left arm, to have her pulse felt. Her face was flushed, she readily swallowed fluids, the right eyelids were almost closed, and were motionless, the right leg and arm were motionless also, and insensible, yet their muscles seemed to be spasmodically contracted.

At the time of this occurrence, a very lively interest was felt, to verify or test the opinion of the celebrated Valsalva, that organic injury of one side of the brain was followed by paralysis of the opposite side of the body.   It had, indeed, been lately the subject of a published epistle.†   On the death of this patient, many learned persons, crowds of students, and others attended the dissection, which lasted many days, and was executed with much care.   As only certain details are connected with what we have now on hand, I shall suppress such as are extraneous to the subject.

Morgagni found, among other things in the abdomen, that the bladder was so distended, as to rise six inches above the pubes, and was filled with a highly coloured lixivious urine, that was squeezed out with difficulty, but was not fœtid. The internal surface of the bladder was inflamed, presenting here and there bloody points, and the urethra, at its upper end, was almost on the point of sphacelation.

" While the skull was sawed through, a quantity of serum came forth; the dura mater was thickened.   The ves-

sels of the pia mater were all filled with' blood, as if they
had been distended by injection.   This blood, like that of
the whole body, was black, and not very fluid.   Under the
pia mater, (probably arachnoidea) and in the convolutions
of the brain, as well as in the lateral ventricles, was found a
transparent water.   The choroid plexuses were not at all
discoloured, although they had vesicles upon them turgid
with water.   On the left plexus, one of these vesicles was
as large as a grape.   The thalamus nervi optici of the left
side was brown.   As I cut the brain into small pieces, I observed that every other part of it was natural and sound;
but that the medullary substance, which was on the external
side of the left thalamus spoken of above, was very soft and
liquified, and was found to be mixed with a certain bloody
fluid, of a colour almost effete; so that nothing was wanting
to make us pronounce it absolutely rotten.   The space of
the brain, which this disorder occupied, was larger than that
which the largest walnut would have taken up; and that
colour of the bloody fluid was most manifest in the middle
thereof.   The cerebrum was not only more hard than the
cerebellum, but even endowed with a wonderful hardness
every where, especially in the whole right hemisphere; and
had only in that place I have mentioned, a kind of bloody
colour, and a loose, ill-compacted substance.   I believe that
this was an apostema sui generis."   Morgagni goes on to
state, that this aposteme happened about the very place
where, according to his observations, organic injuries most
frequently occur.

This case of Morgagni, conforming in the type of symptoms and pathological changes very nearly to what has been
since observed by others, may be considered as an introduction to the study of ramollissement.   It will be proper,
therefore, at the threshold of our inquiry, to trace some of
the leading parallels or discrepancies, between the softening of cerebral matter, and of other tissues, with a view to
ascertain whether it is inflammatory or not.   It is more

than probable that these softened patches of brain, undergo
some preliminary state before they get into that, which we
see in a post mortem examination.   One which, perhaps,
would give the idea of increased consistence and hardness,
had we, as in superficial parts of the body, an opportunity
of feeling it; and which would probably also manifest an
increased hæmatosis or afflux of blood, if we could see it
in life.

   I am strongly disposed, indeed, to view it as that sort of
dissolution of structure, which occurs in large ulcerations on
the surface of the body.   Any one who has witnessed the
progress of such, must remember, that when they occur, and
especially in individuals given up to intemperate bad habits,
and somewhat advanced in life; there is little or no tumefaction of the adjacent parts of the limb, and that the parietes
of the sore are only slightly indurated, slightly swollen, and
moderately injected.   These appearances are continually
preserved as the ulceration extends itself; but when the parts
are examined after death, the edges of the sore are white and
collapsed, so that one might infer from the condition at that
time, that there had been no previous inflammation.   It is
owing, I have no doubt, to the very small quantity of
cellular substance in the brain, and to its soft pulpy structure, that when inflammatory irritations, and the consequent
local afflux of fluids occur; the pulp becomes disorganized
from the predominance of the latter, and is converted into a
soft, fluent putrilage, in immediate contact with the surrounding healthy structure.

   A diminution of cohesion, notwithstanding the apparent
increase of solidity and tenacity upon superficial examination, is one of the most invariable consequences or rather
conditions of an active inflammation.   It is remarkably the
case in cellular substance, which loses thus the most of its
healthy attributes: from being strong, flexible, and elastic,
it becomes so brittle that it tears with little or no resistance,
and the finger may be easily thrust through it.   M. Dupuy-

tren* has founded upon this a very interesting observation about secondary hæmorrhage. It has been proved by him _and Mr. Jones,† that when a ligature is applied to an artery, the internal and the middle coats are invariably cut through, and that it is the external or cellular coat, and the surrounding sheath when it also is included, which holds the ligature on. Ligatures thus placed on healthy arteries remain for ten or twenty days: they then are loosened by the inflammatory softening of the part included, and fall off. But M. Dupuytren asserts, that if the cellular coats be at the time of the application of the ligature, in a state of inflammation, they are cut through almost immediately, and the ligature drops in two or three days. This rule of pathology is so certain that M. Dupuytren says, that provisional ligatures, (ligatures d' attente,) sometimes fall by the inflammation they produce, before the actual ones.

This diminution of cohesion from inflammation is manifested in all the tissues of the body: in the bones, as for example in what is called caries; in the tendons, and aponeuroses; in the glands, as the lymphatic, the liver, the spleen, and others; in the mucous membranes, and especially that of the stomach; in the muscles, where they not only lose the power of voluntary contraction, but are subject to laceration from very inconsiderable violence, and are sometimes deprived almost entirely of cohesion. The same phenomenon occurs in the lungs: they become congested with blood, and are so softened that the finger may be pushed into their substance without difficulty.‡ M. Lallemand has observed, that this test of cohesion becomes an excellent mode of distinguishing an inflammation which has lasted only a day or two, from a considerable congestion which sometimes occurs during the last moments of life. And though in the progress of the complaint the blood combines with the lung, and

---

* Lallemand Recherches sur l'Enceph. p. 86. Paris, 1824.
† Jones on Hæmorrhage.
‡ Loc. cit. p. 80

is followed by suppuration, and consequently the density
and weight of the lung are augmented much; yet the tenacity is still diminished from the healthy standard.

M. Rostan* acknowledges, that many reasons prevail
in inducing him to consider this *softening* as an effect of
inflammation.   Among them are the strongly marked
rose colour, which can only be the result of inflamma-
ry action, and which exists in certain cases; the frequent
existence of fixed pain in the head previous to the disease;
the occasional tumefaction of the adjacent convolutions of
the encephalon, and which, it is supposed, produces coma
by compression; the febrile heat of the skin attended with
thirst, and a full, strong, frequent pulse.   He also asserts,
that softening is often found to surround a sanguineous effusion, as well as a scirrhous or cancerous tumour; and manifests thereby a strong analogy, to what is universally considered as an inflammatory act in the instances of other organs, whose lesions, or disorganizations, having reached
a certain point, are surrounded by a new formation, the result of inflammation.

M. Rostan, however, after stating these as reasons for admitting the disease called ramollissement to be of an inflammatory character, says that it at least is not uniformly so,
because cases occur where a majority of the attending circumstances are not inflammatory, or indicative of such a
state.   For they have no pain, or fever; no tumefaction, or
change of colour in the spot affected; the intellectual, sensitive, and locomotive faculties are not exalted previously to
their depression; and, in fine, the affection occurs in aged
individuals, and in circumstances entirely opposed to the
production of inflammations.   According to his experience,
the colour of the diseased tissue is not changed in a majority
of cases, excepting that it is of a white, more dark and
shining than usual: it is penetrated, then, neither by pus nor

* Recherches sur le Ramollissement du cerveau, Paris, 1823, p. 164

by blood.   In other instances it is of a deep red, like the
lees of wine, and resembles exactly the ecchymosis of scurvy.   M. R. is upon the whole disposed to consider this ramollissement of the brain, as being most frequently from
the attending circumstances, a mode of disorganization resembling most strongly, in its essential characters, the gangrene of old people.   The opinions of M. R., are also held
by Dr. Abercrombie,* who says, " that the ramollissement
is a result of inflammation, I think the appearances described in some of these cases, place beyond doubt.   I have
already stated my belief, that it arises also from another
cause; namely, disease of the arterial system: being thus
analogous to gangrene in other parts of the body, which we
see arising from these two very opposite causes."   M. Lallemand, also, considers the softening of the brain as an inflammatory action, generally of an acute character; but says,
that he has also met with cases, rare to be sure, in which the
symptoms had followed a slow and gradual course, and with
an appearance of mildness unsuited to the idea of active inflammation.†

Colour.—The colour of the cerebral tissue affected with
ramollissement, it would seem is much varied:‡ for it is
yellow, green, rose, red, chesnut, dark white, or like wine
lees, in different individuals, or these several colours may be
congregated in but one person.   They may exist also in different shades, and be variously combined.   Certain attending
circumstances, seem to dispose to particular colours in pre-
ference to others.   The yellowish green appears when ramollissement has followed an ancient attack of apoplexy;
and it is found in the centre of the softened mass.   The
various shades of rose, are manifested around the circumference of a primitive softening, and especially in the convolutions.   The colour of lees is not unusual, and gives to the

* Diseases of Brain and Spinal Cord, Edin. 1828, p. 106
† Loc. Cit. p. 219.   ‡ Rostan, p. 158.

softening the appearance of a scorbutic spot, of a true ecchymosis. It would seem to be an abortive hæmorrhagic effort, and is commonly repeated from space to space, or is
multiplied in spots. One of the most frequent colours is a
milky white.

Consistence —It is extremely difficult to communicate
an idea of compactness or consistence, when the sense of
touch is our only guide, and not an actual measurement of
strength in the body examined. This difficulty is much
increased, when we wish to express a slight departure
only, from the natural standard, having at the same time
due consideration for the varieties depending on age and
temperament. As far then as a fact of the kind can be communicated it is now stated, that the ramollissement of the
brain, has been observed to exist in all the degrees of li-
quidness, from almost perfect fluidity to a firmness, but little short of a natural condition; and, that the middle state
between these two extremes is most frequently met with.
We may be also assisted in recognising these conditions by
bearing in mind, that where temperament and age, influence
in their appropriate manner the compactness of the encephalon, the condition is universal, and the normal colour is
retained; whereas the ramollissement is partial, exists in
one or more spots of variable extent and shape, and is most
commonly attended with a change of colour in the part affected, or in that which is adjacent to it. Moreover the
part does not cut so smoothly as the sound, and by scraping
it with the handle or back of the scalpel, may have its surface readily removed.

Causes.—The causes of this affection are numerous.
Some of the most prominent are a disposition to cerebral
congestion, or what is called an apoplectic constitution; suppressed, habitual evacuations, as those of the hæmorrhoids
and menses; an immoderate use of fermented, or alcoholic
drinks. Depressing moral affections have great influence in
the production of these diseases: such as domestic afflictions

in the loss of relatives or of fortune; the shame and grief inseparable in a sensitive mind, from illicit pregnancy in females. M. Rostan says, that the affection is also more prevalent during great heats, and severe colds; hence he infers, that these states of the atmosphere assist in producing it. Old age seems to give a predisposition, and more especially with women.[*]

Frequency.—It is only within a few years, that ramollissement of the brain has attracted the attention of pathologists as one of its ordinary changes of structure, hence we might be almost tempted to think, that it was a new disease, or at least much more common than formerly.   There is, however, a very easy way of accounting for this state of things. With the exception of Morgagni, who carried such scrupulous exactitude, and minuteness into his cadaverous autopsies, there are none of the older pathologists, who have not committed faults in their observations, by being very superficial and imperfect. This affection would therefore appear to have been unknown to them, whereas Morgagni has left several excellent accounts of it in his dissections.   The pathologists intermediate to Morgagni and the present time, also seem to have avoided the depths of their calling; hence there appears to be what we can scarcely believe in, an interval of many years in the existence of ramollissement. On this subject it is very justly observed,[†] that since the researches of Bayle, of Corvisart, of Broussais, and we may add also of Laennec, consumptions, diseases of the heart, and gastro-intestinal inflammations have multiplied to a most alarming extent, when we compare them with what they were formerly.   Closer inquiry will, however, satisfy us, that this apparent increase has not been in nature, but in our more improved modes of diagnostic; and that asthmas, dyspneas, putrid and nervous fevers, nervous apoplexies, and so on, have disappeared in proportion.   It is the habit of the

<hr>

[*] Rostan. p. 463.   [†] Lall. loc. cit. p. 316

present day, to refer every set of symptoms to the lesion of one or more organs; it was the habit of the former day to consider disease as existing by itself; hence thousands of fanciful forms were attributed to it.

It is now asserted,[*] that softening is the most frequent of cerebral affections; more so, indeed, than apoplexy with sanguineous effusion.   And it is agreed by the most eminent writers, that it exists much more in the old than in the youthful and middle aged.   In forty-three cases quoted by Lallemand, thirty-one were more than forty years old; and in the majority of the remainder, being from ten to forty, the brain had suffered from percussion.   M. Rostan considers it as most unusual among persons under thirty years of age; judging from his personal experience, upon a large population of every age.[†]

Duration.—From the observation of M. Lallemand,[‡] it appears, that about one half of the patients attacked with ramollissement, and who perish from it, die within the first seven days from the commencement of the attack; rather more than a fourth in the second week; about one sixth in the third week; and the remainder at intervals of months. Some individuals, indeed, there is reason to believe, bear this disorganization in its forming stage about them, in a chronic state for years.[§]   This form sometimes occurs where there has been a previous attack of apoplexy, imperfectly resolved, and also in the case of mental derangement. The most essential circumstances in determining the length of an attack, are the *seat* of it, the *extent*, and the mode of treatment.   If superficial, it may last for a very long time, without producing death, and be also extensive; whereas, if it be near the centre of a hemisphere, it kills in a short time, even where small in extent.   M. Rostan[||] has seen a case which had destroyed the whole of a lobe, and killed the patient in two days.

* Rostan, 155   † Id. p 183   ‡ Lallem. p. 217.
§ Rostan, p. 153. || Id p. 154.

It seems to be barely within the reach of possibility for this affection to terminate by resolution.   M. Rostan, however, met with one case,* where, from the symptoms, there was reason to believe that this had occurred, the chief objection to the inference is, that as cerebral congestion is attended with similar symptoms, the complaint may have been the latter, and not ramollissement; it occurred in a female of seventy-six years.   But general experience is in favour of death, being the inevitable lot of individuals affected with softening of the cerebral tissue, in spite of every mode of treatment.

Situation.—In forty-six observations of Lallemand,† sixteen had the Ramollissement in the periphery of the cerebrum in the cortical matter; thirteen had them in the corpora striata, and in the thalami nervorum opticorum; four in the cerebral protuberance, (pons varolii;) eight in the fibrous or white substance; and five with mixed situations. It is then worthy of recollection, that the principal tendency to the disease, is in the ash-coloured substance; as thirty-three out of forty-six patients had it there exclusively, or in parts, where there is a predominance of this substance.   It is evident to the anatomist, that this distribution corresponds with the distribution of vascularity in the brain; as vessels are always more abundant in the ash-coloured substance.   In these cases, many of them had also arachnitis, and it was evident that the inflammation of the cerebral substance was due to that of the arachnoid membrane in contact with it.   There is some little difference of experience about the frequency of its situation in the septum lucidum; M. Rostan has seen it there but once;† whereas, Abercrombie has repeatedly witnessed it there.   My own personal experience tends to a coincidence with that of Mr. A. Unfortunately, I have not kept a full record of observations, but it has for many years been perfectly well known to me,

---

* Id. p. 215.   † Id. p. 161.

that the septum lucidum and the fornix, are frequently reduced into a pulpy semi-fluid state, and especially in dropsy, where there is effusion into the lateral ventricles. Hence,
I invariably avoid dropsical subjects, in a demonstration of
the brain.

This may be accounted for, as cerebral dropsy is a consequence of arachnitis; and, as ramollissement also attends
arachnitis, the parietes of the ventricles will, of course,
(both the white and ashy substance,) where they are lined
by the arachnoidea, be softened, and the fornix and septum
will come in for their share. The different experience of
anatomists on the existence of the commissura mollis, as the
adhesion between the thalami is called, may now be explained on the same principle; it being most generally dissolved, in inflammations attended with ramollissement;
whereas, it is generally entire and perfect, where there has
been no disease of the brain.

The extent of ramollissement varies remarkably: in some
it is not larger than a bean, while in others it invades a whole
lobe or even more.   The middle size is perhaps the most
frequent.   The shape of such affections is indeterminate;
sometimes being spherical, on other occasions oblong, and
again of some other figure.   Frequently, indeed, the limits
cannot be traced in a very precise manner, as the centre is
softer than the circumference, and the latter is blended insensibly into the surrounding healthy structure.   It may
exist at different places in the same hemisphere, and present
in each a different degree of intensity, and also different appearances from the quantity of blood extravasated entering
into their composition respectively.

It is very frequently the concomitant of apoplectic effusion
of blood, and forms for the latter an envelope.   It also attends cancer of the brain, scirrhus, arachnitis, and in fact all
of its pathological conditions.   M. Rostan* says that the ar-

* Rostan, p. 162.

teries of the brain are commonly ossified when this organ is softened. The same excellent authority informs us, that ramollissement is, of all diseases, the most disposed to give rise to a collection of serosity in the ventricles; and he thinks that it occurs precisely on the same principle that effusions occur from other serous membranes when the viscera with which they are connected, suffer from acute or chronic inflammation.*

Symptoms.—The symptoms of ramollissement may be divided into primary and into consecutive, or into a first and second period. I do not propose to dwell on either of these in detail, but in a general manner, merely with the view of completing the subject.

Primary Symptoms.—The most obvious are a fixed excruciating pain of the head, lasting for weeks or even months, remitting occasionally in its violence, and sometimes intermitting entirely. There is vertigo, with a diminution in one or all of the powers of myotility, a weakness in the several faculties of the mind, hypochondriasm, sleepiness. A diminution of the sense of touch; sometimes, however, an augmentation of it, making the slightest application painful. The ears ring, the sight is often perverted and sometimes entirely suspended. In fine, all the animal and intellectual functions depending upon the brain for their proper execution, are put out of their usual train.

Consecutive Symptoms.—The symptoms of the first stage having proceeded for a greater or less time, are at length succeeded by an aggravated form of them. A perfect paralysis of one or more parts of the body ensues; the intellectual and sensitive functions are annihilated, and the patient sinks into an irretrievable coma. Muscular stiffness or convulsion, is uncommon. In some cases this extremity of symptoms comes on at once and abruptly; in others the several individual faculties of myotility, sensation, and intellect, are lost successively and by rather a slow progress.

* Rostan, p. 303.

Mr. Abercrombie relates the case presently to be quoted, of a lady who spent the evening before her death in the enjoy-ment of a social circle, in whom, upon dissection, a very considerable part of a hemisphere of the cerebrum was in a state of softening. I have also met with a case somewhat similar, which will be presented to the reader in due time. The primary symptoms in her had lasted for some years: so little, however, was she aware of their fatal tendency, that she married during their progress.

It has already been stated, that the locality of affections of the brain according to Delaye, Foville, and Pinel Grand-champ, it was supposed, could be ascertained by certain ge-neral signs. As for instance, that when the cortical sub-stance alone was injured, the motility of the muscular ap-paratus of the body was not affected, but only the intellec-tual faculties: and on the contrary, when the white substance was affected, the motility suffered; and that both intellec-tual and locomotive powers became deranged, when both white and cortical substance were impaired.   The inference was hence established, that the cortical matter directed the operations of intellect, and the medullary those of muscular motility.

Should then the assertions of M. M. Gall and Spurzheim, prove correct, we may at a future day, when observations are more multiplied, be able to pronounce with certainty on the part of the surface of the cerebrum that is in a pathological state, by learning what intellectual faculties are deranged or impaired.   In this we shall accomplish for the periphery of the cerebrum, what the pathologists just alluded to have done for its centre; when they declare that in injuries of the cor-pora striata, the inferior extremity of the opposite side be-comes paralyzed, while in those of the thalami nervorum op-ticorum the paralysis is manifested in the pectoral extremity, and that a hemiplegia attends the morbid lesion of both the corpus and the thalamus.

The disease whose symptoms closely resemble those of

ramollissement, are apoplexy, sanguineous congestion, arachnitis, cancer, tubercles, tumours of the dura mater, or from
the internal face of the cranium.   In most organs, and especially in the brain, it is much easier to ascertain that a disease of some kind or other exists in them, that they do not
execute their offices perfectly, than it is to learn the precise
nature of the affection.   General indications of disease are
easily seized upon, but special ones are to be found out only
by the intelligent and attentive.   I may illustrate this by a
familiar comparison: In a machinary consisting of many
parts or wheels, if a part ceases to execute its office, it is readily seen, but it requires a special examination to find out the
nature of the injury sustained by that part or wheel; whether
an axle or one of its cogs be broken, or some other derangement has taken place.   But as, in the human body, we cannot expose to view its internal organs as we would those of a
piece of mechanism; we are constrained to rely entirely upon
symptoms, as indications of a healthy or unhealthy action,
and upon the *mode of access* of these symptoms for distinguishing one affection from another.

In ramollissement of the brain, the symptoms though progressive, seldom follow a regular and continuous march: there
are alternatives of improvements and of relapses, in the intellectual and motive faculties, and the symptoms take time
to evolve themselves. The invasion of apoplexy, on the contrary, is rapid and general; the powers of mind and of motion are precipitated at once into a profound lethargy, and
the discharges of fæces and of urine become involuntary.
A comatose paralytic state, then, is the first symptom of
apoplexy, and the last of ramollissement; in mild cases of the
former, this state recedes, and a solution of the symptoms
occurs; whereas, when ramollissement has advanced far
enough to induce the same state, it seldom or never becomes
ameliorated.

Cancer of the brain is attended with lancinating pains, intermittent at first at long intervals, and then approximating

until they become daily.   In its progress, which sometimes
lasts for years; palsy, epilepsy, and convulsions are evolved,
the skin becomes yellow, and the limbs are the seat of lancinating pains like the head-ach.*   Tubercles and tumours
pressing upon the brain, are principally distinguished by the
chronicity of the symptoms.

The following case of mollescence, already alluded to, the
details of which are given by Dr. Abercrombie,† is almost
unique in the history of cerebral affections, in regard to the
quantity of cerebral substance that was in a state of disorganization, indeed total decomposition previous to death; and
if it did not seem to be presented under circumstances of
sufficient authenticity, might well be called in question. Being rather too long for full insertion, I shall condense it so
as to present the leading features of the symptoms, and of
the dissection.

A young lady between her fourteenth and seventeenth
years, had suffered much from chronic ophthalmia.   In her
eighteenth year, she had paralysis of the face, marked by
the mouth being drawn to the right side, impaired vision
of the left eye, diminished power of contraction in the left
orbicularis oculi, and numbness of the corresponding side of
the face.   For this she was bled generally and topically,
and purged freely; which relieved her in six or eight days.
Some time after, she had a repetition of the attack, which
subsided in the same manner.   Subsequently, she suffered
frequently for a day or two at a time from giddiness, indistinct vision, and vomiting.   In the month of June, 1822,
being then in her nineteenth year, while at the dinner table,
she fell senseless from her chair; her muscles were in a state
of rigidity, (fixidity,) without convulsion; and she remained
in this state for two hours.   Six months afterwards she had
a similar attack, followed by a third in two months, and a
fourth in four months after that again.   From the first of

* Rostan. p 474   † Aber. 178

these paroxysms, her giddiness increased, attended with head-ach, referred to the left temple and to the left ear, and followed by watery discharges from the latter. On the fourth paroxysm, her vision became indistinct: a resort to sea-bathing increased the head-ach, and amaurosis followed. An emetic administered for the latter, was followed by a recurrence of the comatose paroxysms every day, for a fortnight at a time, followed by an intermission for a fortnight. They lasted from half an hour to an hour; her general health, however, continued so good, that she married in February, 1824, about twenty months from the period of her first attack. At this time she was put upon the use of stramonium, with an amendment of symptoms. Two months after marriage she spent the evening with a party in the house of a friend, and the next morning was found dead in her bed.

On examination, it was found that the whole of the left hemisphere, excepting its periphery of cortical matter, was reduced into a soft, pultaceous mass, mixed with portions of a pellucid albuminous substance. What, however, is very remarkable, the left lateral ventricle remained entire in the midst of this destruction of the parts around it; being separated from the diseased mass by a thin septum. On the external part of this hemisphere, lying over the petrous bone, and adhering firmly to the dura mater, there was a tumour the size of a pigeon's egg, composed of a reddish, soft, flesh-coloured matter, and of a semi-pellucid, albuminous substance, in nodules of various degrees of firmness. The right hemisphere was considerably softened on the inner part of the anterior lobe. The left hemisphere seemed to be considerably enlarged, and the right proportionably diminished in size. The cerebellum was healthy, and the optic nerves softer than natural.

It is an interesting fact in pathology, that the lower animals are, like man, subject to ramollissement of the encephalon and of the spinal marrow. M. Dupuy, professor at the veterinary establishment of Alfort, near Paris, seems in the course of five or six years' experience, to have ascertained that very satisfactorily. *

According to his experience, the encephalon is never affected alone in those animals, but is attended with softening of the medulla spinalis at the same time. He has seen twenty cases of the latter, and only two of the former; so that the spinal affection in animals would seem to outnumber the cerebral, as much as the cerebral in man outnumbers the spinal. The ramollissement of the brain occurred in the cortical substance; and of the spinal marrow in the swellings where the fasciculi of nerves to the extremities are given off. In the horse it was more frequent in the posterior swelling, from which the hind legs are supplied with nerves. M. Lallemand thinks that some explanation of these situations may be given by the reflection, that it is not the organ of thought which predominates in animals over the rest of the nervous system, as it does in man.

The colour, consistence, appearance, and qualities of this affection in animals would seem to be the same as in man, and the result of inflammation. The symptoms were trembling of the limbs, weakness, intermittent or continued convulsive movements, a tetanic stiffness of the neck, lower jaw, or extremities, and especially the posterior. The horses presented a remarkable gesture, which, in the phraseology of veterinaries, is called pushing against the wall: supporting the head firmly against a resisting body, and pushing forward with the hind-legs, they withdrew the fore-legs from the ground, and would sometimes remain for an hour in this arched position. When the tetanic spasm was withdrawn, they would then tumble down. They were disposed to renew the position as frequently as they could, until finally they were prevented, by paralysis invading the hinder extremities.

* Lallem. p 508.

CHAPTER XXIII.

IRRITATIONS OF MEDULLA SPINALIS.

PHLEGMASIA

The pathological changes of the medulla spinalis bear a very close analogy with those of the encephalon, as may be supposed from the similitude of structure. They are, however, not so frequently met with. I have, myself, no doubt that this comparative scarcity in part, exists in nature; but I am also satisfied, that if persons were more in the habit of examining the spinal marrow after death, it would be found much more frequently diseased in its membranes or substance, than we at present are inclined to admit. In regard at least to my own experience, I must say, that arachnitis of the spinal marrow is, by no means, a rare complaint in persons of all ages; and frequently exists where the symptoms indicative of it, have either been passed over, or not properly appreciated during life.

Acute inflammation of the substance of the cord, has not been often described. It has been found more usually complicated with mechanical injuries done to the spinal column, and attended with fracture or dislocation of the vertebræ. In a case which I examined in the summer of 1826, where the individual, a robust man, had broken his neck at the junction of the seventh cervical, with the first dorsal vertebra, by being jostled from his cart, and where death occurred

on the third or fourth day after the accident, a good deal of
extravasated blood was found in the cavity of the spine, and
some also in that of the dura mater, of the region injured.
The spinal marrow itself was mashed, or rather, so completely demolished at the seat of the injury, that its life
there, must have been instantly destroyed.   As is usual in
such cases, there was a complete destitution of myotility
and sensibility, in the parts of the body supplied with nerves
from the spinal marrow, below the lesion.

In a case narrated by M. Gendrin,* where the injury had
been inflicted on the fourth and fifth dorsal vertebræ, by the
fall of a piece of timber upon a carpenter; (the examination
being made twenty-six hours after death,) the muscles on
the side of the spinous processes of the region injured,
were red, softened, and infiltrated with blood and serosity.
The fourth and fifth spinous processes were fractured, and
much other injury done to the ligamentous structure of the
vertebræ.   The posterior mediastinum was infiltrated with
pus around the seat of the injury.   The spinal marrow at
that point presented a superficial softening, four inches long
by one line in depth, and having the colour of wine lees.
The right lung was infiltrated in its middle lobe, with a
large quantity of black blood, and had its tissue of a red
violet hue.

In the cases of acute inflammation of the spinal cord, reported by Dr. Abercrombie and Ollivier,† where the affection had arisen without mechanical violence, the tunica
arachnoidea of the cord in the cases generally, had a coating of coagulating lymph upon it, more or less blended with
pus, and in some instances, the latter was found in considerable quantities within the dura mater.   The substance of
the cord itself, was affected to various degrees in different
individuals: in some, it was only somewhat softer than
common, and this in distinct spots; from this comparative-

* Vol i. p. 347
† Traité de la Moelle Épinière, Paris, 1827

ly limited pathological state, it was found in all the gradations, to a perfect diffluent ramollissement for several inches: sometimes confining itself to the anterior columns, and sometimes to the posterior; and on other occasions, affecting both the anterior and the posterior columns.

The testimony of pathologists and writers of the present day, is, I think, decidedly in favour of the acute inflammatory affections of the medulla spinalis, being disposed to end in a softening or melting down, as it were, of the structure. The disease ends fatally in from a week to two months, or more. In some instances, it begins like a rheumatic affection of the back, but generally it ends by a declared palsy, both of touch and myotility, which is more or less general in the limbs, and in the trunk of the body.

Chronic Inflammation.

This affection is productive of precisely the same changes of organization, which occur in the medulla spinalis under similar circumstances. When the irritation is rather mild, and persists for a long time, the tissue of the spinal marrow becomes indurated, and acquires a reddish colour, which is subsequently converted into a deep yellow Sometimes we find the tenacity of the part in proportion to the induration; on other occasions, it becomes more brittle and friable than natural. In the case of a man aged fifty-nine, who had some symptoms of spinal affection from early life, the posterior half of the spinal cord was in this indurated but brittle state, while the anterior half was reduced to a yellowish diffluent pulp.* This case, I think, proves clearly that both induration and ramollissement of a chronic kind may be considered as different stages of the same affection; the induration being finished by a softening in the same way as we see frequently to occur in tumours.

* Gendrin. vol ii p 168

The question is not yet fully settled among pathologists, whether the indurated state of the spinal marrow, without vascular injection, ought to be received as an evidence of inflammation. Upon general principles, I am much disposed to adopt the opinion; for we constantly see a similar change of structure in other organs, and under circumstances of an inflammatory nature, progressing, however, with great slowness. The consistence and hardness to which I here have reference, is about equal to that of the white of an egg, hardened by boiling water. In one case, Bergamaschi * found it of this consistence, with the spinal vessels gorged with red blood. M. Ollivier, in an epileptic girl whom he dissected, found it in a similar condition, but without injection of it or its mucous membranes. M. Portal † has narrated a highly interesting case of this kind as occurring to himself, and in which the inflammatory nature of the affection would seem to have been pretty clearly marked. His words are as follow: "The late Marquis of Causan, of a dry and sensitive temperament, experienced at first formications in the fingers of the right hand, followed by a similar sensation in the foot of the same side. The sensibility of the fingers decreased, but they retained their motility: the insensibility was prolonged to the hand and the foot. These parts became emaciated and cold; and the mischief extended to the hand and to the leg; notwithstanding which, the patient continued to walk. The arm and the thigh of the affected side then went into a marasmus, and the marquis remained in that state for a year, still continuing his exercise, though in his chamber, by means of a crutch. In the mean time, the ends of the fingers and of the toes, on the left side, began to be affected in a way similar to those on the right, and the disease progressed upwards after the same process; the fore-arm and the legs being first affected, and the arms and thighs subsequently.

* Ollivier, loc cit   † Anat Med. vol. iv. p 116

" The marquis was thus forced to keep his bed, being deprived of all motion in the extremities, and in the trunk. He breathed and swallowed easily, and for some time the other functions were properly executed; but gradually the sight dimmed, and finally became extinct; the hearing became hard, and also ceased. The patient still articulated badly a few words, and could swallow a few spoonfuls of broth or of jelly at a time; the pulse was then slow, hard, and unequal. From this grade the malady still progressed slowly. The respiration, from being free became slow; the deglutition was more and more difficult; the pulse diminished to forty, thirty, and even ten pulsations in a minute: finally, the patient died.

"On the examination of the body after death, all its organs, even the brain, were found in a natural state, but that portion of the medulla spinalis contained within the cervical vertebræ, was reduced to a *cartilaginous consistence;* and the membranes of this spot were very red, and much inflamed."

It sometimes happens that the tissue of the spinal marrow, like that of the brain, after it has suffered a long time from chronic inflammation, will be found on death as red as it is in acute inflammation of a few days' standing. This has been observed both where the spinal marrow was irritated by violence,* and where the disease has been spontaneous.† Generally, it will be found that the symptoms indicated at first a slow progress in the malady, and that subsequently they have been rapidly developed, so as to assume an acute character; for example, the limb which previously had been paralytic and motionless, will become convulsed.

---

* Gendrin, vol. ii. p. 174. -   † Portal, vol. iv. p. 116.

Ramollissement of Spinal Cord.

From what has been just stated on the acute and chronic inflammations of the spinal cord, the inference will be readily presented to the mind, that the pathological change called ramollissement, like that of the brain, is a consequence of both chronic and of acute inflammation. It is one of those conditions which the nervous pulp of the brain and of the spinal marrow seems much more disposed to run into, during a state of irritation, than into any other, excepting mere sanguineous congestion. This may arise principally from their peculiar consistence as well as from their peculiar structure.

This affection of the spinal marrow, like those of the brain, is sometimes confined to one half or to one side only, and therefore manifests itself on one side of the body only; but from the smallness of the cord the affection generally lasts in this exclusive way for a few days, and is then transmitted or communicated to the other side also. Being destined to preside over the functions of sentiment and myotility in the trunk and limbs, its derangements are manifested by the lesions of these functions, by their being executed either in excess, in diminution, or by their being perverted. According to M. Pinel, where the ramollissement is inflammatory, there are convulsions, with general phenomena of reaction; but, if it be the contrary, or atonic, M. Foville states that there is first a diminution, and then a complete loss of sentiment and myotility.*

The derangements of the two last are either general or partial in affections of the medulla spinalis, and it is from those states that we are brought to infer the extent and locality of the disease. When it occupies the dorsal and lumbar portions, the trunk, the rectum, the urinary bladder, the genitals, and the inferior extremities, are the seats of the morbid

* Rostan, p. 187.

phenomena: and when it is situated in the upper part of the neck, these phenomena include the thoracic extremities in their range. From this, it will be seen, that the symptoms of disease radiate from the medulla spinalis along the fasciculi of nerves detached from it, to the various points of the body.

The following case will serve to illustrate this subject, and the complications to which inflammation of the spinal marrow is subject.

Mr. Benjamin R. C., aged forty-three, had for many years, twelve or fifteen, been subject to intermittent convulsions, considered to be epileptic; and, when walking, had an awkward, tottering gait. During the last year of his life the convulsions became less frequent; but he finally died in a state of extreme marasmus, evidently connected with them.

Exterior Aspect.—Skin of a leaden colour. Lower extremities dropsical.

Head.—Tunica arachnoidea thickened and opaque in several places: in the fissures between the convolutions, it was separated from the pia mater by water, and at the interior face of the hemispheres, by bubbles of air, possibly from putrefaction. There was an abundance of serum also beneath the arachnoidea around the medulla oblongata. I may mention it in passing, that from this case I learned that it is the adhesion of the tunica arachnoidea to the pia mater, within the first cervical vertebra, which prevents water from passing into the spinal canal from the cranium.

The pia mater was healthy. The cerebrum had its cortical substance softer than usual: the medullary was very plastic, yet tough and soft, and had many points of red blood in it. The lateral ventricles contained each about two drachms of serum; tunica arachnoidea thickened on corpus callosum; marasmus and softening of the fornix;—plexus choroides, large and having several vesicles in it; its veins were filled with dark blood, looking as if it had been stagnated and then soaked in water, for some time previous to death.

The cerebellum was very soft.

The medulla spinalis soft from one end to the other; in the region of the cauda equina it was reduced for an inch into a semi-fluid state.   Its cineritious, and medullary structure parted readily from one another by scraping with a knife handle.   The most posterior fasciculi were very distinct. Tunica arachnoidea somewhat thickened, and opaque in places, and contained about three drachms of serum between it and the pia mater.

The abdomen was natural; and as there had not been any pectoral symptoms, we did not examine the thorax.

This autopsy was made thirty-three hours after death, for Dr. Chapman the attending physician.   There was no perceptible putrefaction, and the body had been kept over a tub of ice; yet as the weather was warm, perhaps it might have assisted in softening the tissue of the brain, and of the medulla spinalis.

A very interesting case of softening of the spinal marrow, and which suits well our present purpose, is narrated by M. Pinel, fils.*   A girl aged 27, in good health, named Maria Brisset, serving as a domestic in a family, was accused of having committed a theft, and though innocent was sent off. Her menses, which had been flowing for three days, were instantly stopped, and she returned to her parents in profound grief for the discredit attached to her.

On the third day afterwards she was found in bed in a state of perfect coma, both in regard to sensation and intelligence.   Being taken to the Hôtel Dieu, her stupor disappeared in a month and a half, but she remained in a state of mania, which occasioned her transfer to the Salpetriere, August 18th, 1818.   The symptoms then were, astonished look, difficult articulation, slow painful answers, which were rarely exact; inertness, but not palsy of all the limbs; almost continual repose, automatic life; sometimes she had ac-

* Rostan, p. 191.

cessions of rage and of impatience. The organic functions were completely and energetically executed. For fifteen months she continued in nearly the same state, only becoming very corpulent. On the 15th of January, 1820, she was suddenly seized with convulsions. The next day she exhibited frothing at the mouth, the eyes turned backwards, grinding of the teeth, tetanic closure of the jaws, profound coma, convulsive jerks of the trunk repeated three or four times a minute. The limbs were immoveable, and did not participate in the convulsions of the trunk.

"The pulse full, frequent, irregular, and tumultuous; the respiration short, embarrassed, and hurried; the alvine evacuations involuntary. The whole body covered with an abundant sweat, of a strong durable smell, and rising in vapour above the patient. For three days the convulsions of the trunk were continually repeated, seeming stronger in the day, and accompanied with a paroxysm of fever, and the other symptoms continued. At the end of this time the patient died."

Autopsy thirty-six hours after death.

Head.—Cranium thick and injected; the dura mater thin, almost diaphanous; the longitudinal sinus gorged with blood; the arachnoid presented in all the extent of the frontal and parietal region, the traces of an ancient inflammation, announced by thickening, by layers of lymph, by a purulent serosity, and close and general adhesions to the cortical substance. The cerebrum and the cerebellum examined with care, offered nothing unusual, only the ventricles contained a little serum, and the cerebral substance was firm.

Spinal Marrow.—The membranes were healthy, but the substance itself was reduced to a yellowish, inodorous, and diffluent pulp, from the fourth cervical to the first lumbar vertebra. In the lumbar region the spinal marrow resumed its ordinary consistence, and was bathed somewhat in a reddish serosity.

The abdominal and thoracic viscera were healthy; the uterus was very small.

Many cases of a similar kind are recorded by pathologists, and I may refer particularly to the writings of M. Rostan,* and to those of Dr. Abercrombie,† but such as I have narrated will be sufficient to illustrate the type of ramollissement of the spinal marrow.

Dissolution and Removal of the Spinal Cord.

Another state to which the spinal cord is subject, is a partial deficiency. I have not met with it myself, but several cases are recorded by medical writers. Mr. Copeland,‡ met with one where the patient, a man, suffered paraplegia, dysuria, obstinacy of the bowels, and a feeling of tightness across his belly, as if a broad band had been bound tightly around it. His health had suffered for a year, and the commencement of his indisposition was attributed to a sprain of the back, from lifting a heavy weight. After a confinement to bed of three months from a perfect paraplegia, he died with gangrenous nates. On autopsy after death, the vertebræ were found in a perfectly healthy state; but within the last dorsal, and the first lumbar vertebræ, the spinal cord was entirely wanting for more than two inches; and the membranes, which there formed an empty bag, were unusually vascular, and much thickened. In Majendie's Journal of Physiology, a case is recorded in which the arms during life had suffered a loss of myotility, but retained their sensibility, and the legs were not affected. This patient, at the autopsy, presented a spinal cord, which had become quite liquid through two thirds of the dorsal, and one third of the cervical region.

* Rostan, from page 186 to 201, inclusively.
† Diseases of Brain and Spinal Marrow, from page 340 to 351, inclusively.
‡ Dis. of Spine

In a child eight years of age, who died of extreme marasmus with caries of the vertebræ, but without loss either of
sensibility or motion of the limbs; Ollivier found four inches
of the cord entirely wanting. Velpau has recorded several
similar cases. These are very singular instances of devia-
tion from the usual routine of symptoms in diseases of the
spine, and are well suited to perplex the pathologist in accounting for them. I am inclined to believe that the cord,
before its entire removal at places, must have gone through
the process of ramollissement and liquefaction described in a
former part of this chapter, and the condition of it is therefore to be referred to that pathological change: this, however, does not account for the anomaly of symptoms.

M. Rullier of Paris, has communicated a very remarkable
case, where the middle third of the medulla spinalis was in a
diffluent limpid state. The individual, aged forty-four, had
the symptoms of the disease on him for ten years: they advanced very gradually until they settled down into a permanent contraction, with aching of the upper extremities. Ho
walked on the Boulevards, however, a few days before death,
and possessed his intellectual and moral faculties unimpaired,
and his passion for sexual intercourse.*

Apoplexy of Spine.

The next affection of the spinal marrow which I think it
useful to describe is apoplexy. The symptoms of paralysis
here, and want of sensation in the part below, come on with
considerable rapidity in many cases, and it may be known
principally by that circumstance. The effusion of blood is,
I believe, much more frequent on the outer side of the dura
mater than within it, and the symptoms would seem to arise
principally from compression of the spinal marrow. This

* Jour. For. Med. Science, vol. iii. p. 593. Phil.

affection is sometimes spontaneous, but more frequently it results from violence as, a blow, a fall, or a strain.   A moment's reference to the anatomy of the spine, will explain to us the greater frequency of extravasation on the outer side of the membranes, than in the substance of the medulla spinalis.   The latter is, when compared with the brain, very deficient in blood vessels, and especially large ones; its natural texture is firmer, and its pia mater is a perfect coat, and possessed of much more strength than the pia mater of the brain: this allows it to support much better such blood vessels as ramify on its surface, and in the substance of the cord.   But on the outer side of the dura mater, loose from it, and adhering to the posterior faces of the vertebræ, exist those numerous veins designated as the sinuses of the vertebral column; other veins also are found on the bony bridges of the vertebræ.   In both cases they have very thin parietes, and are easily ruptured by mechanical violence, or by congestion: they seem to be formed, principally, from the internal membrane of the veins, and to have only a very thin external coat.   Corresponding in office to the sinuses of the dura mater of the brain, they differ from them in this point of structure, that they are too weak to bear much distention without rupturing. Hæmorrhage from these sinuses, then, I believe to be the most frequent cause of apoplexy of the spinal canal.   The following cases will illustrate the consequences of this affection.

" A child aged seven days, September 1st, 1818; was observed not to suck, and appeared as if he were prevented by something which impeded the motion of his tongue. Through the following day he cried frequently, and still did not suck; in the evening he was seen by Mr. White, who found the jaw clinched by spasm, but by very little force it could be opened.   On the third day he was seized with convulsion, which recurred at various intervals, sometimes in the form of tonic spasm of the whole body, and sometimes of violent

convulsive agitation. On the fourth the convulsion continued, and he died in the afternoon.

Inspection.—No disease could be detected in the brain.
In the spinal canal, there was found a long and very firm
coagulum of blood, lying between the bones and the membranes of the cord on the posterior part, and extending the
whole length of the cervical portion.*

It was my misfortune in August, 1828, to lose a child of
three weeks, under similar circumstances Some hesitation
in sucking had exhibited itself, occasionally, almost from
the day of his birth, and seemed to arise from a suspension
of respiration for a few moments at a time. On the eighth
day, these suspensions of respiration became more frequent,
more protracted and obvious, and during their continuance,
were attended with a drawing up of the arms and legs,
with a slight spasmodic motion, and some frothing at the
mouth, together with blackness of visage. When the respiration was restored, it was followed by cries of distress,
like screaming. A lethargic disposition supervened, which,
for the first twenty-four hours would yield to the administration of nourishment; it then became profound, and lasted
so for the next day, 24 hours, when death followed. The
lethargy was attended, during its whole course, by the disorder in respiration, and slight spasm of the extremities.
Towards the last, the intervals of respiration became so long,
and the infant was so perfectly motionless, that on several
occasions, life was supposed by those around to have ceased.

From the simultaneous absence of all my friends, on
whose accuracy, as pathologists, I could rely; an examination
of the body was unfortunately not made: I can only, therefore, deduce the inference, that there must have been some
important lesion of the spinal marrow or brain arising, probably from extravasated blood. While on this subject, I
may state, that the frequent examination of still-born infants,

* Aber. p 362

or those who have died in a few days after birth, has convinced me, that a very common cause of death, is an extravasation of blood; I may indeed say, in so many words,
apoplexy of the brain, and perhaps of the spinal marrow.
Though of the latter, I am not so well assured from actual
observation, probably, from having permitted many opportunities of verifying the opinion, to pass unheeded, in consequence of not having my attention especially directed to
the state of the spinal marrow, as well as to that of the
brain.

This apoplectic state of the brain in children, I have
thought to arise from the same cause which produces the
tumefied ecchymosed scalp, to wit, undue retention of the
head in the pelvis of the mother, and the continued contractions of the uterus driving and accumulating the blood
in it.   The following note I have transcribed from my dia-
ry of dissections.   It was written in 1825, without any
view to a theory, and under no expectation of making it a
subject of publication: it may, therefore, be considered, as an
observation, affected by no other bias than a desire of holding an accurate opinion on a very important subject.   "I
have now examined on various occasions, about seven still-
born children, one of them being a gestation of seven
months.   I have found, invariably, ecchymosis of the cellular substance connecting the integuments of the head, to
the pericranium; generally it was much diffused: and along
with this, I have always found a considerable effusion of
blood under the pia mater and over it, arising from rupture
of its blood vessels.   In some of those cases, the coagulum
of red blood formed a layer over almost the whole of the
cerebrum.   One of the most extensive cases of extravasation had the child's head of unusual dimensions, the horizontal circumference of the cranium being fifteen inches,
and the diagonal one being sixteen and three fourths.   The
labour in this case had lasted twenty-four hours, and was
brought to an end by the administration of one scruple of

ergot, which in fifteen minutes began to take effect. In this case, as well as in another of still birth, where the child was a very fine one, I think it right to state that I had some apprehensions of the dose of ergot having assisted, at least, in the fatal consequences to the child; by causing an incessant violent contraction of the uterus, until the expulsion of the child; and consequently forcing the blood into its head, as the latter passed through the pelvis "

In January, 1825, I examined for Dr. Shoemaker, an experienced accoucheur of this city, a child, aged ten days, of Mr. B. After a very natural delivery and perfect health for a week; this infant was taken with violent crying, difficulty of respiration, and blueness of the face and body. On examination after death, we found the veins of the pia mater congested in the highest degree with blood, and the latter extravasated in spots, under the pia mater, and beneath the parietal bone, between it and the dura mater. The scalp in this case was not ecchymosed, as is usual where blood is extravasated in the cranium. We could only conjecture the period of this pathological condition, to have been contemporaneous with the passage of the child's head through the pelvis.

The preceding cases may be considered as illustrative of apoplectic effusion upon the brain, and perhaps, also, upon the spinal marrow of children; at any rate, there can be no objection to the first reported by Mr White. The following will represent the apoplexy of the spine in adults. " Ollivier reports, that a lady, aged forty, had head-ach and pain of the back; after a few days the pain of the back became very acute, and violent convulsion took place, which was fatal, after continuing five or six hours. All was sound in the brain, but extensive extravasation of blood was found in the spinal canal, which was most abundant about the seat of the pain.

A gentleman, aged sixty-one, had just arrived in Paris, from a long journey, when he complained of pain in his

back, extending from the cervical vertebræ quite to the sacrum.   After a few hours he was seized with paraplegia,
and incontinence of urine and fæces; and he died while the
physician was talking to him, who had been sent for on
the occurrence of the palsy.   There was extensive extravasation of blood in the spinal canal, under the membranes of
the cord.   At the lower part it formed a mass like a bouillie of bullock's blood, in which the substance of the cord
could not be distinguished, as far as the third dorsal vertebra; and above this, where the cord was entire, it was of a
deep red colour, and very soft. *

A gentleman died of a disease which was considered as
apoplectic, but in which he retained his mental faculties to
the last.   No disease was discovered in the brain, but there
was a great quantity of extravasated blood in the spinal canal.†

These cases will be sufficient to · illustrate the affection
with which we are occupied: I have no doubt that it is
of more frequent occurrence than what we suppose, in consequence of the too general neglect of examining the spine
in our autopsies, and that many of the cases of paralysis of
the trunk and limbs, where there is a sudden loss of myotility and sense of touch, with retention of the intellect, depend upon rupture of some of the blood vessels of the spinal canal, and the compression of the spinal marrow.

* Gaulter de Claubray, Jour Gen. de Med. 1828
† Du Hamel Reg. Societ. Acad. Histor. An. 1683, sect. 5, cap. 2, p. 264.
Id 364.

CHAPTER XXIV.

IRRITATIONS OF THE NERVES.

PHLEGMASIA

THE nervous cords, like other parts of the body, are subject to the various grades of inflammation and their consequences; and the ischiatic nerve, from the pelvis downwards,
seems to be especially liable to such attacks. Sometimes the
inflammation is confined to a space of a few lines in length,
but on other occasions it extends for several inches. The
augmentation of local sensibility, and the pain in these cases
are extreme; and there is generally a sense of numbness and
an inability to use the muscles of the part.

The anatomical characters of these inflammations, are a
lively red colour, and a high vascular injection, which becomes the more minute and intense in approaching to the
centre of the phlegmasia. The capillaries which run longi-
·tudinally, are united by a multitude of fine transverse capillaries, which M. Gendrin* says no artificial injection in
the natural state can make evident. The nerve becomes tumefied, its filaments more separated than in the healthy state,
and its interstitial cellular substance infiltrated with serosity.

When the inflammation is very intense, the nerve becomes
of a uniform brown or violet colour, and infiltrated with red
blood. The distinctness of the vascular injection is lost, ex-

* Gendrin, vol ii, p 112

cept upon the boundaries of the phlegmasia.   The nerve becomes harder to the touch, but at the same time its consistence and strength are so diminished that it tears through readily.   Its peculiar texture is lost; it becomes homogeneous,
and resembles a cord of inflamed cellular substance.   In some
of the dissections of persons who had died from inflamed
nerves, reported by M. Gendrin,* pus was found infiltrated
between the fasciculi of nervous cords and also in the surrounding cellular substance along the track of the nerve.   In
these persons the disorganization of the nervous fibrilla was
short of what occurs in the most active inflammations, where
they, as just stated, are converted into a homogeneous mass.

It appears from the experiments of M. Gendrin, that the
inflammation of a nerve, when artificially excited, produces
also an inflammation of the organ to which it is distributed:
thus that of the fifth pair makes the eye inflame; that of the
par vagum, the stomach, but not the lungs; that of the spermatic nerves, the testicles.   But in the extremities the consequences are not the same, but only a serous infiltration, rather inconsiderable, and occurring only when a considerable
length of nerve is affected with phlegmasia.

Sub-Inflammation.

Chronic inflammations of the nervous cords are much less
known than one would suppose: this may arise from the
comparative infrequency of such diseases; but I am also disposed to think that the cases of it have been overlooked or
mistaken when they did occur.   Like acute inflammation,
it may be confined to a spot or be extended for several inches
along the nervous cord.   The pain is excruciating and en-
during; never intermits entirely, but only remits.   The disease has for its anatomical characters, enlargement of the
part affected, augmentation of density and vascularity, indu-

* Gendrin, vol. ii. p. 148.

ration and friability. The cellular substance forming the sheath of the nerve, and holding its fasciculi together, is also thickened, indurated, and becomes infiltrated.

When in London, in 1821, I saw Sir Astley Cooper extirpate a tumour of this kind from one of the nerves of the fore arm, it was about the size of a small nutmeg. He mentioned, that he had, on several other occasions, extirpated similar tumours.

Coutugno* once found an infiltration of the ischiatic nerve, in an individual who had been subject to pain along the course of this organ. In a case reported by Mr. Wardrop, where amputation was performed on a gentleman wounded at Badajoz, to relieve him from violent pains, which he felt along the course of the radial nerve, down to the fingers; this nerve was found tumefied and hard, and the remains of a ball between its filaments above the elbow. It would seem also that this chronic inflammation of nerves is the attendant of large ulcers of the legs. M. Gendrin found it in the saphenus nerve of an old man, attended by varicose ulcers, where the ulceration occupied one half of the length of the lower extremity. This individual had died from apoplexy. Mr. Swant also reports a case of amputation for a large fungous ulcer of the leg in a woman, aged forty-three. On dissection of the limb, the external popliteal nerve, (Nervous Peroneus,) and the internal peroneo Cutaneus were tumefied, and in a state of chronic inflammation.‡

The nerves are found, occasionally, in a state of marasmus. This is especially the case with the optic, where the eye has been lost. It seldom extends beyond the junction of the nerve with its fellow. The nerve in this state is reduced to one third of its common size, is of a drab colour, and has lost all the nervous matter entering into its composition.

* De Ischiade Nervosa. 1770

† Pathol. of Nerv. System, London, 1822   ‡ Gendrin, vol. ii. p. 180.

CHAPTER XXV.

DISSECTIONS ILLUSTRATING THE PATHOLOGY OF THE ENCEPHALON AND MEDULLA SPINALIS.

APOPLEXY WITH FRACTURE OF CERVICAL VERTEBRÆ.

AUTOPSY four hours after death.

Alms House, Oct. 10*th,* 1828.—Dodge, a man aged fifty-six, of intemperate habits, and who had been treated a short time before for mania a potu, fell into the dock, as was supposed, in a fit of intoxication. This occurred on Wednesday evening, the 8th inst ; he was taken out and brought to the Alms House. The symptoms were perfect paralysis of the whole body, from the neck downwards; weak pulse, cold skin: he had enough rationality left to give an account of himself. The head was distorted, the chin inclining over to the right side. The deformity could be removed, but it returned on his being left alone. Some stimulating articles were given, which seemed to recruit his strength at first. The next day he became comatose, and died this day at 12 o'c.

Autopsy at 4 P. M.

Exterior habit full. No putrefaction.

Head.—In cutting up the scalp, much blood flowed from the divided vessels. Dura mater healthy. Tunica arachnoidea opaque, and raised from pia mater on convexities of hemispheres, and elsewhere by serum, bagging it up like a blister. It was remarkably opaque and thickened at the bottom of the fourth ventricle. Just above the left orbitar process of os frontis, there was an indentation of brain large enough to receive the end of the finger transversely. The tunica arachnoidea and pia mater at this point had coalesced, become softened and yellowish, and the adjacent cortical substance seemed also softened; the medullary matter beneath this was harder than elsewhere, approaching to the state of a cicatrix in the brain, perhaps from some old inflammation.

The pia mater of surface and ventricles much congested with blood along the whole right side of falx major, and on the same side of upper surface of tentorium, there was a lamina of recently effused blood in a state of coagulation, covering completely this membrane. It could not be traced to the rupture of any vessel in particular, but seemed rather a transudation, but of this I could not be certain, as there had been no previous injection into the vessels to fill them, for greater satisfaction. The corresponding parts of the left side were free from such effusion, except a spot of a line or two on the flat side of the left hemisphere. Substance of brain of usual consistence. Two drachms of water in ventricles, their arachnoidea being also thickened. Several drachms of serum also at base of brain.

Thorax.—Pulmonary tissue sound, excepting the usual congestion of blood in sudden death. Surface adhering closely universally, on both sides to the thorax and mediastinum, by an old pleuritic inflammation. Heart of common size, but its muscular texture was so weak that I thrust my fingers through the ventricles without difficulty, and lacerated them easily into strips: a great deal of blood had been collected into its right side, which ran out on cutting the large vessels.

Abdomen.—Ancient and close peritoneal adhesion between the whole transverse colon, and the corresponding parietes of abdomen, and also between the latter and the front surface of the stomach. In both cases much of the omentum was engaged in forming these adhesions, and an adhesion also existed between the whole upper surface of the liver, and the diaphragm. Mucous coat of stomach thickened, much corrugated, having much mucus on it, and presenting a rough granulated appearance.   Summits of rugæ, and left end, presented the punctated redness so common in old drunkards. Stomach empty.   Intestines filled with gas.

Spine.—A perfect fracture of the intervertebral matter existed between the bodies of the third and fourth cervical vertebræ, it being torn from both bones into a plate.   The intervertebral matter was also ruptured between the fourth and fifth vertebræ, the ligamentous fastenings of the third, fourth, and fifth, oblique process were torn up, and along with them the periosteum.   The adjoining muscles were infiltrated with blood, and also the whole cellular substance joining the pharynx and upper part of œsophagus, to cervical vertebræ.

On the outer side of the part of the dura mater corresponding to the injured vertebræ there was extravasated blood. There was no extravasation within.   The medulla spinalis was healthy and sound: but opposite to the fractured vertebræ in the centre of the left half, for an inch there was blended with the cortical interior an inconsiderable effusion of blood, so faint that it could only be ascertained as such by comparing it with the cortex above and below.   It seemed also slightly softened.   On the right side it was healthy in the corresponding spot, and as usual.

Puerperal Convulsions.

Oct. 20th, 1824.—I examined for Drs. Hodge and Dewees, the body of a patient who had died of puerperal convulsions, at the full period of utero gestation.   The patient was aged twenty-five, had a vigorous frame, and was in her first pregnancy.   She was ill for thirty-six hours.   The practitioner who had been in attendance before these gentlemen, had administered copious doses of laudanum, the quantity not known.   The night of her death she was delivered by Dr. Hodge with the forceps.

Appearances.—A deep and extensive ecchymosis had formed across the root of the neck, and extended to the shoulders. On the upper surface of the brain, an irregular patch of blood, of two inches square, was extravasated under the pia mater. The extravasation extended to the bottom of the convolutions. The vessels of the brain were turgid with blood.

Having at the time my attention directed to the precise line of reflection of the peritoneum between the uterus and the bladder during the state of pregnancy, with the view to a new manner proposed by Dr. Physick, of executing the Cæsarean operation, I observed that it passed from the lower part of the neck of the uterus to the bladder.

Without difficulty, I dissected the peritoneum from the bladder, raised it from the cervix uteri, and then cut through the latter into the cavity of the uterus. The uterus was about half the pregnant size, being occupied by the placenta, and somewhat distended with gas.

Tetanus.

March 23d, 1828.—J. Davis, aged twelve years, a stout boy in the employment of Mr. W. Fry, printer, in passing through the yard twelve or fourteen days ago, struck the fore part of his right thigh against a rough piece of wood, which made an angular laceration of the integuments, each side of which was about an inch long.

He continued to attend to his duties till Monday, the 17th, when Dr. Chapman saw him: he then had something like sore throat, for which a cathartic was directed. On Saturday morning he came under the care of Dr. Jackson, who found him in a general tetanic state, and prescribed a hundred or more leeches to the spine; but owing to a difficulty in obtaining them, the prescription was only partially executed. He also gave two hundred drops of laudanum at once, with a progressive increase of fifty drops additional, every hour and a half. In the evening, the boy had taken fifteen hun-

dred drops, without any mitigation.   As he had not an evacuation for several days, an injection of spirits of turpentine was prescribed.   This did not act for some time, till at
length, a pinch of snuff was given to the boy, at his urgent
request; the bowels then gave way, and a free purging ensued.   He died in a spasm about nine o'clock, on Saturday
evening.*

Autopsy, eighteen hours after death, assisted by Dr.
Jackson.

The laceration was of the integuments covering the internal edge of the middle of the rectus femoris.   Upon dissecting them up from the fascia, the injury seemed to have
gone to the fascia: the wound was black, owing to a cup
having been applied to it, and its bottom was hardened from
the intermixture of coagulating lymph with fat.   On raising
the fascia from the rectus muscle, I found that the fascia,
though it looked entire, had been perforated, the hole being
now closed; and between it and the muscle a small splinter
existed, half an inch long, and a line or two wide, surrounded by a deposite of coagulating lymph.   The muscle, itself,
bore no mark of disorganization or change of structure; but
at the point alluded to, it felt hard, like a knot, for a space
of six lines in diameter.

Integuments of head bled freely on being cut.   Dura mater much drier than usual—tunica arachnoidea and pia mater
also much drier than common; the latter much congested in
its veins.   Ventricles contained only a little halitus; cortical substance throughout of a deep drab colour, and along
with the medullary very much congested.   Substance of
brain and the nerves firm and hard.   There was a great deal
of vascular congestion along the spinal canal: the parts cut,
on opening the latter, bled very freely.   The spinal marrow and its membranes congested; the former was remark-

---

* The details of this case are more fully communicated by Dr. Jackson,
in vol. iu. p. 321, Am, Jour. Med. Sciences.

ably hard and firm, feeling almost tendinous. There was nothing like inflammation in it, or its membranes, and they were all dry, there being no dropsical effusion.

Thorax.—Heart natural, it contained scarcely any blood, and no coagula; the want of the former was probably occasioned by its being in a fluid state, and much having been lost in the examination of the brain. The left lung was collapsed to one half the size of the other, though elastic; and adhered every where by long, strong, old adhesions, and short ones to the thorax. There was no recollection of a pleurisy having occurred at any time of his life.

Abdomen.—Intestines and stomach extremely distended with gas, and some escaped from the peritoneum: the peritoneum healthy. Liver and spleen healthy. Some parts of the small intestines were much contracted, others collapsed. The colon was lined internally with a thick coat of very fœtid bilious fæces.

The mucous membrane of the stomach in its cardiac half was of a flesh, or light pink sienna colour, the other half pearly yellow: the former part was thickened, and so soft, that it scraped off readily with the finger nail, the latter somewhat softened, but not to any remarkable extent.

Did the congestion of the central nervous system depend upon the laudanum, or upon the disease, or both?

Tetanus.

A carpenter, aged about 26, thick and well set, and rather intemperate, in jumping from the roof of a house upon a scaffold, April 28th, 1828, ran a nail into the left foot; through his shoe. The inconvenience which he suffered from it was not so great as to cause him to stop work. Nearly a fortnight afterwards, May 11th, he was in the river to bathe.

Wednesday, May the 14th, he began to feel some stiffness in the jaws. Dr. Samuel Fox was called in the next day, in the afternoon: he then had perfect opisthotonos with intermittent spasm of the limbs. The course of treatment by the doctor was to cut open freely the skin of the punctured part, and to cauterize it then with caustic alkali. A blister was drawn upon the back of his neck; fifty grains of opium, ten grains at a time, were administered in the course of the night, until he ceased to be able to swallow, and next morning a suppository of sixty grains was given. In the forenoon he was bled 20 ounces; that night, at eight o'clock, he died, May 16th.

May 17th, autopsy in fifteen hours after death, assisted by Dr. Fox.

Part injured.—The nail had penetrated the sole of the left foot, at the anterior end of the fifth metatarsal bone; the incision of the skin still open and ecchymosed. The subcutaneous fat condensed by lymph, interspersed with small spots of red blood; no vestige in it of passage made by the nail. On dissecting this fat away, a hole of two lines diameter was found in the anterior end of the fifth metatarsal bone, which penetrated to its centre, and contained a small bit of sole leather, looking as if it had been cut out with a small punch. The nail had penetrated about three lines on the outer side of the nerve of the little toe, just behind the synovial membrane, so that neither the nerve, the tendons, nor the cavity of the joint, were lacerated by it, and it had stopped somewhat short of the upper surface of the bone. Much pain had been felt at the corresponding point of the upper surface of the foot, and it had been blistered.

Head.—Countenance placid, collection of blood about mouth and face. Scalp bled freely on being cut, and the temporal regions were in almost an ecchymosed state, from the abundance of blood in the veins small and large. Bone and pericranium congested also.

Dura mater healthy; sinuses abounding in blood. Arachnoidea here and there somewhat turbid, probably from his intemperate habits; a little serum beneath it. Pia mater much congested, with some spots of ecchymosis. Cerebrum and cerebellum, when sliced, bled freely from the cut vessels in dots, being both much congested: we thought that they were also somewhat softer than usual, but not universally so. Ventricles healthy, but plexus choroides distended.

Medulla Spinalis.—The vertebral sinuses highly congested, with blood accumulated in them, and partially ecchymosed from their fulness. Membranes healthy, and not unusually occupied with blood. Medulla spinalis itself, about the consistence of the brain, being universally somewhat softer than common.

Thorax.—Heart empty, larger than usual, the lungs almost black behind from congestion of blood; the blood being fluid, it had probably subsided after death, from heart into lungs through pul. artery. Some old pleuritic adhesions on the right side. In left lung some small ossified tubercles near its fissure on surface. Vessels of parietes congested.

Abdomen.—Much flatus; no striking congestion of vessels. Mucous coat of stomach having very little mucus on it, and so soft, that it could be scraped off very readily with the knife handle. No marked injection of it, with the exception of some claret-coloured streaks in the course of its rugæ. Intestines healthy; some hardened fæces in colon. Liver rather small, and of an olive brown.

The abdomen and thorax, were examined before the brain and spinal marrow, but no large vessels were cut.

The impression from this case was, that the brain and medulla spinalis were the suffering organs, though there was no very strongly marked disorganization: the most obvious change being in the undue softness, which, however, was only a little below the standard. Can tetanus differ from other affections, by its being a universal irritation of the brain and medulla spinalis? and, which runs its course in too short a time to admit of much disorganization? Did the congestion depend upon the opium?

Tetanus.

Edwin Bailey, aged 26, of a robust, muscular appearance, came into the Alms House Infirmary, July 12th, 1829, labouring under tetanus, (opisthotonos.)   Ten days previously, he had punctured his foot with a nail: on the fifth day, spasms supervened.   His treatment had been, large quantities of tinctura opii, to the amount, as his friend stated, of ʒi. every half hour.   His treatment in this infirmary, was commenced at noon.   It consisted of bleeding from both arms, to the amount of ℥lvi.; application of ice to the head, previously shaved; and the free administration of brandy.

At 2 o'clock his pulse was 160; ℥xiij. of blood were taken, and brandy given.   At 3 o'clock he died.

Examination eighteen hours after death.

Head.—On opening the cranium, the blood vessels of the pia mater did not appear unusually distended.   Several bubbles of air were seen on the right side; and a few on the left, in the vessels, with some emphysema.

The brain was firm, and congested: at a small distance the medullary matter appeared of a light pink colour: ʒi. of transparent serum was found in each of the lateral ventricles.   The plexus choroides was almost empty of blood; the fornix rather softer than usual: the texture of the cerebellum was firm and natural.

There was a settling of blood on the integuments of the back.

Medulla Spinalis.—The vascularity of the membranes was found in a normal state, the thoracic portion of the arachnoid membrane, turbid, and thickened in spots on the posterior face of medulla: four small, bony and cartilaginous bodies, a line or two in diameter, were seen adhering to the arachnoid membrane.   There was a *sensible softening of the thoracic portion of the medulla,* contrasting very obviously with the cervical and lumbar portions.

This softening was satisfactorily ascertained by pressure, by scraping, and also by tearing the medulla spinalis into strings or slips. The softened portion was of a light pink colour internally, like the brain.

Head and lungs natural.

Stomach enormously large, distended by gas to the amount of two quarts, and containing a pint of mucus and brandy: its mucous coat was entirely covered with a thick, tenacious layer of mucus, mixed with coagulating lymph. The anterior face of mucous coat gangrenous, of a green colour, and diminished consistency.

The same disposition to secrete lymph and mucus was observed in the duodenum.

Liver and spleen healthy. · Intestines healthy.

Place of Injury.—The nail had penetrated the external margin of the sole of the foot, near the cuboid bone, avoiding the fascia, and the puncture could be traced by the tumefaction and ecchymosis surrounding its course upward to the trunk of nervus communicans tibiæ, where it lies at the external side of the foot. The point of the nail seemed here to have stopped in the thickness of the nerve, which was in a state of inflammation.

Mania.

Miss ——, aged nineteen, has for four months been affected with a decided and violent mania, manifesting itself by eccentric notions and conduct on all subjects. Among other things her desire to escape from her friends was incessant; and she on several occasions made attempts at suicide, by plunging a knife at her bosom, by twisting things around her neck, and by sub-mersion. Her mind, previous to this indisposition, was well developed, gay, and vigorous; and was strongly impressed with piety. About eighteen months ago she was thrown from a carriage, and received a contusion on the head; but Dr. Parrish who attended her then, stated that no serious consequences seemed to ally themselves to this accident, and she recovered fully from it.

She had been treated by repeated venesection to a large amount at a time, by cupping and leeching to the head, by blisters over it, and latterly by the application of tartar emetic ointment to the scalp, which had produced the usual soreness of it.

Autopsy twenty-four hours after death.   October 15th, 1828, assisted by Drs Parrish, Otto, and Randolph.

Exterior Aspect.—Marasmus moderate.

Head.—Well developed, and of good shape, forehead full.   The scalp was thickened, indurated to the feel by the irritating applications that had been made to it; cut very easily, and also lacerated easily, so that the stitches in sewing it, were disposed to cut their way out much more readily than usual; it also was watery, as a great deal of serum exuded from it, and was easily torn up from the pericranium.

Dura mater natural.   Pia mater contained in its veins about the usual quantity of blood, probably somewhat more. Tunica arachnoidea healthy generally, but had beneath it, along the gutters, between the convolutions on the top of hemispheres, a collection of serum raising it into serpentine vesications: where it gets beneath the corpus callosum and fornix it was opaque, and also at bottom of fourth ventricle. One of the veins of the pia mater on the borders of the longitudinal sinus, had a cylinder two inches long, of coagulated lymph in it.

Cerebrum.—No change in cortical matter, except it could be rubbed off perhaps with rather more ease than usual. The medullary matter was hard, resisting pressure, but could be lacerated easily, a great deal of serum escaped from its cut surfaces, and these were also thickly interspersed with dots of blood escaping from the vessels.   The corpus striatum appeared larger than usual, and some calibres of blood vessels parallel with one another, and in contact were seen traversing its thickness below: they were at least half a line in diameter, perfectly patulous and round, and about five or six in number. The ventricles contained but a few drops of serum.

The cerebellum was nearly natural. The obvious pathological changes in it were a consistence softer than usual, much softer to the feel, and more lacerable than the cerebrum, and it also contained rather more serum in its interstices than natural, but not so much as the brain: its blood vessels were by no means so numerous and visible.

Other cavities were not examined, as the request of the family was confined to the head, and no other symptoms than those of derangement were manifested.

In this dissection, I considered the sub-arachnoid effusion the partially turbid arachnoid membrane, and interstitial water of the cerebrum, the vascularity, and other abnormal states as pathological; being the result and evidences of irritation in the encephalon. If the greater hardness and the infiltrated state of the brain, and its easy laceration be not an evidence of chronic inflammation, how is it, that the same condition of the scalp, evidently produced by irritating applications to it, should be considered a form of chronic inflammation?

Arachnitis of the Brain and Spinal Marrow, with Pulmonary Consumption.

N. M. a black girl, aged twenty, a domestic in the family of a merchant of this city, was taken unwell about the middle of July, 1827. The symptoms which appeared were a dry husky skin, with not much heat in it; pulse frequent; difficulty of breathing on ascending a flight of stairs; slight head-ach; no appetite; bowels regular; menstruation regular up to the last period; tongue indicating no derangement in the viscera of digestion; a sound of the thorax somewhat flattened on percussion on the right side under the clavicle.

I directed her a diurnal diet, consisting in milk one pint, mixed with water one pint, and bread four ounces, which was continued for one month, with an evident improvement in the symptoms; for she became stronger; the expression of countenance was better, and her breathing easier. I observed, however, the frequency of pulse to continue; it was seldom less than 140, and generally 160 in the minute. As she was extremely diffident, I often charged her with being agitated, but this she denied. There being, however, no local pain, except in the head, and that slight, I must confess that notwithstanding her assertions, I attributed much to agitation.

The symptoms seemed at the expiration of the month to have worn away so completely, with the exception of the state of pulse, that I gave her permission to live more freely, indeed almost as usual, and discontinued my visits. The only medicinal application during this month was a blister upon the upper front part of the chest, which was kept open for some days.

I saw nothing of her afterwards till about the middle of September, and supposed her well: I was then informed to the contrary; and as, in consequence of a newspaper paragraph, the tea of liverwort had begun to excite considerable attention for pulmonary affections, her mistress desired its exhibition in her case. This was conceded, and persevered in for fifteen or twenty days, without the slightest benefit, except that she thought her head relieved by it. About the close of the administration of this remedy, her stomach became exceedingly disordered, and rejected every thing for a day or two, when its extreme irritability ceased, but with an entire loss of appetite.

October 15*th*, 1827.—At this period the symptoms are, one eye turned from its axis, squinting, double vision; articulation rather slow; does not complain of pain in the head; pulse one hundred and sixty; respiration rather easy and tranquil; no pain in thorax. Percussion beneath the right clavicle, produces a heavy fleshy sound. On the application of stethoscope no respiration heard there, but it is heard in other parts of the same lung. Sound and respiration of right lung good. No complaint of abdomen. Loss of appetite. I directed the renewal of the blister to the thorax, and ordered tinct. benz comp. gtt. xxx. three times a day.

A few days after this she became incapable of discharging her urine; the bladder distended and produced the excessive pain, attending that state. Her articulation was broken by sobs and cries, with stuttering and thick speech. The lower extremities became motionless, though extremely painful when touched or moved abruptly; and the other symptoms of cerebral disease increased. The bladder was relieved of a pint and a half of very foetid urine by the catheter, to which instrument I resorted every day afterwards so long as she lived, from the incapability of discharging the urine still continuing, attended with pain and extreme foetor. For two days before death she became comatose, like one under the influence of laudanum, and died, November 4th, 1827, by a very gradual and easy extinction of life.

I examined her twenty-five hours after death, in company with Dr. Meigs, stating to him previously that I had experienced much difficulty in satisfying myself, on the diagnostics of the disease. That I felt assured, from percussion and auscultation, that the right lung under the clavicle was carnified, as in consumption, but that she never had any thing like night sweats from the beginning to the end of her sickness, no local pain, no cough of any constancy, and no expectoration. The symptoms in fact of hectic fever had never been evolved; latterly she had on two or three occasions spit up a very trifling quantity of matter resembling a softened tubercle, but this was all. I also told the doctor, that to account for the symptoms, we, on the principles of physiological medicine, ought to find the brain about the corpora striata and thalami softened or diseased, and also the medulla spinalis in the same way.

Autopsy.—Middle atrophy; with a very tranquil expression of face, frame well developed.

Head.—Dura mater presented the appearance of being half dried on the top of hemispheres. Pia mater congested with red blood. Arachnoidea at basis of brain much thickened by coagulating lymph, identified with its structure; this was more eminently the case about the chiasm of the optic nerves and the inferior part of the third ventricle. The ventricles contained about one ounce of serum; the fornix was in a pulpy, soft state, and the septum lucidum was stretched and resolved here and there into fasciculi of fibres, forming a very imperfect partition between the ventricles. The arachnoidea of ventricles not obviously thickened. Corpora striata softened. An inflammatory adhesion injected with red blood and cylindrical, caused the thalami to adhere; possibly this adhesion might have been the commissura mollis; but if so, it was lower down and farther forward than usual, and much stronger. Substance of brain showed numerous red points of cut vessels. Nothing remarkable about cerebellum, pons, and medulla oblongata; except that wherever the arachnoidea stretched from eminence to eminence it was thickened and inflamed.

Medulla Spinalis.—Dura mater natural; tunica arachnoidea inflamed in its whole length and thickened, adhering very closely to pia mater, and to the roots of the spinal nerves. Texture of medulla softer at places than natural.

Thorax.—Right lung carnified in its upper lobe, and adhering to the thorax where it gave out the flattened sound; raw tubercles in great abundance through its structure, but none of them softened; permeable imperfectly to air in its two lower lobes. Left lung permeable every where, but abounding in immature tubercles from a line to three in diameter; none of them softened. Heart natural.

Abdomen.—Liver healthy, with the exception of a few tubercular masses interspersed in it. Stomach contained a thin, dark-coloured fluid, smelling disagreeably; mucous coat somewhat browned, and the lymphatic glands along its lesser curvature, and in lesser omentum, enlarged and tuberculous; some of them were seen in the thickness of the stomach, along its lesser curvature, from one to two lines broad. Intestines generally healthy, at least the marks of disease were not evident, with the exception of a light slate-colour at their upper part in the mucous coat. Organs of generation generally healthy; the internal coat of uterus injected with blood, and could be raised easily with the point of a knife.

By an oversight I neglected to look at the mucous coat of the ileo-colic junction, and at that of the bladder; which latter organ, at the time of death, contained some of the dreadfully fœtid urine, a little of which escaping by pressure made the room almost intolerable to us.

I consider this case to have been one of the most satisfactory for elucidating the location of disease by the lesion of function, or in other words, for illustrating physiological medicine. Without the squinting, and without the paralysis of the bladder, it would have been very difficult to ascertain what was going on in the brain and spinal marrow.

Chronic Meningitis.

Alms House.—A patient, aged about fifty, of intemperate profligate habits, came into the House for a red scaly eruption all over the body, supposed to be secondary syphilis He was very much emaciated, and extremely low. After being in the House a couple of days, he was suddenly seized with stupor, and died the next day.

Autopsy, May 13th, 1828, twenty-four hours after death.

Head.—Pia and dura mater natural. Arachnoidea turbid universally, and slightly thickened in places, especially about the basis of the cranium. On the convexities of the hemispheres it was raised up from one to five or six lines in diameter, by the deposition of serum between it and the pia mater. The serum had been deposited more or less under the whole of it, and as deep as the bottom of the convolutions of the cerebrum. This character was so strongly marked, that it might, with propriety, be called an external hydrocephalus.

There were two or three drachms of serum in each lateral ventricle, and the arachnoidea in these was also opaque, and somewhat thickened. Encephalon of common consistence generally, with the exception of one or two places, about the bottom of the hemispheres, and the corpora striata, which seemed somewhat softer than usual. The opacity of the arachnoid was visible down the medulla spinalis, as far as it could be seen from the cavity of the cranium.

Thorax.—Slight cartilaginous degeneration of the valves of the heart Some pleuritic inflammation and adhesions: a few crude and small tubercles in the lungs.

Abdomen.—Liver yellow and dry, as in old drunkards. Stomach—Mucous membrane of, somewhat softened, and covered with thick mucus, and presenting the punctated redness of old drunkards. Duodenum—Mucous coat indurated in thin spots, resembling a scirrhous condition of the muciparous apparatus.

Chronic Meningitis, attended with shaking of Limbs, commonly called dumb Palsy, and Paralysis of the Tongue.

Mary Noble, aged about forty, has been a resident of the Alms House since 1823. During this time her complaints have manifested themselves principally by an unsteady tremulous motion in the limbs, and weakness in them. For the last two years her tongue has been so paralytic, that she could not speak, and she has kept almost entirely in bed.

Her senses and intelligence have not been strikingly impaired, and there have not been convulsions at any time, or loss of myotility in the limbs.

Autopsy twenty hours after death. June 14th, 1828.

Exterior Habit.—Emaciation considerable.

Head —Tunica arachnoidea raised on each side, like a large vesication, from all the tops of the hemispheres, and opaque. The water beneath of a light straw colour, and penetrating to the bottom of the convolutions, and separating them a line or more from one another. Cineritious matter of convolutions softened; fibrous matter of the brain plastic but tough, and not so ready as usual, from a sort of agglutation, to submit to tearing in a fixed direction. Thalamus and corpus striatum I thought somewhat tougher or harder than usual. Half an ounce of straw-coloured fluid in each lateral ventricle; tunica arachnoidea opaque under fornix, where it enters. Pons varolii and medulla oblongata, also hardened somewhat beyond what is natural. Cerebellum softer than natural. A small ossification existed under the longitudinal sinus.

Medulla Spinalis.—Membranes healthy, medulla very hard and fibrous, so that by taking it at one end, it was easy to tear off an indefinite number of strips from it, going from one end to the other, like a piece of white oak or of hickory wood.

Thorax.—Heart sound. Right lung collapsed considerably, and a large quantity of gas escaped in a puff from the pleura, when cut into. Lung adhered at places by long filaments to side; had several tubercles in it, with some small pulmonary cavities containing puruloid matter, and of various sizes, from a pea to a nutmeg. The pleura opaque, thickened, rough, and contained a pint or more of purulent, opaque serum. The left pleura was healthy, but the left lung also contained tubercles and small occluded pulmonary cavities filled with puruloid matter, like the right. No symptoms of consumption had been manifested.

Abdomen.—No striking derangement about its viscera

generally. The ileum was injected with blood, and on cutting
it open many ulcers were seen on its mucous coat, with
ragged elevated edges and high vascular injection around as
is usual.   Some few ulcers were in the beginning of the
colon.

Mollescence of Hemispheres of Cerebrum.

Samuel Waggoner, aged sixteen, a resident of the town of
Bellefonte in Pennsylvania, received at harvest time, 1827,
a slight blow at the internal canthus of the left eye.   In a
short time afterwards a tumour began to show itself at the
part; and which, in its progress, protruded the eye ball and
destroyed its vision.   Last winter he was brought to town to
be consigned to the professional care of Dr. Isaac Hays of
the Eye Infirmary.   He was then transferred to the Alms
House, and put under the charge of Dr. Gibson; who, on
Dec. 19th, 1827, in the presence of the clinical class, extirpated the tumour, and along with it the eye ball.   In this
operation, all the contents of the orbit were removed, and a
part of the inferior margin of the orbit, which was in a softened ulcerated state.

The tumour was spheroidal, from two to two and a half
inches in diameter.   Was semi-transparent, traversed by
small ligamentous fibres, and had the consistence of thick
glue, when permitted to cool after being boiled.   It was
principally albuminous, as it coagulated, and became opaque
on immersion in sp. wine.   I did not see Waggoner afterwards till May 1st, when the surgical wards of the house
devolved upon me in the usual routine of arrangement.   The
tumour had, in the mean time, resumed its growth, had
swollen enormously that side of the face, resembled in structure the first one, and was subject to occasional bleeding.   It
was a flattened oval of five inches in diameter, and had a fungous appearance.   It filled up the orbit, had either displaced
or removed the whole anterior parietes of the upper jaw, as

well as of the side of the nose, and also occupied the antrum, and had shoved downwards the left corner of the mouth.

The patient at this time, as might be expected, was weakened and emaciated, his appetite was indifferent. He, however, took his exercise daily, by walking in the ward or in the court; his intellects were good, not obviously impaired, and neither were his senses. He was sometimes sprightly when he could withdraw his reflections from his horrible condition. Considering his case hopeless, I prescribed for two or three weeks, only common cerate dressing, and black drop at night.

In the mean time, the discharges from the tumour became so offensive, that to correct them I directed it to be washed once or twice daily, with pyroligneous acid. Persisting in this application for a week, I was struck in the progress of it, with the tendency of the tumour to slough. It encouraged me to keep on with the acid; and the tumour still diminishing in size, by the detachment continually of large sloughs, I had at length the pleasure of seeing almost the whole of the tumour, with the exception of some deep-seated parts of but small thickness, entirely removed; and, what was quite as unexpected, even the edges of the skin began to cicatrize. The falling off of the tumour left a frightful excavation in the place of the upper jaw; one side of which exposed the left nostril in its whole length, the septum being seen from anterior to posterior margin.

In the progress of the tumour and of its sloughing, Waggoner had pain in the face and also in the forehead, especially the left; and this pain continued with remissions till his death, which occurred June 19th, 1828, at nine o'c. A. M. Till the day before his death, he took his exercise as usual. On no occasion had he a symptom of paralysis partial or general, nor of convulsion, nor interruption to his urine. His senses were perfect and also his intelligence. In my attendance I often directed such questions as might inform me of derangement of the cerebral structure, if any existed, and

invariably the replies only alluded to the pain in his forehead.
The evening before his death he vomited freely, and threw
up some bilious matter.   The want of cerebral symptoms,
the sloughing of the tumour, and the favourable time of his
life excited some conjectures on the possible recovery of the
patient.

Autopsy, June 20th, 1828, twenty-seven hours after
death.

Head.—The centre of the anterior left lobe of the brain
was found resolved into a soft putrilage, equivalent to about
six eighths of the whole lobe.   The periphery of the lobe
enveloped this mass, the bottom of the lobe was not more
than two lines in thickness at most points, and at one point
it was perforated by the ramollissement, and led to an ulceration of the orbitar process of the frontis communicating
with the cavity of the orbit.   The parietes of the ramollissement was six or eight lines thick above.   The whole corpus striatum of that side was dissolved, and the ramollissement consequently invaded the parietes of the left lateral
ventricle.

About one third of the right anterior lobe, bordering
upon the anterior margin of the corpus collosum was also
dissolved in the same way, and about one half of the corpus
striatum of that side.   Adhesion of the pia mater, of an inflammatory kind, existed between the flat sides of the anterior lobes, and thereby the ramollissement of the two lobes
formed a common mass.   The whole of the fornix was dissolved and of the septum lucidum, and a thin lamina of the
under surface of the corpus callosum.   The entire cerebrum
was several degrees below the common consistence, both in
the cortical and medulla substance.   The cortical covering
of the convolutions over the anterior two thirds of the cerebrum, was of a light pea green colour, the remainder was of
the natural colour.

The putrilage, or ramollissement, consisted in bits of cerebral matter, mixed with serum and red blood; its bounda-

ries were not well defined.   In the centre of the mass it
was diffluent, and became, as it receded from the centre, less
and less so, until it blended insensibly with the surrounding cerebral matter.

The cerebellum was sound.

The arachnoidea of the whole base of the brain was
thickened and opaque, and in that state surrounded the
nerves of the base.   On the under surface of the cerebellum, of the pons varolii, and of the medulla oblongata, it
was not only thickened and opaque, but had a coating of
purulent coagulated lymph.

The red inflammation of the pia mater, was very conspi-
spicuous where the ramollissement of the two lobes coalesced, and on the under surface of the left lobe, where its periphery was so thin.   At the latter spot the dura mater was
ulcerated through to the extent of twelve lines or more in
diameter.

Beneath the ulceration of the dura mater, at the side of
the ethmoidal gutter, was the ulceration just alluded to, of
the orbitar process of the os frontis, to an extent equal to the
hole, in the dura mater.   It was not, however, a single hole
in the bone, but several of different sizes, giving it a riddled
appearance, and forming a communication between the cavity of the orbit, and of the cranium.   I am not certain whether any part of the dissolved brain, actually found its way
before death into the orbit through these holes: there was,
however, no impediment, unless it might arise from their
being rather too small.   There is no doubt, that a probe
might have been passed from the orbit into the very centre
of the ramollissement, if the communication had been suspected before death.

The thorax was perfectly sound, and no disease was observable in the abdomen.   The bladder was distended with
urine.

The medulla spinalis and its membranes were perfectly
sound.   I was struck with the facility with which the me-

dulla spinalis, after its membranes were pealed off, could be divided from one end to another into an indefinite number of strings or cords, running parallel with one another like the fibres of a piece of white oak.   I imagine that this test will be found to prove its healthiness when there is a doubt of its being too hard or too soft.

The remarks upon this case are; 1st, that no satisfactory date can be assigned for the commencement of the softening or its cause.   I am induced to consider it as a consequence of the tumour of the orbit, whose development after the operation caused the absorption of the orbitar process of the os frontis and irritation of the adjacent part of the brain, and of its membranes.

2nd.—It is surprising that such cerebral disorganization was followed, neither by suspensions, or derangement of intellect, of the senses, nor of myotility.

3rd.—That the tumour should have sloughed so completely away under the application of pyroligneous acid. Does not this indicate some unknown power in it over such tumours well worthy of farther inquiry and experiment?

4th.—The second progress of the tumour reduced the cavity of the antrum, of the orbit, and of the left nostril into one large excavation, the whole periphery of which was exposed at the time of death.   This tumour, though it shoved the bones opposed to it out of their places, and caused them to drop off; as, for example, all the exterior side of the left nostril, and the parietes of the antrum, above and in front, as well as the left os nasi, and nasal process of os frontis, did yet secrete patches of bone in its own thickness, and formed for itself an imperfect shell at the back and external side of the antrum, perhaps by the distention of the latter.   The septum narium did not give way, but was pushed over to the right side as far as it could go.

Inflammation of the Brain, with Softening of the Cerebellum.

"J. H., a respectable grocei in Southwark, forty-seven years of age, of full habit, inclined to corpulency; head remarkably large, and neck short; after exposure to cold and wet, was affected with violent efforts to vomit, with great pain at the epigastrium, and considerable pain over the eyebrows. He had taken calomel and jalap, Warner's gout cordial, Bateman's drops, and various other spirituous and aromatic drinks. These only increasing the vomiting and pain, had, by the advice of a bleeder, 16 ounces of blood taken from his arm, and eight cups applied to his forehead. Friday, April 11th, I was requested to see him. Found him complaining of intense pain of the head, but particularly at its anterior and posterior parts: great nausea, and constant efforts to vomit, but discharging nothing but a mouthful or two of coloured water, pain at the epigastrium, not increased upon pressure. Head hot; temporal and carotid arteries throbbed violently; face and lips of a purplish hue; pulse full, slow, and somewhat tense; bowels constipated; tongue furred and moist; slight redness of point and edges   I immediately drew off from the arm 20 ounces of blood; directed cold to be kept constantly applied to the head, and, to abate the irritability of the stomach—R. Sub-mur. hydrarg. gr. x. div. in pil. No v. One to be taken every hour. *Afternoon.*— Vomiting and nausea entirely ceased; pain of head continues unabated; tongue somewhat cleaner; all the other symptoms the same as in the morning; drew off from the arm 20 ounces of blood, continue cold to head, and direct the compound senna tea to open the bowels.

"*Saturday, April 12th.*—Pain in head much abated; the bowels had been copiously opened; the discharge being of a dark colour; head still hot; pulse smaller, softer, quicker; tongue dry and brown in the centre; gastric uneasiness gone; slight suffusion of the eyes; intellect good; directed sub-mur.

hyd. grs. iij. every third hour; cold to the head to be continued. *Afternoon.*—Head painful and hot; pulse as at last
visit; bowels continue regularly open. Directed a blister to
the nape of the neck; head to be shaved, and cold applica-
cations to be continued.

"*Sunday, April* 13th.—Blister has drawn; head less painful; cooler; intellect good; pulse more natural; bowels open.
The head has not been shaved, according to the directions of
yesterday. Continue cold to head. *Afternoon.*—Pain of
the head returned with great violence; pulse quick and frequent, tense—left eye appears more protuberant than right;
skin rather hot; tongue dry and brown, with difficulty protruded. The head has not yet been shaved, and for the last
twelve hours the cold to the head has not been kept applied
with sufficient regularity; ordered leeches to temples.

" *Monday, April* 14th.—Leeches had not been applied
until this morning, and then only twelve. The patient, however, appears somewhat better. Ordered, to open bowels,
comp. senna tea; sinapisms to lower extremities; leeches to
temples repeated.

" *Tuesday, April* 15th.—Patient much worse; lays in a
half comatose state; when roused, answers regularly to questions, then falls back into stupor; eyes suffused, pupils contracted, but dilate readily on the admission of light; pulse
contracted, quick, and tense. Directed vss. sixteen ounces;
cold to be continued to head; and an enema, to open the bowels. Dr. Klapp was at this date requested to see the patient
with me. *Afternoon.*—Good deal of the tenderness of epigastrium; other symptoms as in the morning. Directed fourteen cups over the stomach; blisters to calves of legs; continue cold to head. *Evening* —Patient worse, stupor; hot
head; suffused eyes; pulse quick and tense; picking at bed-
clothes; breathing slow and irregular, but no shorter; during
the night great restlessness and delirium; at seven o'clock
had fifty leeches applied to the anterior part of the scalp, at
which part the pain was most complained of; the remainder

to be covered with a blister. It may be mentioned, that when the patient was directed to-day to protrude his tongue, he invariably forgot to draw it in, until directed to do so.

"*Wednesday, April* 16*th.*—Patient better; head cooler; pulse softer and more regular; blister begins to draw; bowels constipated; calomel x. grs., to be taken and followed by comp. senna tea.

"*Thursday, April* 17*th.*—Continues better; returns rational answers, when roused; bowels have been fully acted upon; pulse regular: the discharges from the bowels are fœtid, very dark-coloured. Continue senna tea. Sense of hearing rather dull.

"*Friday, April* 18*th* —Continues apparently better; pulse regular; head cool; complains of blister on the head; bowels, during last night, copiously opened; discharges still black and fœtid, and large in quantity, skin dry; tongue moist; slightly furred; protruded with ease, and fully; appears inclined to sleep, but desires something to eat; directed a few spoonfuls of thin gruel, and R sacc. limonis recent. ʒis. carb. pot. q. s. ad sat ; aq puræ; ʒiv spir. nitr. dulc. ʒiss. M. Table spoonful to be taken every hour; sinapisms to the feet, the blisters on the head to be dressed.

"*Saturday, April* 19*th.*—Patient perfectly rational, with the exception, that when directed to present the right hand, he invariably presents the opposite, and vice versa; in the same manner, when directed to draw up one leg, it is always the opposite which he moves; if the arm or leg, intended, be touched, it is still always the opposite which is moved. There are many circumstances which lead to the belief that the genital organs experience a good deal of excitement; skin natural in temperature; tongue slightly furred, pulse rather quick and frequent; patient has entire command over all his muscles, so far as respects the mere circumstance of putting them in action. Continue medicine. *Afternoon*— 4 *o'clock.*—Restless; breathing rather hurried; tongue dry, and dark-coloured in the centre; some degree of muttering,

5 5

delirium. 7 *o'clock.*—More composed; pupils somewhat dilated; dress head with ung. lyttæ vesicat. 10 *o'clock.*—Stupor has returned; the motion and sound of lips in breathing same *as in a person smoking;* when roused, answers exactly to questions; but is averse from being disturbed.

" *Sunday, April* 20th.—Same state as last night. 4 *o'clock, P. M.*—Respiration laborious, unequal dilatation of pupils; strabismus; left side paralyzed; pulse frequent, weak. 7 *o'clock.*—Stertor; rattling noise in throat; both pupils widely dilated. 7 *o'clock.*—Death without convulsions.

"*Post Mortem Examination,* twenty hours after death.— Scalp and bones of the skull of uncommon thickness; dura mater engorged with blood; on cutting around this membrane, and attempting to separate the falciform process, found an unnatural adhesion, laterally, between this and the surface of the brain, a portion of which latter was removed, adhering to the falx before it could be drawn out from fissure; tunica arachnoidea, on upper surface of brain, thickened, opaque; considerable effusion of serum beneath it; on cutting into the medullary portion of the brain, its surface was covered by innumerable minute points of blood. The cortical part of cerebrum of a much darker colour than natural. Six or eight ounces of serum in the ventricles, and at the basis of brain; plexus choroides loaded with blood; rest of cerebrum natural; at the basis of brain, arachnoid membrane much thickened by the effusion of coagulable lymph; presented a jelly-like appearance; *at the posterior and inferior part of cerebellum softening to the size of about a dollar, and of some depth; the substance of the cerebellum being reduced to the consistency of thin starch;* the lower portion of the medulla oblongata, or rather the commencement of medulla spinalis, appeared contracted in size, and much denser than natural. Dissection allowed to be carried no farther."

The preceding case occurred to Dr. D. F. Condie, and was communicated to me by him, with permission to use it as I thought best

Secretory Irritations of the Arachnoidea and Pia Mater.

Hydrocephalus, in an acute state, generally runs its course in from seven to eleven days, at least we have the very satisfactory observations of M. M. Parent et Martinet for advancing this opinion, and it is marked by those disordered actions of the locomotive, sensitive, and intellectual apparatus which distinguish other cerebral affections.

In it there is a peculiar expression of surprise or of stupor in the face; the pupils are either dilated or contracted, the eye is injected, turned from its axis, and rolls about continually; sometimes there is a paralysis of the eyelids. The face is in a state of trismus, or of convulsion, and injected. Head-ach, delirium, coma, and stupor are amongst the most frequent and satisfactory symptoms The locomotive apparatus may be affected in a variety of ways: sometimes there is a state of contraction, with a local or general rigidity; on other occasions a general or local paralysis. Sometimes there is a restlessness amounting only to inquietude, and at other times there is a convulsion either partial or general. The stomach is affected with nausea and vomiting, the circulation is disturbed as in other severe affections, the respiratory functions, except there be a complication, present nothing peculiar.

On the dissection of patients who die from acute hydrocephalus, we find redness of the arachnoid membrane, with a thickening, opacity, and increased density of its structure, exsudations of various kinds on its surface, as purulent, seropurulent, gelatinous; and layers of coagulating lymph. We moreover find an effusion of serum beneath the arachnoid in the cellular substance, uniting it to the pia mater, and also in the ventricles This serous effusion seldom goes beyond an ounce, but sometimes it reaches to six ounces.

With these facts before us touching acute hydrocephalus,

or in other words acute arachnitis, showing how formidable
and rapid is its progress: and how complete is the subversion
which it produces of all the moral and of the physical faculties connected with the brain; we are put to great difficulty
in reconciling with it, the phenomena of chronic hydrocephalus, and in believing that the two are the same disease.

Chronic hydrocephalus sometimes begins during uterine
life, and expands the head of an infant to the size of that of
an adult. I once met with it in this state, where it produced
a laceration of the cervix uteri and the death of the mother;
the cranium is now in the anatomical museum.   Most commonly, however, it begins in a few months after birth, and
goes on to increase for years, until finally the head is swollen into an enormous mass, which the individual is incapable of supporting, and he therefore is confined to a recumbent posture.   The disease having reached a certain point,
will remain stationary for a long time;-but generally it ends
by some slight violence, accident, or exposure, giving rise to
symptoms of acute hydrocephalus and the patient dies rapidly
under their influence.   In these cases of chronic hydrocephalus, the ossification of the cranium is incomplete, the sutures and the fontanelles remain open much beyond the usual
time, and if nature finally succeeds in putting a complete
bony case around the brain, it is commonly by the aid of
some extra pieces   The brain itself is not augmented in
quantity; but by the large secretion of water into its lateral
ventricles, it is distended into a thin sac, whose parietes are
sometimes not more than a line or two thick.

Cases of an almost incredible accumulation of water are
reported.   Frabicius Hildanus, for example,* narrates one
which lasted for fifteen years, where the head measured an
ell in circumference, and was found to contain eighteeen
pints of water, and I have myself seen in Edinburgh a cranium, which, judging from its extraordinary size, I should

* Dict. des Sc. Med , vol xxii. 248

suppose, had contained at least ten or twelve pints   The grand source of surprise in these cases is, that vitality should continue long enough to allow of such an extremity of disease, in an organ generally so essential to life.   In what light then, are we to view chronic hydrocephalus?—surely not as an inflammation, for if it were such, we should then have the general derangement and prostration of mental and physical functions usually dependent upon an inflammation, and it would be impossible for the disease to advance to such an extreme.   It appears to me to be one of the purest examples of a secretory irritation: merely that slight exaltation of action, whereby the exhalents of the arachnoid membrane, pass off their serous fluid rather more rapidly, than it can be absorbed; and the irregularity between exhalation and absorption being kept up for years, finally produces an immense excess of the former, as in chronic hydrocele and ascites.   The analogy goes indeed still farther; for as hydrocele and ascites do exist without disease of the generative and digestive organs, so chronic hydrocephalus being a pure meningeal affection, the essential features in the structure of the brain, are but little, if at all impaired; and the stretching of it out has no greater effect upon its organic functions, than an extra dilatation of the stomach would have upon digestion. The following case will at least serve to illustrate the position which this affection should hold in our pathological doctrines; and for the opportunity of instruction which it afforded me, I am much indebted to Dr. J. K. Mitchell, who attended the patient in his last illness.

Chronic Hydrocephalus.

Autopsy, December 14th, 1828, eighteen hours after death.   Weather moderate.

Master M., aged eight and a half years, had his head no larger than usual at the period of his birth.   At the age of six weeks, symptoms of hydrocephalus were manifested, for which he underwent an active treatment which was continued for some time.   As he advanced in age he began to walk; his head continued to grow inordinately; his stature was not much affected, and he reached almost the size which is common to boys of eight years.   He could walk, run, and participated in the amusements common to childhood; was sent to school, where he learned very readily the subjects usually taught; was remarkably smart, sprightly, and intelligent in his conversation; was very fond of music, and learned readily a variety of tunes; his memory was also excellent.

For a long time after birth, the sutures of the cranium were open, and the fontanelles unusually large; the ossification was, however, finally completed, and the cranium became firm.   The size of his head was so great that he attracted much attention; and he was apt to fall, especially forwards, from readily losing his equilibrium.

Dec. 12th, 1828, he fell against a door, and bruised his forehead on the left side considerably.   In an hour afterwards he vomited, became very sick, and took to bed, and died the next evening about nine o'clock.   The subsequent day, at three P. M. we proceeded to examine his head.   Its dimensions were as follows: the largest horizontal circumference of the cranium, measured around the frontal and parietal protuberances, twenty-eight inches; peripheral distance between meatus auditorii externi, nineteen and a half inches; peripheral distance from root of nose to occipital protuberance nineteen and a half inches.

Diameters measured with Callipers —Antero-posterior, 9 3-10 inches.—Between parietal protuberances, 7 1-2 do.—Between temples, back part, 7 do.—From chin to vertex, 10 do.—Between meatus auditorii externi, 5 do.

The bones of the cranium were of the thickness common to children of his age, and the sutures firmly fastened, the sagittal was continued to the root of the nose.   There was an os triquetrum on each side of the coronal suture, but no other supernumerary pieces. The integuments of the head were thin and stretched.

The dura mater adhered firmly to the cranium, especially along the sutures. The pia mater was vascular; no pathological state was perceptible in the arachnoidea, either internally or externally. The convolutions were much shallower than usual, being about a third the common depth.

The lateral ventricles, together, contained *five* pints of limpid, transparent serum, and were distended into perfect bags; the thickness of the cerebrum around them varied in places from four to eight lines. Having made a long cut from the above into each lateral ventricle, I found the medullary surface of the ventricles disposed to separate itself from the contiguous part of the cerebrum. The corpus callosum was thinned to about one line, and stretched to the breadth of an inch and a half, and its raphe was semi-diaphanous. Beginning, therefore, at the corpus callosum, we peeled the upper circumference of the lateral ventricle off, as one would tear off paper from a wall: we continued to trace the layer along, and stripped off in the same way the lower circumference of the same ventricle, the layer coming off successively from the hippocampi, and from the thalamus; we found this layer continuous with the fornix, which was raised up in the progress of this peeling process. I endeavoured to strip, by the same process, the surface of the tubercula quadrigemina and the valve of the cerebellum, by the continuation of structure with the surface of the thalamus, but it failed.

The process was executed on both lateral ventricles with equal facility; so that a medullary layer, one line in thickness, was stripped off completely from the whole periphery of each lateral ventricle, beginning at the corpus callosum and ending at the internal side of the thalami. It is worthy of specific notice, that a cineritious layer of the same thickness, and continuous with the other, came off from the surface of the corpus striatum.

The septum lucidum was wanting in great measure, there being a free communication of the lateral ventricles of some inches in diameter between the corpus callosum and the fornix.   The margin of the imperfect partition formed by the septum was rounded, and had no appearance of laceration.

The cineritious substance of the cerebrum was softened, and followed the pia mater in stripping off this membrane. But the cineritious substance could not be detached clearly from the sub-cineritious medullary substance, in consequence of their intimate coalition.

Taking then the thickness of the cerebrum into view, from its surface to the surface of the lateral ventricles, there were evidently made out three layers of matter, the external cineritious, then the sub-cineritious medullary layer forming the convolutions and their bases, and then the layer of medullary matter forming the periphery of the ventricles. These two layers of medullary matter seemed perfectly distinct from one another, 1st, By the almost spontaneous separation which they made when it first attracted our attention, and then the perfect facility with which the ventricular layer was stripped off universally from the other.   2dly, In examining the vascular arrangement, it appeared that the adjacent surface of each had their capillaries branching out distinctly, as is the case with contiguous but distinct membranes elsewhere.

The capillaries of the encephalon were generally congested with red blood.   The cerebellum, pons, crura, and the base of the encephalon were healthy.   There was no sub-arachnoid infiltration any where, the convolutions being close and compacted.

The examination was not extended beyond the head.

For preparations of peripheral layer of ventricles, see Anatomical Museum.   This was the only part we were permitted to bring away.

I am indebted to Dr. Mitchell, for the following personal history of the patient, in a letter to myself.

"William M. was born in Philadelphia, on the 4th of June, 1820, the fourth child of his parents. Although his entrance into the world was tedious, no remarkable difficulty attended his birth, nor was there at first perceived any peculiarity in his conformation. When about six weeks old, incessant cries and a distressing restlessness indicated the existence of pain; and in a few hours he became incapable of drawing nourishment from his mother, making many fruitless essays with a smacking sound. A physician, after examining his mouth, and dividing the *frenum linguæ,* expressed some fears of the occurrence of disease of the brain. Severe and protracted diarrhœa soon followed, and a very manifest enlargement of the head confirmed the opinion of the medical adviser.

"After a variety of treatment, the general health of the child was restored, and continued unimpaired until about a month before his decease, which happened on the 13th of December, 1828, when in the ninth year of his age. During the whole of this period of nearly eight years, his head continued to enlarge without being connected with the slightest head-ach, or any functional derangement whatever. The bones of the cranium became firmly united, and the fontanelles closed in his fifth year.

"When fifteen months old the child spoke well, and at eighteen months was able to sing a variety of musical airs with tolerable correctness; and always exhibited a strong predilection for music.

"Nearly four years elapsed before he was able to balance himself on his legs, and he was not a confident walker until five years of age. Indeed, the great weight of his head rendered him always very liable to falls, and caused him frequently to impinge upon his forehead. Sometimes, when at school, he fell backwards from the form.

"His intellectual faculties generally were very respectable, and his powers of observation rather remarkable. But his memory both of language and sentiments, was such as to

create surprise in those who took the pains to converse with
him.   The following example of his powers of recollection
may not be amiss: A customer of his father having been
absent two years, returned, and, on his entrance into the
shop, saluted as an acquaintance its inmates; but they had
forgotten him.   On turning to little M——, the latter immediately called him by name, inquired kindly about him,
and then told him that he had not been to see them for two
years.

"Of a grave and quiet temperament, he preferred the society of his seniors, and took little interest in the common
pastimes of childhood.   Only sedate children were agreea-
ble to him.

"For so youthful a person, his sentiments and affections
were of a lofty character.   Seeing the distress of his mother,
when commercial affairs took his father to Europe, the child,
then five years of age, said, 'Father will soon be back; if he
don't come again, I will be a husband to my mother, and
will work for her, and take care of her when she is old.'

"For two years before his death, little M—— became affected by religious impressions, which grew stronger and
stronger until his death.   Often advising others, he presented in his own conduct a fine exemplification of his principles, being distinguished among the children of the family
and the school, for love of truth and general sincerity of
character.   At length, even while in full health and vigour,
he spoke of death as a thing to be desired; and, when dying,
expressed pleasure at the approaching crisis.

"On Sunday evening, several weeks before his decease,
he was seized with severe nausea and vomiting, which having
subsided, returned on the following Sunday, and so on with
weekly intervals, until, on Friday, the 12th of December, a
severe fall, followed in eight or ten hours by like symptoms,
terminated his existence.

"During his short illness, he referred all his pain to his
stomach, and never complained of head-ach or vertigo.   His

pulse became gradually slower and more feeble, the temperature of the surface declined: but his mental faculties, and
his affections, remained unchanged until he was in *articulo
mortis.*

" The singular nature of this case, together with the curious anatomical facts disclosed by your *post mortem* exa-
amination, induced me to make a minute inquiry into the
history of the subject of it, previously to the period at which
I was called to visit him, which I now beg leave to convey
to you."

*Chronic Hydrocephalus, and Tumour on Cerebellum
producing Hemiplegia, Blindness, Deafness, Loss of
Touch, &c. &c.*

Mrs. Rebecca D., ætat. about thirty, the mother of two
young and healthy children, and of a good constitution, was
taken in the spring of 1827, with symptoms of paralysis after some slight indisposition.   I saw her in August, and the
symptoms were then, intermittent loss of vision in left eye,
slow winking on that side, difficulty of hearing, and of articulation, loss of taste on left side of tongue, pain in the back
part of the head, incessant roaring in her left ear, mouth
drawn to right side.   Diminished myotility in left upper
and lower extremity, and inclination of the body to that side
when sitting; in walking across the room with assistance,
she invariably swerved from the straight line towards the
left side, so that her motion became diagonal to the left.

She also complained of pain in the bladder, especially on
making water; and whilst I was examining this organ a few
days afterwards with a catheter, she was suddenly seized
with an epileptic fit, to which, under the name of faintings,
she had been subject for several months, having had attacks
upon any sudden emotion even when a girl.

Her functions in other respects, were healthy, and her
menses regular.

I treated her by adopting repeated leeching to the temples, bleeding from the arm, blisters on back of neck, and on temples; light nutritious diet, with some ligneous teas, as sarsaparilla, valerian, and from time to time, from three to five grains of blue mass or cathartic pills of aloes and calomel daily. She improved so much under this treatment in four or five weeks, that she ceased to occupy her bed habitually, improved in flesh, could, by clinging to the furniture, take her turns around the bed room, and finally got down stairs. The several symptoms stated, all got better, excepting the roaring and pain in the head.

With occasional slight changes for better or for worse, she passed through the winter. In the March of 1828, the symptoms being stationary, Dr. Parrish was joined in consultation, and upon his suggestion, rust of iron was taken to the amount of eight or ten grains three times a day, and an issue was permanently fixed on each side of the head after she had been twice blistered all over it. This treatment was persisted in for two months without benefit; her mouth became sore from the steel rust, and she complained of its heating her stomach.

In the progress of this part of the treatment, I observed for the first time, though the symptom might have been constantly present, that there was a loss of sensation in the skin of the left side of the face, from the middle line backwards, and that the left conjunctiva was also torpid, so that it, like the skin, might be scratched with the end of a straw without her feeling it

Her epileptic paroxysms during all this time recurred irregularly at intervals of ten, fifteen, or twenty days In the latter part of June, 1828, she went into the country by advice, and was absent till about the end of August. On her return, the symptoms were for the most part aggravated. She had become thinner. her stomach rejected frequently its contents; I thought that this might arise from emetics of twenty grains of ipecacuanha each, having been administered

to her in the early part of the summer three times a week
for four or five weeks in succession, just before she left the
city. The value of this opinion will, however, be seen from
the dissection. The blindness of the left eye, which formerly had been only intermittent, now prevailed incessantly,
with occasional blindness of the right also, the deafness of
the left side had increased with the noise and pain in her
head at the back part; insensibility of left side of face the
same; to this was added a diminished myotility in it, keeping it almost stationary when she talked; left side of tongue
insensible to taste, mouth drawn somewhat to right side, myotility of left extremities also diminished, but no want of sensibility in their integuments.

Her menses had now been suspended for four months, and
her bowels were disposed to constipation; there was a more
frequent recurrence of the epileptic paroxysms.

From this period, (August 28th,) till the day of her death,
(October 19th, eleven o'clock P. M. in an epileptic fit,) the
symptoms increased regularly and gradually, total blindness
supervened for a month previous to death; she could no
longer sit up out of bed with any comfort, her articulation
became thick and slow, her swallowing difficult and slow,
and when the food was down it was frequently brought up
again involuntarily; and what was remarkable, the process
was a sort of ruminating one, for she could immediately after swallow with an appetite, and digest well, this leads us
to infer that the mucous coat was sound in its office, and the
muscular alone irritable. Her epilepsies occurred three or
four times or oftener in the day, sometimes not so often.

The night before she died, she became conscious of the
presence of a candle in the room, by its light, but she could
not distinguish objects. Her intellects never failed; they
remained good to the last, excepting that sort of indifference
and dulness which always attends a long sickness and soli-
tude.

Her bladder at various times during my attendance, conti-

nued irritable, but for a few weeks before she died, she ceased
to complain of it.   About the middle of September, it was
ascertained that the interruption to her menses proceeded
from pregnancy.

By a very gradual process she approached her last moment,
becoming weaker and weaker, until life was finally extinguished in the epileptic paroxysms of the evening of the
19th.

Autopsy on the evening of the 20th, twenty hours after
death—present Drs. Parrish and Pancoast.

Exterior Aspect.—No putrefaction, countenance placid;
middle marasmus; no settling of blood in face.

Head.—Scalp bled freely, on being cut across from ear to
ear.   Bones of middling thickness.

Membranes.—Dura mater of healthy colour and texture,
but drier than usual along the middle line of the head; for
half an inch or an inch from longitudinal sinus, on either
side an unusual number of granular bodies like the glands of
Pacchioni, and supposed to be so; they pitted deeply the
bones; in the sinus they were not unusually abundant or
large. . Arachnoidea and pia mater healthy, but they also
seemed half dried, and the vessels of the pia mater were not
unusually turgid; indeed they were rather collapsed.   These
membranes adhered very closely to one another, there being
no sub-arachnoid effusion; they also adhered to the dura
mater along the longitudinal sinus more than usual, seeming
to stick to it.

The texture of the cerebrum was healthy, except that it
seemed rather more collapsed and flaccid than usual.   Its
ventricles contained together six ounces of a clear transparent
serum, and were very much distended by it, the corpus callosum being lifted up considerably from the fornix, and the
septum so thin that it was almost torn.   The fornix adhered
more than usual to the velum interpositum, and the latter
was turbid or opaque where it passes into the ventricles.   The

ventricles communicated freely. No thickening of their arachnoidea was perceptible, nor distention of their vessels.

Cerebellum.—It was universally very flaccid, so that it could not retain its shape, but flattened itself by its own weight. On the under surface of its crus of the left side, there was a flattened oval tumour which originated from the crus, and had grown to the size of a hen's egg, extending itself forwards upon the side of the pons, and flattening it in. This tumour consisted in a congeries of cells of various sizes, the walls of which were in a semi-cartilaginous state; and some of them contained serum, others a tuberculous-like matter, and others again a red, spongy, bloody matter. The most familiar comparison of it, is with the ovarium in the beginning of its cellular dropsies. This tumour had raised up in its development, a part of the lateral substance of the cerebellum, and the corresponding pia mater and arachnoidea; its first aspect was more like a cyst than any thing else, on the side next to the crus of the cerebellum.

The tumour had disturbed the position of all the nerves, from the fourth to the ninth inclusively, because in its development they had to pass along its under surface, and were both displaced and stretched by the circuit they had to perform. The trigeminus was absolutely torn off, except a few filaments, from the attachment of its root at the pons, and was there almost absorbed; and the remainder of its filaments were separated and pressed into a flat fasciculus. The medulla oblongata was pushed to the right side by this tumour, and bent.

Thorax—Pleuræ.—Adhesions between right superior lobe and thorax; in other respects healthy.

Lungs—Generally sound and healthy; settling of blood at their posterior parts. Right superior lobe contained half-a-dozen separated tubercles, the largest six or eight lines in diameter. They were of that dry, crumbling, cheese-like kind, which look like old crude tubercles aborted, and which are not attended with derangement of the contiguous pulmonary structure, but merely push it aside. *Heart*—Natural size, firm, and healthy.

Abdomen.—Peritoneum healthy. Stomach—mucous coat empty, and of a sienna colour, except about the antrum pylori, where it was more of a pink colour. Small intestines healthy. Large intestines healthy; contained but little flatus, but filled with hard, dry, compacted fæces, which extended itself for some inches into ileum.

The uterus was up to the umbilicus, had pushed up the intestines, and was next to the abdominal parietes, triangular, and contained a fœtus of about six months, lying across the abdomen, the head to the left corner, and the buttocks to the right corner. The collection of fæces seemed to have arisen from the uterus pressing on the rectum, as her common position was on the back.

Congenital Hydrocephalus forming a Cyst on the back of the Head.

June 29th, 1829.—Mrs. H., wife of a shoemaker in Philadelphia, was brought to bed of a female child, by Dr. Marsellis after the full term of gestation. There was nothing unusual during the latter, except a fall of the mother about a fortnight before her confinement. The child was nearly the size of an eight months' one, and had appended to the occipital region a tumour larger than the head itself.

I saw it, for the first time, two or three days after its birth. The tumour was at that time soft and fluctuating, about nine or ten inches in circumference, and of a spheroidal shape: it was connected, by a pedicle of an inch or more in diameter, to the posterior fontanelle. The fontanelle was the same diameter, and nearly square; and the pedicle of the tumour, having a fibrous feel, seemed to pass through the fontanelle from the interior of the cranium. There was just below this pedicle a small cyst, which contained half an ounce of fluid. The cranium was of little more than half the common size;

the forehead very flat and receding, and the eyes and face projecting and large, as they commonly seem to be in anencephalous cases. The anterior fontanelle nearly closed.

The occiput was also small, and very much flattened on its under surface.

The integuments of the tumour around its pedicle were the common hairy scalp, but the remainder of them were bare smooth skin, thinner at some places than at others, and having at the former the condition of cicatrices. A soft, fleshy mass was felt, half the size of a common fist, in the centre of the tumour, and this mass seemed to spring from the interior of the cranium. The tumour was somewhat excoriated at places, and had here and there thin scabs upon it. On one occasion a scab gave way, and a quantity of serum flowed out. It was red, and hotter than other parts of the child's body.

The child, in its actions and general condition, resembled other children of the same age: it sucked, it cried, and threw its limbs about. Handling the tumour, or squeezing it, seemed to give pain. Its stomach and bowels were in good order.

Taking all the circumstances together, I immediately concluded this to be a case of congenital hydrocephalus, which had occurred in the lateral ventricles of the brain, before the ossification of the cranium had advanced much, probably about the fourth or fifth month of uterine life; and that the posterior parts of the hemispheres had been protruded backwards, and, by the progress of the disease and the natural growth of the head together, had been converted into cysts containing serum,—that the character, in short, of the disease corresponded with spina bifida. I therefore determined to treat it by evacuating the water.

I introduced, for some days in succession, several acupuncturation needles, and drew off at a trial, through the holes, two or more ounces in a very gradual way, of a thin straw-coloured serum; this, for the time, produced a diminution of the tumour, but it would again become plump in twenty-four hours. The fluid at last became too thick to flow through such orifices, and I then resorted to my lancet, which was plunged in obliquely for half an inch, on each side of the tumour, as there appeared to be two cysts. By such means I evacuated these cysts daily. On one occasion, after an intermission of forty-eight hours, I drew off nearly half a pint of serum.

While this process was occurring daily, the tumour was kept moistened with brandy and water, as a refrigerant mixture: an 'inflammation, in the mean time was evidently existing in it, being exhibited by the red, vascular injection of its integuments, by its heat, and by its tenderness on pressure.

On the 10th of July the infant had a convulsion of some minutes; the next day it had another, and also for succeeding days: on the 14th it ceased to suck; that day and the next it had many convulsions, and became pale, with frothing at the mouth. It died on the fifteenth, at 5 o'clock, P. M. having lived seventeen days.

July 16*th*, 1829.—Autopsy sixteen hours after death. Weather warm.

On exposing this tumour, it turned out to be what I had supposed, a congenite hydrocephalus, which had shoved the posterior lobes of the cerebrum out through the posterior fontanelle. The dura mater of the tumour was identified with its integuments; its pia mater was highly inflamed, injected, and adhered universally to the integument. Each posterior lobe was distended into a spherical sac, containing purulent serum, and having its inner surface in a softened disorganized state. The connexion of the sac of the left side with the corresponding lateral ventricle was traced by a probe and finger, passed from one into the other. But on the right side the sac was insulated, the lateral ventricle of that side being closed by a universal adhesion of its contiguous surfaces.

The anterior and middle lobes of the cerebrum and the cerebellum, were in situ, and were not inflamed; they were of the usual consistence in infants of that age, and were connected to the dilated posterior lobes by a narrow isthmus passing through the posterior fontanelle. Pons and medulla oblongata healthy.

No other part than head examined.

[Since the preceding form went to press, I have ascertained through a friend who took the actual measurement, that the circumference of the tumour was *twelve and a half* inches, instead of nine or ten.]

Dissection of an Anencephalous Fœtus, (Female,) August 17th, 1826.

This fœtus appeared to have been carried for six months. It had no neck, properly speaking; for the base of the head rested upon the upper surface of the thorax, the integuments of the face going directly to the front of the breast. The whole posterior half of the spinal canal from one end to the other was deficient, as well as the integuments; in lieu of the latter, was a thin, loose membrane, looking like a cicatrix, and having the transparency of the deciduæ. On the membrane being slit open from one end to the other, a total deficiency of spinal marrow was observable: the roots of the nerves, however, remained and adhered to this membrane; from which I inferred that it was actually the relics of the membranes of the spinal marrow. Some of these roots were imperfect, but they nearly all had the anterior and the posterior fasciculi.

The vault of the cranium was wanting down to the very base—the foramen magnum was defective at its posterior part, from the want of occipital bone behind—the orbitary processes of the os frontis wanting, as well as this bone ge-

nerally, whereby the eyeballs were exposed above.   There
was no brain—the only vestige of it was a small flattened
sac, collapsed upon the base of the cranium, and having a
roughness on its internal periphery resembling granulations.
The sac I took for the membranes of the brain, and the granulations for the processes of the pia mater.   The nerves
of the basis of the brain adhered to the bottom of this sac,
and then went through their respective foramina.

There was nothing wrong in the abdomen or thorax
which caught my attention.

INDEX TO PLATES.

PLATE 1 faces,   -   -   -   -   page 117.
———— 2 ————   -   -   -   -   164.
———— 3 ————   -   -   -   -   171.
———— 4 ————   -   -   -   -   299.

EXPLANATION OF PLATES.

PLATE I

Its object is to illustrate the general colour of the gastro-enteric mucous membrane in health and in disease.

FIG. 1. A section of the left half of the stomach of a rabbit described in Experiment 5th, page 121. It is of a lake colour approaching vermilion. The deepness of its tinge, shows its state of hæmatosis during digestion.

FIG. 2, Is a section of the right half of the same stomach, of a dull pearl, showing the difference of the tinge or state of hæ-matosis. This arises probably from digestion, being chiefly executed in the left half of the stomach.

FIG. 3, Represents the mucous coat of the stomach of a gentleman who died suddenly from an ossification of the coronary arteries of the heart. The case is narrated at page 122, Observation 2nd. The mucous coat is here of a bright brown, or light, warm, sienna colour, which may be considered as the state of the stomach immediately subsequent to digestion, as the individual had taken a glass of cream a few hours previously.

Fig. 4. The intestinum jejunum of the same case—it is seen to be of a deeper tinge than the stomach, its state of hæmatosis being augmented by its containing the articles passed off from the stomach.

Fig. 5, Represents the state of the mucous coat of the stomach in acute gastritis, see Observation 5th, page 147. Its blood vessels were in a state of extreme congestion, with spots of extravasation into the mucous coat; besides which it was in a black and almost sphacelated condition in many parts. The severity of the irritation may be judged of, from the clots of blood which were found in the stomach.

Fig. 6, Represents the state of the cardiac part of the stomach, in a case of gastritis of twenty days' continuance, in which the acuteness of the irritation had subsided considerably: see Observation 7th, page 148. The ramiform appearance, a.a.a., represents the veins occupied as they were with blood. The blotches of blood now almost removed are seen at b.b.b.b.

Fig. 7, Represents a chronic gastritis, see Observation 9th, page 153. The dilated tortuous state of the blood vessels is here very evident. a. Shows the appearance of the black spots of extravasated blood.

Fig. 8, Is the mucous coat of the colon of the same individual; the appearance of the slate-coloured patches diffused over it is well represented.

Fig. 9, Is a portion of the small intestine of the same individual; it shows the sooty appearance of the peritoneal coat from chronic inflammation.

PLATE II.

Represents the appearance of the mucous membrane of the stomach, where an acute inflammation followed a chronic one, from intemperance: see Observation 17th, page 164.

Fig. 1. *a.a.* The dilated varicose veins of the mucous coat near the cardiac orifice, in the midst of black, slate-coloured spots. These veins filled with blood, and not terminating in larger trunks, but branching out at both extremities, so as to have no regular termination, in which respect they resemble the diploic sinuses of the cranium.

b. The deep pink colour and ramiform punctated injection of the stomach generally.

Fig. 2. A section of the mucous coat taken from near the pyloric orifice, and showing the same state of inflammation.

PLATE III

Represents the appearance, from inflammation, of the muciparous follicles of the intestinal canal in children.

Fig. 1. A section of the colon in Case 5th, page 184. The numerous dots spread over its surface, some of which are indicated from the letter *a.*, show the state of the mucous follicles, their enlargement and vesicular condition. This state is previous to ulceration.

Fig. 2. A section of the colon of a child who died from decided cholera infantum: see Case 2nd, page 178. The letter *a* indicates some of the tumid mucous follicles: they resemble the preceding, except in being rather more distinct.

Fig. 3. A section of jejunum from Case 1st, page 176, of cholera infantum. The mucous follicles are also seen here very distinctly enlarged, and also ulcerated. *a.* Points to an ordinary erythemoid ulceration of the mucous coat, whereas *b.* shows the ulcerated tumid mucous follicles.

Fig. 4, Is a section of colon from the same subject: the ulceration of the mucous follicles is there still more distinct: *a.* points to some of them.

PLATE IV.

The drawing here was taken from the Case of Croup, narrated at page 299.

a. Tongue.   *b.* Trachea.   *c. c.* Tonsil glands.   *d.* Larynx. *e. e.* Bronchia.

The larynx, trachea, and bronchia being slit open, a perfect and entire lining, *f. f. f.*, of coagulating lymph is seen extending from the superior margin of the glottis to the lungs.

INDEX.

A

	Page
Abdomen, dissections of,	191
Abscess of Neck,	50
Abscess of Lungs,	240
Acephalocysts,	365
Acute Gastritis following a chronic one,	164
Acute Gastritis, case of,	147, 152
Adipose Secretions,	58
Alimentary Canal in Consumption,	254
Animals subject to Mollescence of Brain,	387
Anencephalous Fœtus,	451
Aorta, rupture of,	125
Aortitis, a case of,	317
Apoplexy of Brain,	408
Apoplexy of Spine,	399
Arachnitis, case of,	419
Arsenic, a case of death from,	297
Ascites, case of,	194
Atrophy of Lungs,	227

B

Bayle's division of Phthisis,	244
Brain, Pathology of,	351

C

Cancer of Brain,	364
Cartilaginous state of Brain,	364
Carditis,	270
Cases of Cholera Infantum,	176
Cellular Tissue, Irritations of,	45
———, Phlegmasia of,	46
———, Sub-inflammation of,	53
———, Secretory irritation of,	56
———, Nutritive irritation of,	58
Cervical Vertebræ, fracture of,	408
Cholera Infantum,	171
Cholica Pictonum,	203

	Page
Chronic Pericarditis,	264
Chronic Gastritis,	148
Chronic Catarrh,	304
Chronic Inflammation of Brain,	358
Chronic Gastro-Enteritis with Tubercular Mesenteric Glands,	167
Complications of Pulmonary Consumption,	252
Colon, colour of,	122
———, Exsiccation of,	203
Congenital Hydrocephalus,	448
Congestion of Muc Memb from suffocation,	132
Corvisart,	260
Croup, a case of,	299

D

Dehtescence,	28
Dissolution of Spinal Cord,	398
Diseases of Heart, cases of,	314
Disease, general considerations on,	9
Disease Progress of,	11
———, Termination of,	13
———, Prognostics of,	15
———, Treatment of,	17
———, Forms of,	18
Diagnostic,	14

E

Emphysema of Lungs,	233
Empyema, cases of,	228
Encephalon, Mollescence of,	371
Encephalon, Irritations of,	351
Enlargement of Heart, a case of,	314
Erysipelas,	52
Erythemoid Inflammation,	82
Epiglottis, Ulceration of,	302
Experiments on Nervous System,	330

	Page
Experiments on Muc Memb.	119
Extra Uterine Fœtus,	216
Excavations, Pulmonary,	249

F

False Membranes,	74
Fever,	43
Fever, a case of,	198
Fistulous Abscesses,	100
Fungiform State of Mucous Membranes,	114

G

Gangrene,	29
Gangrene of Muc Memb.	104
Gangrene of Lungs,	241
Gastric Irritation, cases of, 155,	156
Gastritis, Acute, cases of, 147, 152, 163,	164
Gastro Intestinal Mucous Membrane, colour of,	117
Gastro-Enteritis, Chronic, a case of,	153

H

Hæmorrhages,	30
Hemiplegia, case of,	443
Heart, Dilatations of,	276
———, Induration of,	273
———, Irritations of,	260
———, Ossifications of,	279
———, Vegetations of,	195
———, Mollescence of,	271
———, Rupture of,	297
Hernia, cases of,	208
Hunter's notion of a Nervous System,	328
Hunter, on Perforations of Stomach,	105
Hydro-Pericarditis,	266
Hydrothorax, case of,	313
Hydrocephalus, Chronic, cases of,	435
Hypertrophy of Lungs,	227
Hypertrophy of Heart,	278
Hydatids of Brain,	365

I

| Indurations of Heart, | 273 |
| Induration of Encephalon, | 358 |

	Page
Indurations of Medulla Spinalis,	392
Inflammation, Chronic, of Medulla Spinalis,	391
Inflammatory Indurations of the Brain,	355
Inflammation Internal, of Heart,	317
Irritation,	22
———, Forms of,	26
———, Phenomena of,	28
Intemperance, State of Stomach from,	145
Intus-Susception of Intestines,	207

L

Le Gallois's confirmation of opinions,	331
Lymphatic Glands, suppurations of,	102
Lumbar Abscess,	217
Lungs, cadaverous condition of,	223
Lungs, Irritations of,	223

M

Mania, a case of,	417
Materia Vitæ diffusa,	328
Medulla Spinalis, Irritations of,	389
Measles, a case of,	310
Measures used in France,	109
Medulla Spinalis, experiments on,	331
Medulla Oblongata, experiments on,	334
Meningitis, case of,	423
Metastasis, case of,	319
Mollescence of Heart,	271
Mollescence of Mucous Membranes,	105
Mollescence of Stomach in Infants, cases of,	158
Mollescence of Stomach, cases of,	112
Mollescence, Extensive, of Cerebrum, a case of,	426
Mollescence of Cerebellum, a case of,	431
Mollescence of Brain, account of,	371
Mollescence of Stomach in adult,	316
Morgagni's account of Mollescence of Brain,	372
Mucous Membranes, Irritations of,	78

Page

Mucous Membranes, Sympathies of, 79
———————, Phlegmasia of, 81
———————, Chronic inflammation of, 94
———————, Ulcerations of, 99
———————, Gangrene of, 104
———————, Mollescence of, 105
———————, Fungus of, 114
———————, Appearance of, 117
———————, Natural colour of, 119
———————, Passive Congestion of, 128
———————, Red inflammation of, 135
———————, Follicular inflammation of, 171

N

Nervous System, general pathology of, 326
Nervous System, dissections of, 408
Nervous System, effects of its diseases on other parts, 343
Nervous Irritation, 34
Nervous Palpitations, 269
Nerves, Irritations of, 405
———, Sub-inflammation of, 406
Nutritive Irritation, 36

O

Œdema of Lungs, 238
Œsophagus, Stricture of, 197
Ossification of Coronary Arteries, 122
Ovarium, Suppurated, a case of, 213

P

Palsy, a case of, 424
Passive congestion of Mucous Membranes, 128
Peripneumony, 238
———————, a case of, 303
Perforations, 77
Pericarditis, 261
Peritonitis, Acute, cases of, 191

Page

Phlegmasia, 28
Phlegmasia of Encephalon, 351
Phlegmasia of Medulla Spinalis, 389
Philip's, Wilson, contradiction to experiments, 340
Phthisis Pulmonalis, account of, 243
Phthisis Pulmonalis, cases of, 305
Physick, Dr., on Yellow Fever, 143
Pleuritis, cases of, 310
Pneumo-Pericarditis, 268
Polypi of Heart, 284
Pseudo-Membranous Inflammation, 87
Puerperal Convulsions, 410
Pus, 30
Pustular Phlegmasia of Mucous Membranes, 91

R

Rœderer and Wagler on Cryptæ, 92
Ramiform Injection, 97
Red Inflammation of Mucous Membranes, 135
Resolution, 29
Rostan on Mollescence of Encephalon, 376
Sanguineous congestion of the Brain, 351
Scirrhus, 29
Scirrhus of Stomach, 200
——————— of colon and Rectum, 201
Secretory Irritation, 35
Serous Membranes, Irritations of, 60
———————, Sympathies of, 61
———————, Phlegmasia of, 63
———————, Pseudo-membranes, 67
———————, Secretions from, 66, 75
———————, Adhesions, 69, 75
———————, Sub-inflammation of, 72
———————, Tubercles, 74
Shivering, 43
Slate-coloured spots, 95
Softening of Brain, 371
Spinal Cord, Mollescence of, 394

	Page		Page
Stomach, Consistence of,	108	Tuberculous Infiltration,	247
————, Thickness of,	108	Tumours,	56
Sudden Death from agitation,	314	Tumour on Cerebellum,	443
Sub-inflammation,	32		
Suppuration,	29		
Sweating,	43	**U**	
Sympathies of Nervous System,	343	Ulcers of Mucous Membranes,	99
Sympathies,	37	Ulceration,	29
		Umbilicus, discharges at,	206
T			
		V	
Tetanus, cases of,	411		
Tubercles,	243	Valves of Heart, Ossifications of,	289
Tubercles of Brain,	366	Ventricles, Ossifications of,	283

FINIS.